The Biology of Child Health

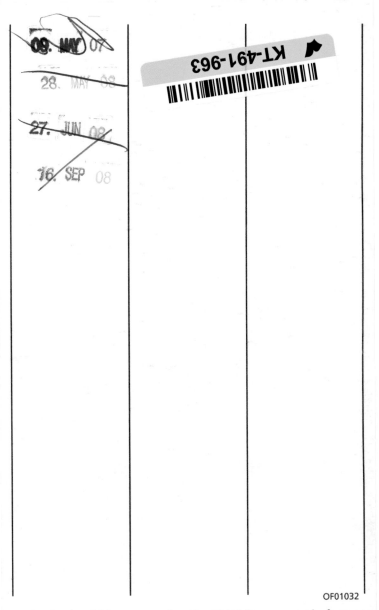

The Biology of
Child Health

A Reader in Development
and Assessment

Edited by
Sarah Neill and Helen Knowles

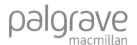
palgrave
macmillan

First published 2004 by
PALGRAVE MACMILLAN
Houndmills, Basingstoke, Hampshire RG21 6XS and
175 Fifth Avenue, New York, N.Y. 10010
Companies and representatives throughout the world

PALGRAVE MACMILLAN is the global academic imprint of the
Palgrave Macmillan division of St. Martin's Press, LLC and of
Palgrave Macmillan Ltd. Macmillan® is a registered trademark
in the United States, United Kingdom and other countries.
Palgrave is a registered trademark in the European Union and
other countries.

ISBN 0–333–77636–4

This book is printed on paper suitable for recycling and
made from fully managed and sustained forest sources.

A catalogue record for this book is available from the British Library.

10	9	8	7	6	5	4	3	2	1
13	12	11	10	09	08	07	06	05	04

Printed in China

Contents

List of Illustrations

Tables

Figures

Boxes

Foreword

It is with enormous pleasure that I write the foreword to this book to all who are interested in the care of children and young people. It is an essential addition to the existing body of child development knowledge, which is a prerequisite to skilled care across a range of practice fields.

Is it, I believe, difficult to identify and manage the care of a child or young person, whose development is interrupted (for whatever reason), if the normal stages of development are not within the practitioner's repertoire to use a guide for assessment.

Each chapter of the book has been written by experienced individuals who are aware of the need to ensure that an individual child or young person's total needs must be recognized, particularly when they are ill. Although this book focuses on biological development, the authors also acknowledge the importance of the psychosocial needs of the child.

I commend the book and hope that it provides an additional source of information to ensure a complete understanding of child development.

Elizabeth Fradd
Director of Nursing
Commission for Health Impovement
April 2003

Acknowledgements

I would like to thank all the many people who have been involved with this book since its inception: the chapter authors, the staff at Palgrave Macmillan, my work colleagues at De Montfort University and University College Northampton. I am grateful for all the effort that has gone into the book and the encouragement I received during what has been a lengthy project. In particular I would also like to thank my husband for his unfailing support and his tolerance of the time it has taken from our evenings and weekends. Finally a special thanks goes to my co-editor, Helen Knowles, for all her hard work without which the book would never have been completed.

Sarah Neill
April 2003

The publisher and authors would also like to thank the organizations and persons listed below for permission to reproduce material from their publications.

Elsevier Science for Figure 2.7 from Hinchliffe and Montague, 1996, *Physiology for Nursing Practice*, Figure 3.2 from Fitzgerald and Fitzgerald, 1994, *Human Embryology;* Figures 3.3, 3.4, 3.5 and 5.3 from Hinchliffe S, *et al.*, 1987, *Physiology for Nursing Practice;* Figure 3.8 from Betz, Hunsberger and Wright, 1994, *Family Centred Nursing Care of Children;* Figure 5.5 from Whaley and Wong, 1999, *Nursing Care of Infants and Children;* Figures 7.2 and 7.4 from Moore and Persaud, 1993, *Before We Are Born: Essentials of Embryology and Birth Defects* 4th ed © Mosby; Figure 7.3 from Thompson and McFarland, 1993, *Mosby's Clinical Nursing* 3rd ed; Figure 8.3 from Hazinski MF, 1992, *Nursing Care of the Critically Ill Child* 2nd ed; Figures 8.4 and 8.5 from McDonald and Avery, 1987, *Dentistry for the Child and Adolscent* 5th ed; Figures 9.6 and 9.7 from Larsen, 1993, *Human Embryology;* Figures 10.1 and 10.2 from Staines N, 1999, *Introducing Immunology* 2nd ed. **Professor Hugo Devlieger** for Figure 5.4 from his thesis 'The Chest Wall in the Preterm Infant' © 1987 Hugo Devlieger. **The Institute for Neuro-Physiological Psychology**, for Figure 4.4 adapted from Beuret LJ, 1995, in Goddard, 1990, *A Developmental Basis for Learning Difficulties and Language Disorders,* © 1990 Sally Goddard Blythe, INPP Monograph Series 1/90. **Lippincott, Williams and Wilkins** for Figure 3.1 from Sadler, 2000, *Langman's Medical Embryology* 8th ed. **Oxford University Press** for Figure

2.8 from Gardner, RJM, and Sutherland GR, *Chromosome Abnormalities and Genetic Counseling* 2nd ed, © 1989, 1996 Oxford University Press; and Figures 3.9 and 4.3 from Sinclair and Dangerfield, 1998, *Human Growth After Birth* 6e. **Pearson Education Inc**. for Figure 7.5 from Marieb, E, 2004, *Human Anatomy and Physiology* 6th ed and Figure 7.8 from Martini, F, 2004 *Fundamentals of Anatomy and Physiology* 6th ed. **WB Saunders** for Figure 4.2 from Moore, K, and Persaud PNV, 2003, *The Developing Human: Clinically Orientated Embryology*. **Worth Publishers** for Figure 3.6 from Bloom FE, and Lazerson A, *Brain, Mind and Behaviour* © 1985, 1988, 2001 Educational Broadcasting Corp., used with permission from Worth Publishers.

Every effort has been made to obtain necessary permission with reference to copyright material. The publisher and authors apologize, if, inadvertently, any sources remain unacknowledged and will be glad to make the necessary arrangements at the earliest opportunity.

Notes on the Contributors

Editors

Sarah Neill, MSc, PGDE, BSc (Hons), RGN, RSCN.
Senior Lecturer in Children's Nursing, University College Northampton, UK.
Sarah Neill has a background in a wide range of clinical posts in children's nursing, followed by ten years as a lecturer, primarily for pre- and post-registration children's nurses, where she has specialized in the teaching of biological aspects of child health.

Helen Knowles, MSc, BSc, RGN, RHV.
Helen Knowles is currently working on quality improvement programmes within a Primary Care Trust. She has a background in nursing and health visiting, with a breadth of experience both in practice and higher education, where she was involved in teaching biology to student nurses.

Chapter authors

Dr Simon Langley-Evans, BSc, PhD, PGCHE, RNutr.
Lecturer in Nutritional Biochemistry, University of Nottingham, UK.
Simon has over 15 years' experience of research and teaching in UK universities. He is a nutritionist, specializing in fetal development and has published extensively on the early life origins of adult disease.

Dr Sue Price, Consultant Geneticist, Northampton, UK.
Following her medical degree from Manchester University, Susan trained in paediatrics for eight years. An interest in genetics and fetal malformation led to a Diploma in Clinical Genetics and subsequent accreditation as a Clinical Geneticist. She has been an NHS consultant in Northamptonshire since 1998.

Lorraine Bowden, Lecturer in Nursing, King's College, London, UK.

Sandy Oldfield, BSc (Hons), MSc, RSCN, RGN, RNT.
Senior Lecturer in Children's Nursing, Oxford Brookes University, UK.
Sandy Oldfield has been teaching in higher education for fourteen years and has a clinical background in paediatric surgery. Her main teaching area is child development and her academic background in biology and psychology has led

to interest in integrating these disciplines in teaching and practice. Her primary research interest is stress, coping and adjustment of children and families.

Ah-Fong Hoo, Clinical Nurse Specialist, Portex Respiratory Unit, Great Ormond Street Hospital NHS Trust & Institute of Child Health, London, UK.
Prior to her current post, Ah-Fong Hoo was a practising midwife and neonatal nurse for fifteen years. Her research interest is the application of knowledge of respiratory physiology, and interpretation of results of lung function tests in infants and young children, to strengthen the scientific basis for prevention and treatment of respiratory disease in early life. She has several publications.

Alexandra Lewandowska, Lecturer/Researcher in Children's Nursing, University of Nottingham, UK.
Alexandra's lecturing responsibilities include all aspects of nursing at DipHE, Degree and MSc level. She has been an honorary research fellow at Melbourne University, Australia and a Florence Nightingale Scholar at the Florida Atlantic University, USA. Alexandra's current research interests include how parents learn complicated nursing procedures.

Dr Craig Smith, Consultant Neonatologist, Nottingham, UK.
As well as his work as a Consultant Neonatologist, Craig is an honorary clinical teacher and a Royal College of Paediatrics and Child Health tutor. He has an interest in the provision of medical education and has published research on the coordination of breathing and swallowing in infants.

Barbara Novak, Lecturer in Applied Biological Sciences, City University, London, UK.
Barbara has a long standing clinical background in paediatric cardiothoracic and intensive care nursing. Her academic commitment is to the Applied Biological Sciences where she teaches within the disciplines of embryology, physiology, pharmacology and pathophysiology amongst others. Her research interests span across issues within the applied biological sciences and philosophy of education. She has numerous publications.

Julie Wilcox, Practice Educator, Great Ormond Street Hospital NHS Trust, London, UK.
Julie Wilcox works as a Practice Educator in a paediatric unit specializing in gastroenterology, metabolics and endocrinology. She has a background in paediatric nurse education and a specialist interest in paediatric nutrition.

Agnes Kanneh, Lecturer in Applied Biological Sciences, City University, London, UK.
Agnes Kanneh's current interest is in paediatric pain theory and pharmacological principles. Previous research activities include nurse–parent communication

and the relationship between childhood physical growth and the control of asthma. Her ongoing aspiration lies in facilitating students' conceptual understanding of biological sciences theory, its relevance and application to practice. Publications include neonatal physiology, infant nutrition and paediatric pharmacological principles.

Edward Purssell, MSc BSc RGN RSCN
Lecturer in Nursing, King's College, London, UK.
Edward is a Lecturer specializing in paediatrics and infectious diseases, and currently works at King's College London and the Paediatric Infectious Diseases Unit at St George's Hospital, London. He has a particular interest in antibiotics and antibiotic resistance, paedatric HIV and vaccination.

Introduction

This book is intended for readers who wish to gain insight into the biological development of the child and is particularly suitable for those involved in health care. While there are a number of texts that focus on the psychosocial and gross functional development of the child, there are far fewer resources that address biological aspects of the development of children and the effects of this development on their health. Such material is spread across a wide range of texts and other publications and is therefore not easy to access. This leads to students of child development feeling more knowledgeable about the psychosocial development of a child rather than integrating this with the child's biological development.

The potential outcome of this is health care practitioners who are more skilled in meeting these psychosocial needs of the child and family than in promoting the physical health of the child. To give an example: if the practitioner does not understand the limited development of the renal system, too much fluid may be given which the body is unable to excrete, resulting in overhydration and cardiac overload. By contrast a lack of understanding of the child's cognitive development may result in explanations about care that are too complex for the child to be able to understand. This may lead to children feeling anxious about events as they do not understand what is to happen. Clearly while the former may have more serious outcomes, the latter is also undesirable. This book is intended to try to redress the balance between the current emphasis on the psychosocial to a more comprehensive approach. Although the book does not explore the child's psychosocial needs, it is not intended that they should be ignored. Rather this book should be used in conjunction with other texts to provide the student with a more rounded understanding of the development of the child.

It was the experience of teaching child health care students about the biology and physiology of child health that stimulated the editors to embark on the development of this book. We knew from our own clinical experiences how our own knowledge and understanding of biological systems and processes had helped us to develop our clinical care and were anxious to put together a book that would help convey this understanding. We felt that if students had a greater understanding of biological development not only would they have the satisfaction of knowing why they were giving such information or care, but would also be able to impart this understanding to the child and the family, potentially also improving the quality of care at home. A detailed understanding of the biological development of the gastrointestinal tract, for example, leads to a much more complete understanding of the process of weaning and how to help parents care for their offspring at this stage of development.

We have drawn together material on a range of different areas of developmental biology from preconceptual influences on child health to genetics and the development of various body systems. Inevitably the chapters reflect the availability of information about the developing child with our knowledge of the very early embryological development being probably more advanced than that of the growing child, where research is, of course, much less easy to conduct. The chapters focus primarily on the biological development and how biological processes differ from those in the adult. It is assumed that the reader has some understanding of normal adult physiology. Chapters vary in the detail that they contain about the effects of possible errors in development, but all have an important focus on the assessment of the child in health.

How to use this book

The book has been laid out specifically with your learning needs in mind. To this end each chapter begins with a set of learning outcomes which you can expect to achieve when you have read the chapter. Within each chapter several further techniques have been used to facilitate learning. These include:

- boxes containing text on key points raised within the chapter, and
- icons 🖐 in the margin which indicate text where the biological knowledge is applied to a clinical example.

At the end of each chapter you are encouraged to review your learning by answering a series of review questions. Each chapter also concludes with suggestions for further reading to enable you to either develop your knowledge of the underpinning theory or to investigate the topic to a deeper level. Finally each chapter has its own reference list.

CHAPTER 1

Before Life Begins: Preconceptual influences on Child Health

Dr Simon Langley-Evans

Contents

Learning Outcomes

At the end of the chapter you will be able to:

- Identify parental factors, before pregnancy, that can positively promote good health in children.
- Demonstrate awareness of factors in the lifestyle of prospective parents which may have a negative impact upon child health.
- Discuss how preconceptual healthcare can be promoted and the ways in which childrens health and well-being will be enhanced by that care.

Introduction

For many centuries the main priority of doctors and midwives dealing with pregnancy and childbirth has been to ensure the survival of the mother and child. In Victorian times and the earlier part of the twentieth century death rates among pregnant women were as high as 5–6 per 1000 births and the then high infant mortality rates of 160–200 per 1000 births were similar to what we now see in the developing nations of Africa. Advances in medical care, hygiene, housing and diet have transformed the priorities of obstetric care. Maternal deaths associated with childbirth are now extremely rare, at a rate of less than 0.1 per 1000 births, and infant deaths are only 6.6 per 1000 live births, even among the most socially disadvantaged groups in the United Kingdom (Office for National Statistics, 1997).

With the changing emphasis of healthcare in pregnancy, more attention has focused on maintaining good health for the mother and for the developing baby. Most recently it has been realized that factors that may have an apparently minimal effect on the fetus while in the womb, may in fact have a major influence on the baby's risk of health problems in childhood and adult life (Barker, 1998). Despite the growing awareness of the need for promoting a healthier lifestyle in pregnant women, our ability to recommend suitable diets, levels of exercise and other behaviours is very much limited by a lack of knowledge. Most dietary advice for pregnancy, for example, consists of a list of 'don'ts' rather than constructive information on how to maximize the growth and well-being of the baby.

This chapter will focus on the period before life begins; the preconception period. Until relatively recently, the importance of the preconception period in influencing the health of a child had been ignored. It is now clear that preparation of both mother and father for healthy pregnancy is an essential element of healthy human development. While many pregnancies are unplanned, a significant number of couples plan to have children at particular stages in their lives and may spend several months, or years, in attempting to conceive. The material covered in this chapter will consider the parental factors which may be important in achieving conception, in maintaining healthy pregnancy and in maximizing the short- and long-term health of the resulting infant. As shown in Table 1.1 these factors can be divided into lifestyle factors, socioeconomic factors, environmental factors and physical factors. This chapter will concentrate upon lifestyle and physical factors.

The Goals of Preconceptual Advice

The central aims of preconceptual assessment, advice and care are to promote the concept that babies are in general the product of two healthy parents (Health Committee, 1991; Reynolds, 1998). By increasing the awareness of prospective parents of the need to improve and maintain the health of both

Table 1.1 Important Parental Factors in Preconceptual Care

Parental factors		Examples
Behaviour:	aspects of the parents' lifestyle that they can control	Diet Smoking Alcohol Drugs
Environment:	influences of the home and workplace on health	Working conditions Exposure to pollutants Housing quality
Physical:	health conditions that may influence the well-being of the developing baby	Obstetric history Genetic disorders General health issues Physical activity Age
Social:	the circumstances in which the parents live	Financial security Access to health care

partners prior to pregnancy, it is intended that fertility will be increased, and hence conception aided, and that the risk to the baby of death or abnormality will be minimized.

Promotion of Conception and Fertility

Infertility is an increasing cause for concern among couples. One element of preconception advice should focus on steps that may be taken to enhance fertility and the chances of successful conception. For men this will include strategies for increasing sperm numbers and quality. Among women, the emphasis is more wide ranging, as, in addition to the production of healthy mature eggs it is necessary to ensure a suitable environment in the uterus to support a developing embryo.

Avoidance of Fetal Abnormalities

The development of the fetus involves rapid cell growth and division and during this period the child is extremely vulnerable. A wide range of fetal abnormalities (also termed congenital defects) may occur, which may prove to be lethal, e.g. anencephaly, or disabling after birth, e.g. spina bifida. While some of these abnormalities may be hereditary (defects that are inherited with the genetic material from one or both parents), others may occur due to exposure to harmful substances in the environment, or due to the lack of particular nutrients. Children whose mothers took the drug thalidomide in the

1960s, as a treatment for morning sickness, suffered disability as the drug impaired the normal growth and development of their limbs (Brent and Holmes, 1988). More recently, it has been noted that low intakes of the B vitamin folic acid, in the diets of pregnant women, during the first 12 weeks of gestation, is associated with higher risk of spina bifida (Medical Research Council Vitamin Study Research Group, 1991).

Fetal Growth

Low weight at birth is considered to be one of the greatest risks facing an infant. The growth of a fetus is primarily controlled by factors over which the parents have no control. Fetuses whose growth is slower than the 10th centile (i.e. the slowest growing 10 per cent of all fetuses) are termed Intrauterine Growth Retarded (IUGR) fetuses. IUGR fetuses are more likely to be born prematurely, are more likely to die in the neonatal period (first 28 days after birth) and infancy and are more likely to be hospitalized for a period of time after birth (OPCS, 1992).

The rate of fetal growth is determined by the genetic inheritance of the individual, but can be slowed by maternal factors. A small woman for example will slow the growth of a fetus intended to be genetically large (see Figure 1.1). Diet is another factor that can constrain the genetically determined growth of the fetus. Studies of populations exposed to famine in the developing world and during World War II have indicated that although the effects are slight, a poor diet will slow the growth of a developing fetus (Lumey, 1992).

Research that began in the early 1990s has revealed that the effects of low birthweight on the health and well-being of the developing fetus and infant may be more far reaching than the immediate risk of prematurity, neonatal illness and death. Studies by Barker and colleagues (Barker, 1998) indicate that a baby born with low birthweight has up to twice the risk of death from coronary heart disease or stroke 50–60 years later, when compared to a baby of average size and additionally has up to eight times the risk of developing adult onset diabetes.

Promoting optimal fetal growth may thus be of prime importance in reducing risk of disease in later life. As shown in Table 1.2 different attributes at birth can be related to periods of abnormal growth at particular stages of pregnancy (Barker, 1998; Langley-Evans, 1997). The different organs of the human fetus all develop, grow and mature during different stages of gestation. The heart, for example, develops in the early embryonic period and as early as six weeks into the pregnancy already has four chambers and is beating. The heart then grows rapidly along with the overall increase in the size of the baby. Other organs, such as the kidneys, are formed early in gestation, but much of their growth and maturation takes place in the later period. The time of rapid growth for an organ, during which its' cells divide, enlarge and become

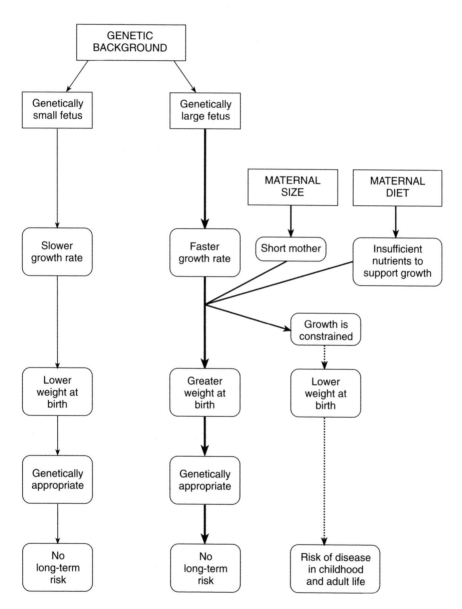

Figure 1.1 Factors Influencing the Rate of Fetal Growth

Table 1.2   Timing of Fetal Growth Retardation and Long-term Consequences

Timing of undernutrition or other insult	Body shape at birth	Long-term disease risk
Early gestation	Low birthweight Symmetrically small	High blood pressure
Mid-gestation	Low birthweight Long and thin	High blood pressure Diabetes Coronary heart disease
Late gestation	Normal birthweight Short in relation to head circumference	High blood pressure Asthma and eczema Stroke Coronary heart disease

specialized is termed a critical or vulnerable period. If the developing fetus encounters an unfavourable environment during such a critical period, for example a poor supply of nutrients, or exposure to tobacco smoke, then that organ or group of organs may not grow, develop or mature according to its genetically determined plan. This may result in a permanent change to its structure and function that is known as programming (Barker, 1998). The links between low birthweight and heart disease and large head size and asthma are examples of programmed disease. One aim of periconceptual advice may be to optimize the maternal stores of nutrients and hence provide an ideal environment for fetal development to reduce these programming influences.

The long-term health of a baby may be programmed by factors present before conception. Observations made in many parts of the world indicate that the size of a baby at birth (and indirectly future risk of heart disease, high blood pressure and diabetes) relates to maternal height and weight in very early pregnancy, or before conception (Barker, 1998). Women who are underweight before conceiving are believed to have suffered from long periods of poor nutrition. As a consequence they are likely to hold poor body stores of nutrients such as the B vitamins or key minerals such as zinc, which are needed to aid normal fetal growth. In contrast, women who are overweight or obese before conceiving appear to produce larger babies, presumably due to rich reserves of energy in the form of body fat. Remarkably, studies of young rats suggest that their blood pressure may be partly explained by the diet their parents experienced during *their* fetal life (Langley-Evans *et al.*, 1998).

Warner and his colleagues have investigated early fetal influences on later allergic conditions (Warner *et al.*, 1997). This work suggests that pregnant women, particularly those with allergic tendencies themselves, may expose their developing fetuses to allergens (the components of food, dust, pollen, cat hair, etc.), in the second trimester of pregnancy and that this somehow sensitizes the child and establishes allergies long before birth. It remains to be seen whether allergen avoidance both before and during pregnancy is of any advantage in reducing the incidence of childhood allergies and asthma.

Preparing Men for Parenthood

Most research that has considered the impact of the preconception period upon child health has focused on the preparation of women for pregnancy. However, the process of conception and the beginnings of life are equally dependent on the male contribution. It is relevant to consider how male health can influence the outcome for the child. Table 1.3 summarizes the main issues relating to men and preconceptual advice.

Sperm Development

The sole contribution of the man to the developing fetus is genetic material in the form of sperm. Figure 1.2 summarizes the process of sperm production from the male germ cells, which are present at birth, through to mature spermatozoa. At birth the testes of the male infant contain germ cells that are termed spermatogonia. These cells are located in the cell layers of the seminiferous tubules which make up the coiled interior of each testicle. When full sperm production begins at puberty, a series of cell divisions occur every 90 minutes within the testes, driven by the production of the hormone, testosterone. The first cell division follows the process of mitosis and produces two

Table 1.3 Key Preconceptual Issues for Men

Key issues	Comments
Maintaining healthy reproductive function e.g. sperm production, erectile function	Essential for conception
Healthy diet	Maintains healthy sperm production
Avoidance of potentially harmful chemicals	Teratogens in the workplace may harm child
Maintain immunity to infections	Ensure no exposure of partner to rubella in pregnancy
Supporting partner	Provision of social support and easing cessation of smoking, alcohol use and dietary change

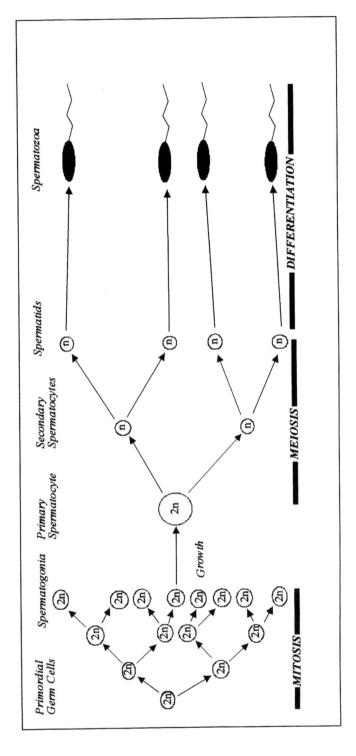

Figure 1.2 Production of Spermatozoa

Note: The Mature spermatozoa are produced through cell divisions to multiply the number of spermatogonia (mitosis) and then through cell divisions (meiosis) to halve the number of genetic material. 2*n* represents the full complement of 46 (23 pairs of) chromosomes present in normal human cells. *n* represents the 23 unpaired chromosomes that are found in human gametes (sperm and eggs).

primary spermatocytes from every active spermatogonium. Cells in the human body contain genetic material held on 46 chromosomes, which associate in 23 pairs. Spermatogonia and primary spermatocytes have the same quantity of genetic material as other cells within the body. An embryo receives half its' genetic material from the father and half from the mother. If the gametes (sperm and egg) which fuse to form the embryo contain the full 46 chromosomes the embryo would inherit 92 chromosomes and would thus not be a viable human. In order to produce gametes appropriately the primary spermatocytes divide through the process of meiosis, which reduces their genetic material by half. The products of meiosis are four spermatids for every dividing primary spermatocyte, thus eight spermatids, with 23 chromosomes, are produced from each spermatogonium that becomes active. The final step of sperm production is the differentiation of the spermatids to form mature sperm, with a tail for swimming through the female reproductive tract.

Male fertility depends heavily on both the quantity and the quality of the sperm produced. Normally a man will produce 2–4 ml of semen per ejaculation and this will contain 40–80 million spermatozoa. Of these a high proportion may be abnormally formed (70 per cent) and only 40 per cent will be described as motile, that is having the ability to swim through the female reproductive tract towards an ovum in the fallopian tube.

Male fertility in the western world is currently giving some cause for concern as over the last 50 years sperm counts have declined by 2.1 per cent per year, every year. Thus the current generation of men considering parenthood produce only half the active sperm capable of fertilization that their grandfathers produced (Lutz, 1996). The reason for the fall in male fertility is unclear, but some researchers have blamed so-called hormone-disrupters. The production of normal sperm is governed by the male sex hormone testosterone, produced within the testes. Agents in the environment may prevent the normal actions of this hormone and components of paint, plastics, cling-film, detergents and pesticides have all been proposed to promote male infertility in this manner. Perhaps most importantly over the 50 year period over which sperm counts have fallen, many women have adopted the oestrogen-based contraceptive pill and excrete large amounts of female hormones into our water supplies. When ingested by men, or even boys, this may have a feminizing effect and reduce sperm counts. Sperm numbers and quality have been noted to be poor in men working in crop production and exposed to pesticides and herbicides. Equivalent workers in organic production where there is no use of such agents have markedly better semen quality (Jensen *et al.*, 1996). This has been taken by advocates of organic food as evidence that men should follow an organic-based diet to maximize fertility, but it would seem too early to endorse this view.

Clearly the avoidance of environmental agents that may harm fertility may be important for would-be fathers, but sperm counts and function may also be improved through dietary change. Diets that are low in protein, energy and zinc may reduce rates of sperm production, so supplements of particularly the latter, may be advisable if the normal diet is a poor provider (Prasad, 1991). In the United Kingdom protein and energy requirements would almost always be met within the diet of a normal male. Some studies have suggested that increasing intakes of the antioxidant nutrients, (selenium, vitamins A, C and E) may improve the fertility of men with poor sperm counts or quality (Hawkes and Turek, 2001).

Exposure to Harmful Agents

Mutations of DNA (genetic errors) in sperm or egg cells may be passed on to children who may later develop inherited diseases which had previously not been observed in a family. Such mutations may contribute to abnormalities in the fetus, or the early onset of serious disease later in life. Mutations are often caused by exposure to radiation or harmful substances in the environment. These substances are termed teratogens and it is clearly of importance for men to minimize exposure for their own health, as well as those of future children. Frequently exposure to teratogens occurs in the workplace.

Support for Partner

As will be seen later in this chapter, much of the advice given to women preparing for conception and during pregnancy concerns diet and lifestyle. Where significant changes to lifestyle are made by the woman, for example giving up smoking and alcohol, it is important for her to be supported in making the change by her partner. Similarly it is important to appreciate that any change in diet requires tremendous willpower and successful change is more likely to be achieved if the prospective father also adopts a more balanced and healthy diet.

Preconceptual Care for Men

In practice, the majority of men will receive no advice or healthcare prior to conceiving a child and in general men are more reluctant than women to seek general medical advice or attend community well-person clinics. The exceptions to this will be those who are suffering from fertility problems with their partner. These individuals are likely to be highly motivated having taken steps to have fertility treatments and counselling.

In preparing for parenthood men should be advised to give up smoking, limit alcohol consumption, avoid unnecessary medication and consume a healthy balanced diet. Ideally exposure to possible teratogens in the home and occupational environment should be avoided and it would be appropriate to update immunizations against infections that may harm a developing fetus, for example Rubella (German measles).

Preparing Women for Parenthood

For women the emphasis of periconceptual advice is directed not just at successful conception, as with men, but also the development and maintenance of a suitable environment within the womb for the healthy growth of a baby. Many women will become pregnant without receiving any preconceptual advice from health professionals. In most cases this does not seriously disadvantage the health of the baby. There are, however, some groups of women whose pregnancies are considered to be high-risk and who should be targeted with effective periconceptual advice (see Table 1.4). This advice should include consideration of the medical condition and drug usage of the mother-to-be, but will largely focus upon the maintenance of good health through improvements in diet and nutritional status.

Diet

Although it is clear that a woman's dietary needs alter during pregnancy, surprisingly little is known of the changing requirements for nutrition during pregnancy compared to pre-pregnancy. As a consequence the dietary advice given to pregnant women is often vague and unspecific. In general pregnant women are instructed to follow a diet that is well balanced and consistent with guidelines on healthy eating (HEA 1994). It is recognized however, that changes in women's diets should ideally be made before conception rather than during pregnancy. Many aspects of healthy nutrition and metabolism depend upon stores of nutrients in addition to the day-to-day quality of the diet, and this means that adjustment of the diet in the preconceptual period may be of considerable benefit to both mother and baby during pregnancy.

Folic acid

Folic acid is one of the B vitamins, with green vegetables and pulses providing the richest natural sources (see Table 1.5). Folic acid exists in a variety of chemical forms, collectively known as folate. Folate plays a critical role in normal cell division and deficiencies are associated with anaemia in adults and birth defects in children. A large proportion of the population may consume only low levels of active folate, partly because large quantities of the folate-containing vegetables have to be eaten to meet the recommended levels and also because folate is unstable. With long-term storage and overcooking the folates in food are either destroyed or change to forms that are not absorbed and utilized by the body (Gregory, 1997).

Table 1.4   High-risk Pregnancies: Women who Should be Targeted for
Preconceptual Advice

High-risk group	Nature of risk
Underweight women	Problems conceiving, risk of preterm delivery and other complications of pregnancy
Overweight or obese women	Problems conceiving, risk of diabetes and high blood pressure in pregnancy
Previous history of complications	Miscarriage, low birthweight and premature delivery likely to recur
Adolescents	Low maternal weight gain, low birthweight, risk of premature delivery
Women over 35	More frequent caesarian and other complications, e.g. diabetes, high blood pressure, higher risk of fetal mortality and abnormalities
Women on low income	Higher risk of premature delivery and low birthweight
Smokers	Higher risk of spontaneous abortion and low birthweight
Women with eating disorders	Anorexia and bulimia are associated with problems conceiving
Women with medical conditions (diabetes, genetic disorder, bowel disorders)	Higher risk of premature delivery, high blood pressure, major complications of pregnancy, caesarian section and low birth weight. Diabetes may cause macrosomia (very large infants)

Folic acid is particularly important in pregnancy as low intakes have been associated with risk of neural tube defects (NTD). NTD include anencephaly, in which the baby fails to develop a brain and dies, and spina bifida (Joint Department of Health, Expert Advisory Group, 1992). Spina bifida is one of the most common fetal abnormalities seen in Britain and occurs when the spinal cord fails to close in the fourth week of embryonic life. This leaves it exposed to the outside environment, resulting in paralysis, incontinence, and frequently, learning disabilities. The condition affects approximately 0.3 children per 1000 live births. A large research trial, published in 1991, revealed that among women who had already had a child with NTD, daily folic acid

Table 1.5 Key Sources of Folic Acid

Food	Average portion size (g)	Folate per portion (µg)
Liver (lambs)	40	95
Bovril	9	95
Brussels Sprouts	90	100
Spinach	90	80
Wholegrain bread*	90	105
Cornflakes*	40	100
Branflakes*	40	100
Oranges	160	50
Orange juice	200	40
Green beans	90	50
Cauliflower	90	45
Potatoes	180	45
Broccoli	45	30

Notes:
*foods fortified with folate (added in production process).
1. Pregnant women and women intending to become pregnant should not eat liver or liver products.
2. Recommendations for folate intake: Women intending to become pregnant should consume 400µg folate per day for three months prior to conception and for the first three months of pregnancy.

supplementation prior to conception and throughout pregnancy could protect against neural tube defects (Medical Research Council Vitamin Study Research Group, 1991).

One of the main functions of folic acid in all individuals is the formation of new red blood cells. Individuals who are deficient in folate develop a condition called megaloblastic anaemia, in which the cells from which red blood cells are formed fail to divide. The neural tube closes at a time in gestation when the fetus is also forming an extensive cardiovascular system and producing red cells. Folate deficiency at this time may lead to NTD due to competition for the nutrient between the developing vasculature and nervous system. Supplements of folate may prevent NTD by overcoming this competition between the two localized systems.

The current recommendation for women with previous history of a pregnancy with NTD is to consume 4mg of folate as a daily supplement. In 1992 the Government issued recommendations that all women considering having a child should consume more folate-rich foods and take folate supplements at a dose of 400µg per day. This dose is ten times less than that recommended for women with previous history of NTD, but is still beyond what could be achieved through a normal diet (Department of Health, 1993). Advice to take folate supplements is a cornerstone of preconceptual care for women. Neural tube defects such as spina bifida occur before most women are aware of pregnancy and so it is necessary to begin the supplementation three months before conceiving and to continue for the first 12 weeks of pregnancy. Consumption of multivitamins in pregnancy is not considered safe and women should purchase or be prescribed folic acid alone. It is not necessary for women with no prior history of NTD-associated pregnancy to continue supplements throughout pregnancy.

Awareness of the importance of folic acid in pregnancy rose among women of childbearing age over the last few years of the twentieth century, due to mass-media campaigns and also food labelling to highlight rich sources of folate. Following the Department of Health's advice to take folic acid supplements in preparation for pregnancy and in the first 12 weeks, sales of folic acid supplements increased by 100-fold over four years (Kadir *et al.*, 1999). This suggests that the message has succeeded in changing women's behaviour. Other studies, however, indicate that only 30 per cent of pregnant women actually took folic acid supplements over the same period and this is backed up by the finding that between 1992 and 1996 there was no appreciable decline in the number of NTD (Alberman and Noble, 1999). Although women may buy supplements as advised they may not remember to take them regularly. As 40 per cent of pregnancies are unplanned, the taking of supplements in preparation for pregnancy is not always practical. Unfortunately the advice given by health professionals may have been less effective than mass-media campaigns, largely due to a lack of awareness at all levels of the primary care team (Pearce *et al.*, 1996), highlighting the need for improved education and training in nutrition among all groups of health professionals.

It is becoming clear that the best way to reduce women's risk of having children with NTD is to add folic acid to commonly consumed foods. This is a process known as fortification and is currently used to improve our intakes of iron in cereals and vitamin D in dairy foods. In 2000 the US government passed a law requiring folic acid to be added to all flour-based foods. Over a 12 month period this resulted in a decrease in cases of spina bifida and anencephaly of almost a third. More recently the UK Food Standards Agency recommended that a similar policy should not be adopted, but the strong reaction this produced from experts in the field (Oakley, 2002) may mean a US-style fortification policy is introduced in Britain in the near future.

Vitamin A

Vitamin A, in contrast to folic acid, is a nutrient for which pregnant women are advised to reduce intakes. Vitamin A is a term that covers quite distinct chemicals in the diet. The plant form of vitamin A, which is abundant in red and orange fruits and vegetables (especially carrots), is ß-carotene. The form of vitamin A active in the human body is retinol, which is found in meat, liver, kidney, milk and dairy produce. The ß-carotene and similar compounds in the diet can be converted within the human gut to active retinol (Buttriss 1997).

Animal experiments have shown that in pregnancy, vitamin A is a teratogen. High doses lead to abnormalities of the brain, skeleton and eyes. In humans the consumption of supplements, which are between eight and 240 times greater than normal dietary intakes, has been demonstrated to increase risk of birth defects (Martinez-Frias and Salvador, 1990). As a result the Chief Medical Officer for the UK advised in 1990 that women who are pregnant or considering pregnancy should avoid rich sources of preformed vitamin A. As retinol can be stored for long periods in the liver, care should be taken in the use of vitamin supplements as part of preconceptual care. No risk to the fetus is associated with the consumption of the plant forms of vitamin A (carotenoids).

Until relatively recently pregnant women were urged to consume high intakes of liver in order to bolster iron reserves and avoid anaemia. Animals and humans store more than 90 per cent of their retinol in liver and as such it is now recommended that pregnant women avoid offal. The vitamin A content of animal livers has risen dramatically with changes in animal feeding practices and 100g can contain 40,000μg, more than 50 times the recommended level in the diet.

Zinc

Zinc is a mineral that is essential during pregnancy for the normal development of the embryo (Buttriss 1997). In the well-nourished British population, however, the severe zinc deficiency required to produce these effects is unlikely to occur and there are no recommendations for pregnant women to take zinc supplements. High dose zinc supplements may not be safe, not least because they deplete the body's stores of copper and iron. Building up zinc stores before conception is unlikely to be of benefit, since the body cannot store the mineral.

Caffeine

Another element of the diet that may be a cause for concern in pregnancy is caffeine, a natural plant product present in large quantities in tea, coffee and soft drinks. It is able to freely cross the placental barrier between mother and fetus and may thus have effects on fetal development. There are some indications that caffeine is a teratogen and increases risk of miscarriage and low birthweight, but large trials of over 12,000 women suggest no adverse effects (Klebanoff *et al.*, 1999). With continuing controversy in this area it may be appropriate to advise pregnant women to reduce intakes of caffeine-containing drinks, or switch to decaffeinated equivalents.

Caffeine is not stored in the human body and so preconceptual changes may be only really necessary as a means of breaking established drinking habits. Weinberg and Wilcox (1990) suggest that caffeine may reduce fertility and report that conception rates among women were halved by drinking the equivalent of one cup of coffee per day. However, other researchers have not confirmed these findings and the reality of any adverse effect of caffeine remains unresolved.

Weight Before Conception

It is normal for considerable weight gain to occur during pregnancy. Over the whole 40 weeks of pregnancy the average woman will gain 12.5 kg. It is of vital importance that this normal weight gain is allowed to occur and women should never attempt to lose weight during a pregnancy (Campbell, 1991). Inappropriate weight prior to conception should, however, be an issue dealt with as part of preconceptual advice. Women who are underweight or over-weight may well have difficulty in conceiving. Underweight attributable to poor nutritional intakes or excessive physical activity can lead to the loss of normal menstrual cycle activity (ammenhorrea), as is frequently noted in female athletes and girls with eating disorders such as anorexia nervosa (Stewart, 1992). This is due to a loss of the secretion of oestrogen from the ovaries and follicle-stimulating hormone from the pituitary gland. Obesity may also result in abnormal levels of the sex hormones oestrogen and proge-strone, which will effectively prevent ovulation or implantation of a fertilized egg. To maximize fertility it is recommended that women's body mass index (BMI: weight [kg]/height[m]^2) falls within the ideal range (20–25). Overweight women should not attempt to lose weight at the same time as trying to conceive a baby. Weight loss can lead to temporary infertility and dieting to lose weight is not advised in the 2–3 months before conception (Naeye, 1979).

Smoking and Alcohol Consumption

Almost a third of women, in the UK, between the ages of 16 and 45 are smok-ers and many of these women will continue to smoke while pregnant. There is evidence to suggest that smoking reduces fertility in women. Smoking has been also linked to miscarriage, fetal abnormalities and is a known cause of low birthweight. Some studies have suggested that babies of women smoking 20 cigarettes per day will be on average 200g lighter than those of non-smokers. The babies of smokers are also significantly more likely to be born prema-turely, which carries major risk of death or disability (Macleod-Clark and Maclaine, 1992). Advice to stop smoking, or at least reduce the number of cigarettes smoked, should be a major component of preconceptual advice.

There are clear associations between the consumption of alcohol during pregnancy and fetal abnormalities. Alcohol is a teratogen that can cause malformations of the heart and lungs, nervous system defects and facial abnor-malities (Spohr *et al.*, 1993). The levels of alcohol required to produce terato-genic effects are still unclear. Light drinking (1 to 2 units of alcohol per day) has not been reported to have any harmful effects on developing fetuses, but increasing this to 4 units per day greatly increases risk. Women who are moder-ate to heavy consumers of alcohol will clearly need to reduce their intake for pregnancy and should receive appropriate advice as part of preconceptual care.

Furthermore, the most likely time for alcohol to induce malformations in the baby will be in the very early, embryonic phase of pregancy. This is the time when the organs are formed and are vulnerable to teratogenic actions. At this time alcohol may cause irreversible damage before the woman is aware that she is pregnant.

Infections

In addition to HIV infection, mentioned above, there are a number of bacterial, viral and yeast infections that may be harmful to the developing fetus if contracted during pregnancy. Rubella, or German measles, is of particular relevance to preconcepetual care and will be considered here. Rubella infection during pregnancy is associated with stillbirth or miscarriage and abnormalities in the fetus. Congenital Rubella syndrome may leave the child deaf, blind or mentally retarded. All women considering pregnancy should be screened for immunity against Rubella. Most women will have been immunized while at school or acquired immunity through infection. Where screening reveals a lack of immunity it will be necessary to vaccinate before conception and then to allow three months following the vaccination before ending the use of contraception.

Medical Conditions

There are a number of medical conditions which, if present in the pregnant woman, may have an adverse effect upon the developing baby. Most of these are not the concern of preconceptual counsellors, for example pregnancy related high blood pressure, or will be dealt with by other specialists, for example genetic counselling for families with a history of inherited disease. Diabetes, however, is a condition which may be present before conception and have a significant effect upon the baby.

Diabetes occurs in 10–15 people per 1000 of the population under the age of 65. Diabetes may be type 1, where the individual has to control blood glucose levels through insulin injections, or type 2, where insulin is not normally required. Women with type I diabetes may have difficulty in controlling blood glucose levels in pregnancy. The changes to the rate of metabolism in pregnancy may result in high blood glucose (hyperglycaemia), which can be damaging to the mother, but also spill over into the fetus. High glucose levels in the fetus cause the production of insulin which leads to abnormally high rates of growth (macrosomia) and can lead to lung, heart and nervous system defects (Jovanovic-Peterson and Peterson, 1992).

For an insulin-dependent diabetic considering pregnancy, advice is needed on the management of glucose levels before conception. The diet for pregnancy must be based upon frequent and small meals to prevent the glucose level rising too high after eating and to avoid intervals between feeds when the glucose level falls too low. It is advised that this preconceptual advice on diabetes management is followed up with specialist diabetic antenatal clinics through the pregnancy (Oakley, 1989).

Preconceptual Assessment and Advice

In reality the majority of women will become pregnant without any preconceptual advice from health professionals and will depend upon health promotion literature and media campaigns to raise awareness of the issues covered by this chapter. Most women who do receive advice from primary health care teams will be in one or more of the groups considered at high-risk of pregnancy-related problems shown in Table 1.4. For such women the priorities for advice fall into the broad categories of weight, diet, smoking and alcohol use, although other issues are clearly of importance (see Table 1.6).

Table 1.6   Key Preconceptual Issues for Women

Key issues	Comments
Maintaining healthy body weight	BMI below 20 or over 30 may prevent conception and is considered high risk in pregnancy
Healthy diet	Folic acid supplements essential Reduce vitamin A intake Reduce caffeine intake
Avoidance of potentially harmful chemicals	Teratogens in the workplace may harm child Stop smoking Reduce alcohol intake Avoid non-prescription drugs
Maintain immunity to infections	Check immunity to Rubella

Review Questions

1. What are the main goals of preconceptual advice for both men and women?
2. Low weight at birth is perceived as a risk to health in childhood and later life. What are the main factors that determine the rate at which a fetus grows?
3. Describe the factors that may impact upon male fertility.
4. What are the dietary priorities for women in the preconception period?

5. Describe the risks associated with the use of alcohol and tobacco in pregnancy.

Further Reading

Maternal age and its relation to risk in pregnancy is an issue that has not been addressed in detail in this chapter. Pregnant women over the age of 35 are considered at higher risk of low birthweight infants or fetal abnormalities. An aim of preconceptual advice is clearly of importance within this group. Adolescent pregnancy is a major issue in the UK today, and is also considered a high risk for both mother and infant. Review the main issues that contribute to risk in the under 16s.

Since 1978 the organization Foresight has been involved in the promotion of preconceptual health. Foresight funds research into the links between male and female health before conception and the health and well-being of the fetus and child. Foresight publishes materials to aid health professionals in providing patients with appropriate advice. Their address is: Foresight, 28 The Paddock, Godalming, Surrey, GU7 1XD.

The use of folic acid supplements before and during pregnancy is one of the key issues in preconceptual care. Given the dangers of vitamin A toxicity it is essential that nutritional supplements are used with care in early pregnancy. Investigate this issue further with reference to nutrition textbooks and, in particular, Buttriss (1997). Further information on this may be obtained in a series of factfiles and information packs produced by the National Dairy Council, which are available free of charge from: National Dairy Council, 5–7 John Princes Street, London, W1M OAP.

References

Alberman, E and Noble, JM (1999) Food should be fortified with folic acid. *British Medical Journal*, 319, 93.

Barker, DJP (1998). *Mothers, Babies and Health in Later Life*. London: Churchill Livingstone.

Brent, RL and Holmes, LB (1988) Clinical and basic science lessons from the thalidomide tragedy – what have we learned about the causes of limb defects? *Teratology*, 38, 241–51.

Buttriss, J (1997). *Vitamins, Minerals and Health*. London: National Dairy Council.

Campbell, DM (1991) *Maternal and fetal nutrition*, in DS McClaren *et al.* (eds), *Textbook of Paediatric Nutrition*. London: Churchill Livingstone, pp. 3–20.

Department of Health (1993) *Pregnancy, Folic Acid and You*. Heywood: Health Publication Unit.

Gregory JF (1997) Bioavailability of folate. *European Journal of Clinical Nutrition*, 51, suppl. 1, S54–S59.

Hawkes, WC and Turek, PJ (2001). Effects of dietary selenium on sperm motility in healthy men. *Journal of Andrology*, 22, 764–72.

Health Committee (1991) *Maternity Services: Preconception, vol. 1*. London: HMSO.

Health Education Authority (1994) *The Balance of Good Health*. London: HEA.

Jensen, TK, Giwercman, A, Carlsen, E, Scheike, T and Skakkebaek, NE (1996) Semen quality among members of organic food associations in Zealand, Denmark. *Lancet*, 347(9018), 1844.

Joint Department of Health, Expert Advisory Group (1992) *Folic Acid and the Prevention of Neural Tube Defects*. Department of Health, Scottish Office Home and Health Department, Welsh Office, Department of Health and Social Services Northern Ireland.

Jovanovic-Peterson, L and Peterson, CM (1992) Pregnancy in the diabetic woman: Guidelines for a successful outcome. *Endocrinology and Metabolism Clinics North America*, 21, 433–56.

Kadir, RA, Sabin, C, Whitlow, B, Brockbank, E and Economides, D (1999). Neural tube defects and periconceptual folic acid in England and Wales: A retrospective study. *British Medical Journal*, 319, 92–3.

Klebanoff, MA, Levine, RJ, DerSimonen, R, Clemens, JD and Wilkins, DG (1999) Maternal serum paraxanthine: A caffeine metabolite and the risk of spontaneous abortion. *New England Journal of Medicine*, 341, 1639–44.

Langley-Evans, SC (1997) Fetal programming of immune function and respiratory disease. *Clinical and Experimental Allergy*, 27, 1377–9.

Langley-Evans, SC, Dunn, RL, Jackson, AA (1998) Blood pressure changes programmed by exposure to maternal protein restriction are transmitted to a second generation through the germ line. *Proceedings of the Nutrition Society*, 57, 78A.

Lumey, LH (1992) Decreased birthweights in infants after maternal in utero exposure to the Dutch famine of 1944–45. *Paediatric and Perinatal Epidemiology*, 6, 240–53.

Lutz, D (1996) No conception. Masquerading as sex hormones, chemicals ubiquitous in our environment could threaten our children's ability to reproduce. *The Sciences*, Jan/Feb, 12–15.

Macleod-Clark, J and Maclaine K (1992) The effects of smoking in pregnancy: A review of approaches to behavioural change. *Midwifery*, 8, 19–30.

Martinez-Frias, ML and Salvador, J (1990) Epidemiological aspects of prenatal exposure to high doses of vitamin A in Spain. *European Journal of Epidemiology*, 6, 118–23.

Medical Research Council Vitamin Study Research Group (1991) Prevention of neural tube defects: results of the Medical Research Council vitamin study. *Lancet*, 338(8760), 131–7.

Naeye, RL (1979) Perinatal mortality rates of overweight, normal weight and underweight mothers related to weight gain. *American Journal of Obstetrics and Gynaecology*, 135, 3.

Oakley, C (1989) A midwife for women with diabetes. *Nursing Times*, 85, 36–8.

Oakley, GP (2002) Delaying folic acid fortification of flour – Governments that do not ensure fortification are committing public health malpractice. *British Medical Journal*, 324, 1348–9.

Office for National Statistics (1997) *Health of Adult Britain, 1841–1994*. London, Stationery Office.

OPCS, Office of Population Censuses and Surveys (1992) *1990 Mortality Statistics Perinatal and Infant: Social and Biological Factors*. England and Wales. Series DH3 Number 24, London: HMSO.

Pearce, HR, Smith, NA, Fox, EF and Bingham, JS (1996) Periconceptual folic acid: Knowledge amongst patients and health care workers in a London teaching hospital. *British Journal of Family Planning*, 22, 20–1.

Prasad, AS (1991) Discovery of human zinc deficiency and studies in an experimental human model. *American Journal of Clinical Nutrition*, 53, 403–12.

Reynolds, HD (1998) Preconceptual care: An integral part of primary care for women. *Journal of Nurse Midwifery*, 43, 6.

Spohr, HL, Willms, J and Steinhausen, HC (1993) Prenatal alcohol exposure and long-term developmental consequences. *Lancet*, 341(8850), 907–10.

Stewart, DE (1992) Reproductive functions in eating disorders. *Annals of Medicine*, 24, 287–91.

Warner, JA, Jones, AC, Miles, EA, Colwell, BM and Warner, JO (1997) Prenatal origins of asthma and allergy, in ST Holgate (ed.), *The Rising Trends in Asthma*. Chichester: Wiley, 220–8.

Weinberg, CR and Wilcox AJ (1990) Caffeine and infertility. *Lancet*, 335(8692), 792.

CHAPTER 2

Inheritance and Child Health

Dr Sue Price

Contents

- The Components of Inheritance
- Mechanism of Genetic Disease
- Assessment
- Review Questions
- Further Reading
- References

Learning Outcomes

At the end of this chapter you will be able to:

- Compare and contrast different types of cell division.
- Describe the normal human chromosome complement.
- Describe the relationship of DNA (deoxyribonucleic acid) to chromosome structure and analyse its role as a genetic molecule.
- Describe common examples of chromosome abnormality.
- Critically analyse the implications of dominant, recessive, X-linked and multifactorial inheritance for families.
- Describe the methods of assessment available and integrate this with an understanding of the mechanism of genetic disease.

Introduction

Following verification of the true chromosome complement in man in 1946, and the discovery of the structure of DNA (deoxyribonucleic acid) in 1953 (Watson and Crick, 1953a, b), there has been a rapid rise in our understanding of genetic disease. The characterization of the entire human genome – all the genes in a cell – will give us a new understanding of functional biology and disease mechanisms. Genetic abnormalities account for half of early pregnancy losses. About 2 per cent of neonates have a chromosome or single gene abnormality, and there is often a genetic basis for the 2–3 per cent of newborns with major congenital malformations. Altered genes cause 50 per cent of childhood deafness, blindness and learning disability (Mueller and Young, 1998).

This chapter describes the components of inheritance, how errors can occur during the transmission of genetic material from one generation to another and approaches to the assessment process in relation to genetic disorders.

The Components of Inheritance

Chromosomes and DNA

The nucleus of the cell contains the chromosomes and hence most of the genetic information in the cell. Chromosomes can be seen with a microscope in the nucleus of cells (See Figure 2.1). The chromosomes contain tightly

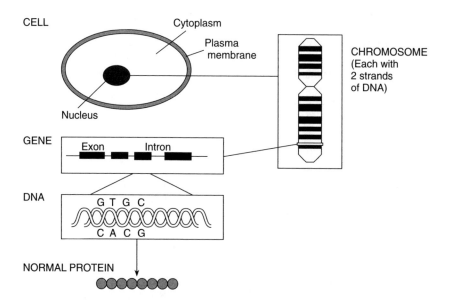

Figure 2.1 The Organization of Genetic Material Within the Cell

packed DNA (deoxyribonucleic acid), molecules which encode genes. A gene is the segment of DNA which specifies the code for the RNA (Ribonucleic acid) sequence that will direct the synthesis of a specific functional polypeptide. Genes thus control activities within the cell.

The tightly packed DNA molecules are arranged as follows. The fundamental unit of DNA packaging in the chromosome is the nucleosome. A nucleosome consists of a central core of eight histones (proteins) around which 146 base pairs of DNA is coiled in 1.75 turns. A small bridge of DNA links one nucleosome to the next. This 'string of beads' is further coiled to make a chromatin fibre, which can be seen using electron microscopy. When fully packaged the chromatin fibres form loops around a scaffold of acid proteins (Figure 2.2).

The normal human chromosome number is 46 (Figure 2.3) made up of 23 pairs, or homologues, (Figure 2.4). One pair determines the sex of an individual – a male has an X and Y chromosome, and the female two X chromosomes. The other 22 pairs, termed autosomes, are numbered one to 22 based on size.

Each chromosome has a constriction, called the centromere, either centrally on a chromosome or near to one end. This divides the chromosome into a shorter 'p' and longer 'q' arm. The centromere has an important role in cell division.

A karyotype describes the number and shape of chromosomes for an individual. They can be described using a standard system of symbols where the number of the chromosome is written first, followed by the sex chromosome constitution and then any abnormality.

The Structure of DNA

DNA fulfils the two main requirements for a genetic molecule:

1. a method of coding information; and
2. an ability to replicate.

DNA consists of two chains of nucleotides lying parallel, but in opposite directions, held together with hydrogen bonds (Figure 2.5). The structure resembles a ladder twisted into a helix. Each tread of the ladder is made up of two nitrogenous bases facing each other joined by a hydrogen bond. On the outer edge at each side is a sugar joined with a phosphate to the rung above.

There are four possible nitrogenous bases – adenine (A), guanine (G), cytosine (C) and thymine (T). Each base can only bond with one other – C must pair with G and A with T. Therefore the sequence on one side of the ladder determines that on the other. A series of three nucleotides along a strand of DNA is called a codon, and different sequences within a codon designate different amino acids. Only about 3 per cent our total DNA is coding

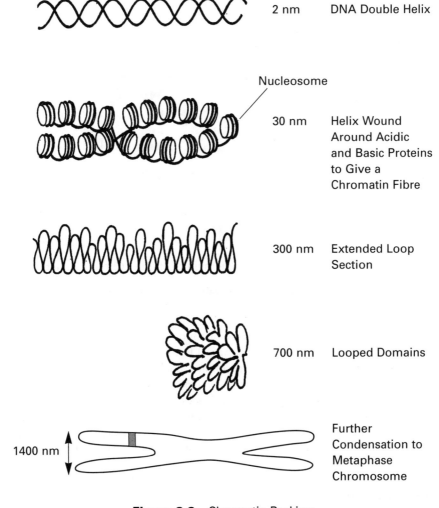

2 nm   DNA Double Helix

Nucleosome

30 nm   Helix Wound Around Acidic and Basic Proteins to Give a Chromatin Fibre

300 nm   Extended Loop Section

700 nm   Looped Domains

1400 nm

Further Condensation to Metaphase Chromosome

Figure 2.2 Chromatin Packing

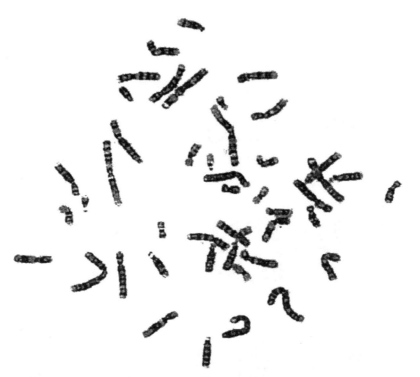

Figure 2.3   The Normal Complement of Human Chromosomes

Source: Karyotypes kindly provided by Juliet Alexander of Applied Imaging International.

sequence (Mueller and Young, 1998). The term gene is usually used to specify the coding sequence of a specific string of amino-acids that will form a protein (see transcription and translation). A typical human gene (see Figure 2.6) will begin with a promoter region that can influence whether or not a gene is used. An initiation sequence is then followed by a variable number of exons (coding sequences) and introns (non-coding sequences) followed by a 'stop' codon.

The structure of the sugar molecules means that each strand (the verticals of the ladder) has a direction. One end is called 5' (five prime) and the other 3'. DNA can only be synthesized or read in one direction going from 5' to 3'.

DNA Replication

DNA replication is required for cell division. At the completion of replication each new section contains one strand from the original helix with a new complimentary second strand. During DNA synthesis the helix is 'unzipped' by a helicase enzyme and each strand acts a template – attracting the four different nitrogenous bases (with sugar and phosphate group attached) in the correct sequence – which are then joined together by another specific enzyme

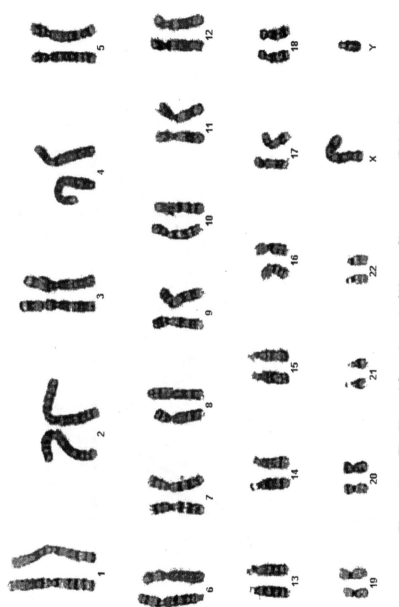

Figure 2.4   The Normal Complement of Human Chromosomes (Paired)

Source: Karyotypes kindly provided by Juliet Alexander of Applied Imaging International.

28

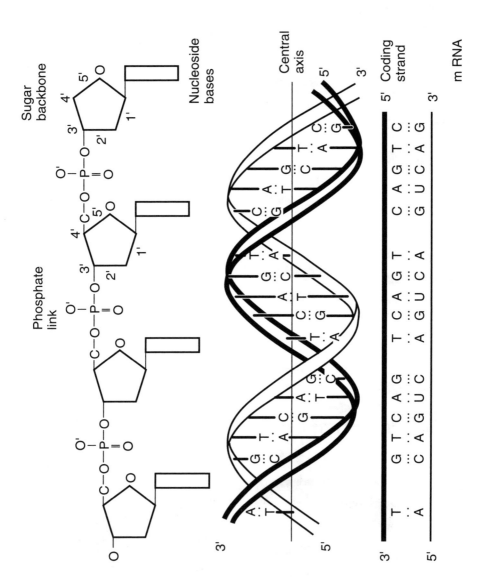

Figure 2.5 The Basic Structure of DNA

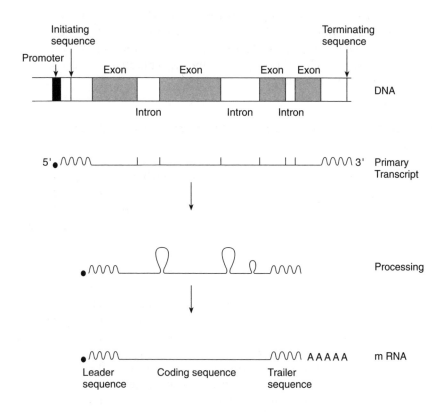

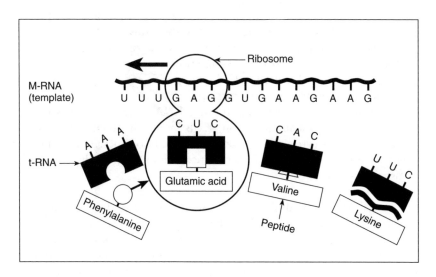

Figure 2.6 The Path of a Typical Gene through Transcription

(DNA polymerase). Replication is initiated at specific points along a strand leading to 'replication forks'. The process can only proceed in the 5' to 3' direction so one strand, the leading strand, can progress smoothly, whereas the second strand, called the lagging strand, is replicated in small sections, which are then joined together.

Transcription and Translation – The Mechanism for Protein Synthesis

Cells use the information coded in the DNA as a blueprint to produce the innumerable proteins needed for the body's structure and biochemical processes. Transcription and translation describes the mechanism that the body uses to read this blueprint accurately. Figures 2.6 show the stages involved.

1. The information coded in one of the DNA strands is used as a template to specify the sequence of the single stranded ribonucleic acid, RNA, in a process known as transcription. Transcription is similar to DNA replication but RNA uses uridine instead of thymine at these base positions. The DNA has sequences called promoter regions, which guide the RNA polymerase to sites for transcription initiation.
2. This first transcript (called the 'primary' transcript) is further processed to remove non-coding regions of genes, introns, and elements are added which protect the molecule in the cytoplasm. This transport molecule is called messenger RNA (mRNA).
3. Messenger RNA leaves the nucleus and is taken to ribosomes. These are small spherical structures in the cytoplasm that consist mostly of RNA and have a key role in the translation of the information contained within the mRNA into functional proteins. Translation is the process by which information on the mRNA is used to build the specific amino acid sequence that determines the protein and its function.
4. Also within cytoplasm are small transfer RNA molecules with sequences that correspond to a single codon. Each binds with their corresponding amino acid in the cytoplasm and takes it to the ribosomes. The amino acids align themselves on the mRNA template and join to give polypeptides thus constructing proteins.

Different cells transcribe different DNA sequences depending on their function. The DNA molecule should not be thought of as a static structure, but one that can react to the environment by altering which genes are transcribed. Hormones and growth factors influence transcription in specific cell types by triggering movement of transcription factors. Gene expression can also be influenced at RNA level if the primary transcript can be 'edited' in different ways to make different products depending on the circumstances.

Cell Division

New cells can only be made from existing cells in the body. There are two types of cell division – mitosis and meiosis (Figures 2.7 and 2.8). Mitosis is involved in new cell formation for body growth, renewal and repair, and producing cells with the same chromosome number as the original cell. Meiosis only occurs in the egg or sperm producing cells of the female or male gonads respectively, and only once between generations. It produces male and female gametes which have half of the normal chromosome number (a haploid cell) as they have a single copy from each chromosome pair i.e. 23 in all.

Mitosis

Mitosis is a process lasting 1–2 hrs. In preparation for cell division DNA synthesis occurs. Two chromatids are held together at the centromere and the chromatin is fully packaged. At this point the chromosomes can be seen under a microscope. Each chromatid has an original DNA strand with its newly synthesized strand. Crucial to cell division is the formation of the mitotic spindle. This is where microtubular fibres extend from both poles of the cell towards the equator. The chromosomes use the spindle to line up along the equator, and as the cell divides the chromosome breaks at the centromere with each new cell receiving one chromatid.

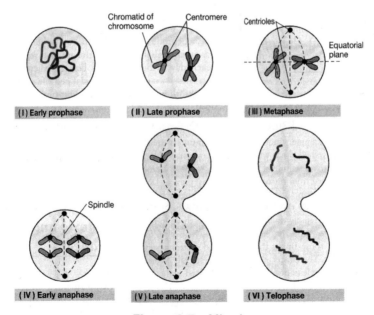

Figure 2.7 Mitosis

Source: Reprinted from *Physiology for Nursing Practice*, Hinchliffe & Montague, copyright 1996, with permission from Elsevier.

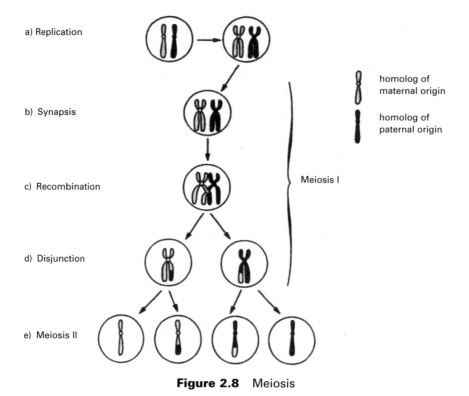

a) Replication

b) Synapsis

c) Recombination

d) Disjunction

e) Meiosis II

Meiosis I

homolog of
maternal origin

homolog of
paternal origin

Figure 2.8   Meiosis

Source: From *Chromosome Abnormalities and Genetic Counseling, Second Edition* by RJM
Gardner and GR Sutherland, copyright 1989, 1996 by Oxford University Press, Inc. Used by
permission of Oxford University Press, Inc.

Meiosis

Meiosis is divided into two main sections I and II. The chromosome number
is *halved* in meiosis I since no prior DNA synthesis occurs. Early in meiosis I,
the maternal and paternal chromosomes form into corresponding pairs and at
this point there is recombination with exchange of reciprocal fragments. The
points at which crossover occurs, the chiasmata, perform the secondary function of holding the pairs together. At cell division each cell receives a maternal *or* paternal homologue. A further division called Meiosis II then occurs
which is similar to mitosis.

Box 2.1   Protein Synthesis

DNA contains information that allows the cell to synthesize proteins. It
does this by transcribing the information code to a segment of RNA which
then moves to the ribosome outside of the nucleus where the amino acids
are combined in a specific order to produce a functioning protein.

Cells have the capacity to respond to hormones and growth factors by initiating transcription of DNA and thus the eventual production of particular functioning proteins. In this way the body is able to respond to the changing environment by increasing and decreasing the levels of functioning proteins.

Mechanisms of Genetic Disease

Only one of each pair of chromosomes is passed from a parent to a child. When gametes form there is a possibility that errors may occur so a pregnancy starts with a different chromosome pattern or genetic code at a specific locus not present in either parent. The normal inheritance pattern allows prediction of the transmission of a genetic disease in a family.

Chromosome Abnormalities

Where a chromosome anomaly is detected it may be present in all body cells or only in a subset, giving a mosaic pattern. Chromosome anomalies form three main groups:

- numerical, where there are abnormal numbers of chromosomes
- structural, where chromosomes have been broken or rearranged
- uniparental disomy, where the usual inheritance of chromosomes from both parents has been disturbed.

Numerical abnormalities

These fall into three groups – polyploidy, aneuploidy and mixoploidy.

1. Polyploidy means that there are extra copies of the *whole* chromosome complement. A pregnancy with triploidy has three copies of each chromosome, giving a pattern of 69XXX, 69XXY or 69XYY, and will occasionally progress to term. Some cells in the body are naturally polyploid, e.g. regenerating liver cells prior to division. Nulliploidy, where there are no chromosomes, is normal in red blood and squamous skin cells which are without nuclei.
2. Aneuploidy results in either the gain or loss of a *specific* chromosome termed trisomy or monosomy respectively. Cancer cells often have various aneuploidies. Aneuploid cells arise as a result of non-disjunction. In meiosis I this would be failure of the paired homologues to separate, or, in mitosis and meiosis II, failure of sister chromatid separation. Occasionally chromosomes can also be lost if they do not migrate properly toward the

poles at cell division. Table 2.1 gives examples of the common human aneuploidies.

3. Mixoploidy describes the situation where two or more different karyotypes are identified on analysis. This is called mosaicism if the cells derive from one zygote. This can arise if there is non-disjunction not in the first mitotic division after meiosis but in a subsequent one. Mosaicism with a normal cell line will tend to ameliorate the phenotype. A phenotype is the way that the genetic inheritance is expressed in the body.

Table 2.1 Examples of Autosomal Trisomies and Sex Chromosome Anomalies

Anomaly and Aetiology	Birth Incidence	Clinical Features
Trisomy 21 (Down's syndrome) 95% nondisjunction 1% mosaic-variable phenotype 4% unbalanced translocation	1/700	Upslanting palpebral fissures, speckled irides, small nose, flat facial profile, brachycephalic skull, single palmar creases, short 5th finger. IQ usually <50. Congenital heart disease (40%), duodenal atresia, cataracts (2%), epilepsy (10%), hypothyroidism (3%), leukaemia (1%)
Trisomy 18 (Edwards syndrome) Nondisjunction Occasional mosaicism	1/3000	Low birth weight, small chin, prominent occiput, low set ears. Clenched hands, overlapping index and 5th fingers, rockerbottom feet, short sternum. Low survival past 1yr, little developmental progress. Cardiac and renal malformations common
47XXY (Klinefelter syndrome) Extra X maternal in 60%, paternal in 40% 15% mosaic	1/1000 males	Long limbs, gynaecomastia, scoliosis. Poor development of secondary sexual characteristics, infertility. Adult onset diabetes (8%), mild learning disability (20%)
45XO (Turner syndrome) Nondisjunction in either parent. 75% maternal X present. 60% have 45X, others have an isochromosome of Xq or a deletion of Xp 15% are mosaic	1/5000 females	Neonatal excess skin fold at neck or peripheral lymphoedema. Proportionate short stature. No adult growth spurt without hormone therapy. Streak ovaries. Broad chest, widely spaced nipples, wide neck, increased carrying angle at the elbow. 20% have congenital heart disease. Horseshoe kidneys. May become hypertensive.

Structural abnormalities

Structural abnormalities arise when chromosomes become broken and rearranged. The resultant karyotype may be balanced, with no net gain or loss of material, or unbalanced. Where there is a single break the terminal portion is usually lost at cell division, because it has no centromere, giving rise to a deletion. Table 2.2 gives examples of the common human deletion syndromes.

Table 2.2   Examples of Chromosome Microdeletion Syndromes

Syndrome	Chromosomal location	Clinical features
Wolf–Hirschhorn Syndrome	4p16.3	Ocular hypertelorism with broad or beaked nose giving 'Greek' helmet appearance. Growth retardation, microcephaly, cleft lip/palate, severe learning disability, seizures.
Cri du chat Syndrome	5p15.2-p15.3	Low birth weight, poor growth, cat-like cry, round face, epicanthic folds. Severe learning disability, microcephaly, congenital heart defects in 30%.
Williams Syndrome	7q11.23 (elastin gene)	Learning disability with characteristic chatty personality. Classical facial features include stellate irides, anteverted nares and sagging cheeks. Hypercalcaemia. Congenital heart disease
WAGR Syndrome	11p13 (WT1 and PAX 6 genes)	Wilms' tumour 50%, aniridia, growth retardation, genital anomalies, moderate to severe learning disability

Where there are two breaks in the chromosome the intervening section may be:

- lost – an interstitial deletion;
- inverted and reinserted at the same point, giving an inversion;
- moved to a different place in the same or another chromosome, creating an insertion; or
- formed into a ring. If the ring contains a centromere it can continue in cell divisions. There will be a variable loss of material from the ends of the chromosome involved.

Balanced chromosome rearrangements, or those with insignificant markers, can be inherited within families (see below). However most unbalanced abnormalities occur as single cases. Chromosome patterns that appear the same under the microscope will involve different amounts of gain or loss of material at gene level, and may have very different physical features.

Marker chromosomes, small extra fragments of chromatin, are sometimes seen. They may be familial, and the clinical significance is very much dependent on the content of the marker. Techniques such as chromosome painting, have helped to determine the chromosome of origin of such fragments.

Translocations

Reciprocal translocations are common. They occur when there is a two-way exchange of chromosome material between two non-homologous chromosomes – that is each chromosome involved is from a different pair. Where there is no apparent loss of material at the breakpoints, and an individual has a normal phenotype, the karyotype is balanced. However translocations can be lead to unbalanced gametes and can cause infertility or miscarriage, or result in liveborn children with an unbalanced chromosome pattern.

For chromosomes where the centromere is near one end (13, 14, 15, 21 and 22) a separate type of translocation, termed a Robertsonian translocation, can occur (Figure 2.9). Essentially the two chromosomes involved fuse around the centromere to give one composite chromosome. The overall pattern may be balanced in a parent, but gametes with an unbalanced chromosome amount can arise, particularly where Chromosome 21 is involved. This gives an affected couple a higher risk of conceiving a pregnancy with Down's syndrome.

Uniparental disomy

Uniparental disomy occurs when a child has both chromosomes of a particular pair from one parent. Where there is non-disjunction for a chromosome pair in meiosis I in one parent, the result is trisomy for that chromosome. If the second parent's chromosome is lost, the term uniparental heterodisomy is used since both chromosomes in the pair from one parent will be represented. Uniparental isodisomy occurs where the error is in meiosis II and the individual has two copies of the *same* chromosome from one parent. Uniparental disomy can cause genetic disease because we now understand that, *for certain genes*, expression can be altered depending on whether inheritance has been on the maternal or paternal chromosome. This phenomenon is known as imprinting (Hall, 1990). There are many theories surrounding the biological function of imprinting. It seems that imprinting may be involved in regulation of growth in the embryo (see Figures 2.10 and 2.11).

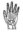 Example of imprinting

Two syndromes, Angelman (AS) and Prader-Willi (PWS), are both associated with deletions of 15q12 that look identical on chromosome analysis. However

37

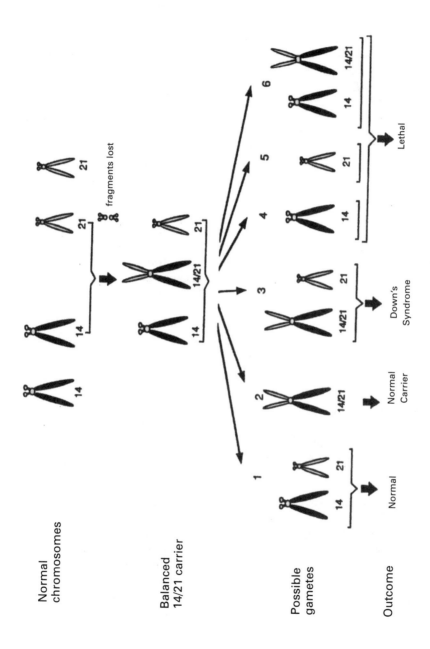

Figure 2.9 Examples of Roberstsonian Translocation

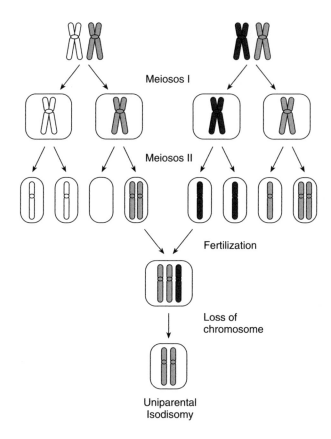

Meiosos I

Meiosos II

Fertilization

Loss of
chromosome

Uniparental
Isodisomy

Figure 2.10   Non-disjunction at Meiosis II Giving Rise to Uniparental Disomy

in PWS the deletion can be shown to be on the paternal and in AS on the maternal chromosome 15 and the two syndromes have very different physical features:

Angelman Syndrome (AS)

- severe learning disability
- few if any words
- growth retardation
- unsteady gait
- epilepsy
- inappropriate laughter
- often very fair colouring

Prader-Willi Syndrome (PWS)

- moderate learning disability
- severe hypotonia in infancy
  hypogenitalism in boys
- progression to obesity in
  childhood
- abnormal eating behaviour
- risk of diabetes in later life

The two patterns can also occur if there is uniparental disomy for chromosome 15 following initial non-disjunction with loss of the maternal or paternal complement

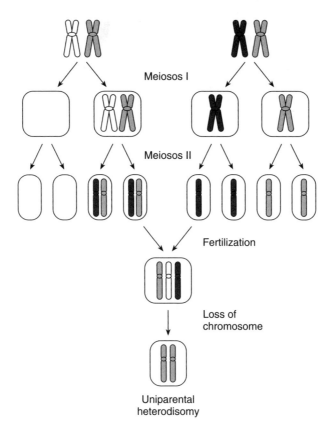

Figure 2.11   Non-disjunction at Meiosis I Giving Rise to Uniparental
Heterodisomy

Genetic Disease at Gene Level

Human cells probably contain around 35,000 genes. This genetic complement is called the 'human genome'. Some are necessary only for embryonic
development. Since genes direct the production of all cell proteins, an altered
gene can often have a profound effect on cell growth and function. By the age
of 25 years, 5 per cent of the population will have a disorder caused by a
genetic change. Various complex methods have been used to place specific
genes in their correct chromosome position and to sequence their code.
Knowledge of the correct sequence allows the study of alterations, or 'mutations', within families as a cause of disease. Mutation can be caused by exposure to harmful X-rays or chemicals, but most occur as errors in DNA
replication and repair.

In general terms, a mutation may mean that no protein product is
produced, or that the product has little or no function. Sometimes, if a protein

forms part of a complex structure, such as collagen, an abnormal protein may be more disruptive than no protein at all. Alternatively the product may function in an abnormal way with a gain in function. Mutations may not be in the gene itself but in regulator regions such as the promoters, or at the junction of an intron (non-coding sequence) and exon (coding sequence) affecting mRNA formation. The following section describes various types of mutation with examples.

Mutations within a gene may be:

- Deletions;
- Duplications;
- Insertions;
- Inversions; or
- Substitutions.

Deletions

A deletion is a loss of part of the genetic code. About 60 per cent of individuals with the X-linked condition Duchenne muscular dystrophy (DMD) can be shown to have a deletion of exons within the dystrophin gene. For these families simple genetic tests can detect female carriers and offer prenatal diagnosis if requested. The DMD gene is one of the largest described, and other mutations have proven far more difficult to detect.

Another well-known example would be deletion of the phenylalanine codon at position 508 in the cystic fibrosis gene (ΔF508) which accounts for about 75 per cent of mutations in this gene in the UK. In the general population 1 in 20 people is a carrier of Cystic Fibrosis. The effect of a deletion depends not only on its size but whether it is 'in frame' – that is a whole number of codons are removed. This may allow transcription after the deletion. If the reading frame is shifted so the code is read out of sequence, the misread sequence may code for 'stop' and the result is a shortened product.

Large deletions may involve more than one gene and give rise to contiguous gene deletion syndromes. This is suspected when a recognized single gene disorder is associated with atypical learning disability, or other disease, caused by loss of additional nearby genes. One example would be the extension of a dystrophin deletion into neighbouring genes on the X chromosome causing chronic granulomatous disease and retinitis pigmentosa as well as Duchenne muscular dystrophy (DMD).

Duplications

The effect of any additional genetic material will depend on its position within a gene and any effect on the reading frame. Type I Hereditary Motor and Sensory Neuropathy (HMSN) is a dominant condition often caused by a duplication in a myelin protein gene. Overproduction of the protein product seems to be harmful and can present in childhood with pes cavus (claw foot, with excessive arches) and diminished reflexes.

Insertions

Over the past few years a special type of insertion, which leads to an 'unstable' or 'dynamic' mutation, has been described. In various places in the genome there are repeated copies of a triplet sequence such as CAG or CCG. The number of repeats at these sites will vary between individuals within a normal range but in excess of this range it is called an 'expansion'. Triplet expansions have been increasingly documented as a cause of disease, particularly neurological conditions. Expansion of a CAG repeat in the Huntington's disease gene leads to a gain in function. Massive expansions of CGG in the FMR1 gene cause the fragile X syndromes FRAXA and FRAXE by silencing their promoter.

In general, disease severity increases with expansion size, and the expansions are unstable with a tendency to increase from one generation to the next. This phenomenon is called anticipation.

Inversions

Sometimes a section of a gene may be inverted. Over 50 per cent of severe Haemophilia A is caused by a rearrangement in the Factor VIII gene caused by a small inversion on the X chromosome.

Single base substitutions

Single base substitution means that one amino acid will be replaced by another. This may be silent if the amino acid is of similar structure and charge, but if a particular amino acid has a pivotal part in the finished structure of the protein the protein product may well have altered function. A well-known example would be the change from GAG to GTG at the sixth position of the beta-globin chain which substitutes valine for glutamic acid and causes sickle cell anaemia if inherited from both parents.

Other Genetic Mechanisms that can alter Function

Gene expression can be altered by events affecting chromatin structure. A translocation, where there is chromosome rearrangement, may disrupt a gene at the point where the chromosome breaks. Another example would be an event that moves a gene further away from a promoter or enhancer, or moves a gene into a position where it is silenced. This is likely to be the mechanism in the dominant condition Facio-Scapulo-Humeral dystrophy (FSH), which causes progressive weakness of muscles of facial expression, shoulder and hip joints. A deletion of a non-coding repeat sequence at the tip of 4q moves the gene nearer to the telomere (the tip of the chromosome) and it is not expressed.

Box 2.2 Determinants of Genetic Disease

There are many ways in which genetic disease can arise. These can lead to the following types of errors with the genetic components of the cell:

- Variation in the number of sets of chromosomes;
- Variation in the number of chromosomes;
- Abnormalities so that pieces of chromosome are missing or repeated or in the wrong order;
- Both copies of the chromosome can come from the same parent; and
- Mutations at the level of the gene, which influences the ability to produce functional proteins.

Some of these problems are incompatible with life; others can cause major disability

---

Patterns of Mendelian Inheritance

The normal characteristics that we inherit from our parents follow the same patterns as altered genes through the process of meiosis. Figure 2.12 identifies the symbols used in constructing a pedigree and these diagrams help to describe the patterns of inheritance that are commonly found in families.

In the simplest case, the presence or absence of a genetic disease is determined by a change in a gene at a single locus. About 5000 single gene diseases are known. The pattern of inheritance depends on which chromosome is involved (an autosome or sex chromosome) and whether the change is dominant or recessive.

At each autosomal locus there are two alleles making up the genotype (the genetic constitution of an individual). One allele is inherited from the mother and one from the father. An allele is one of several alternative forms of gene or DNA sequence at a specific chromosome location (locus).

If only one altered gene results in the disease this is called a dominant change, and an individual carrying this change is a heterozygote. If an individual has one change with no ill effect they are called a '*carrier*' for the condition and the change is said to be recessive. There are five basic patterns of inheritance derived from dominant and recessive changes on autosomal and sex chromosomes (see Table 2.3).

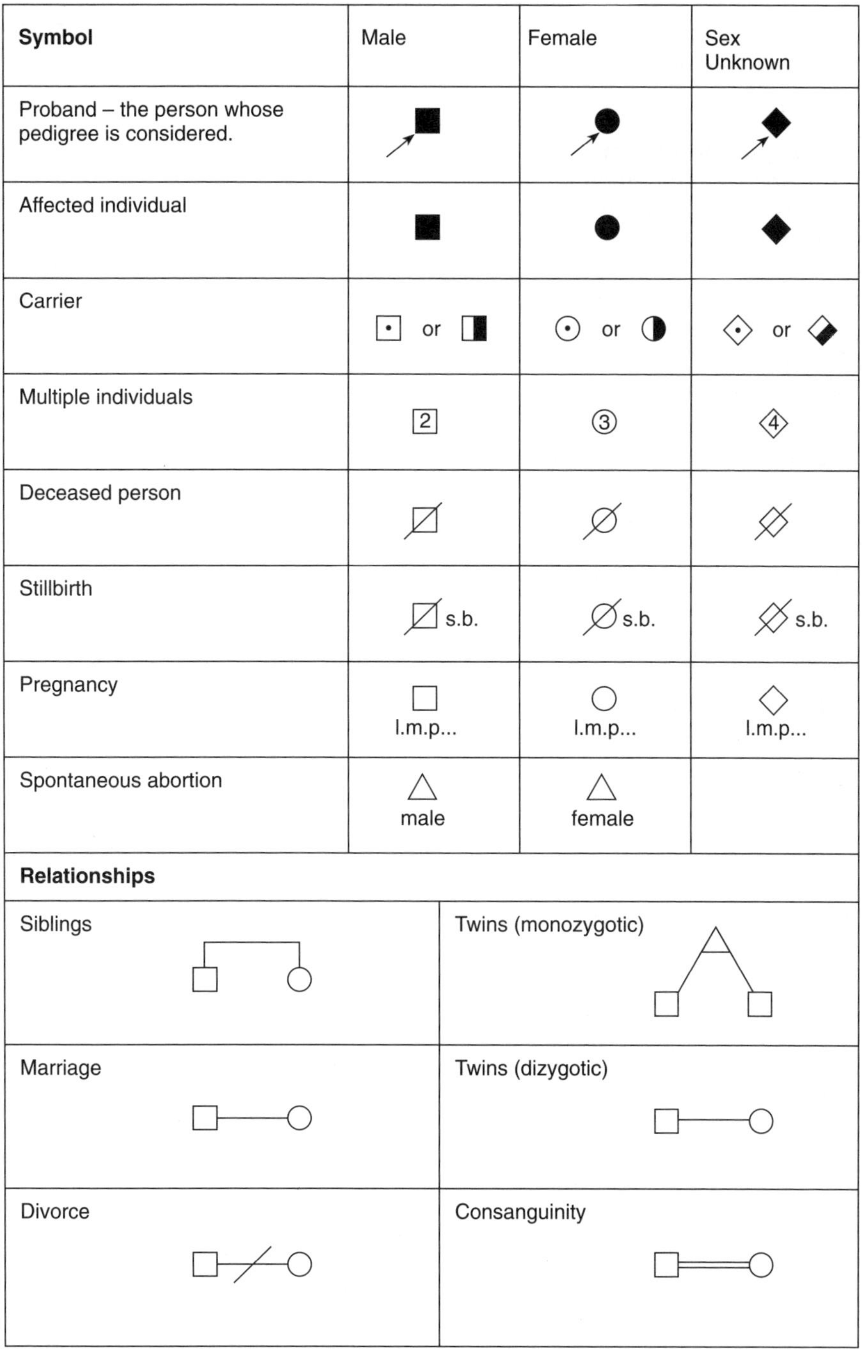

Symbol	Male	Female	Sex Unknown
Proband – the person whose pedigree is considered.	▪	●	◆
Affected individual	■	●	◆
Carrier	⊡ or ◧	⊙ or ◑	◇ or ◈
Multiple individuals	2	③	④
Deceased person	⊘	⊘	⊘
Stillbirth	⊘ s.b.	⊘ s.b.	⊘ s.b.
Pregnancy	□ l.m.p...	○ l.m.p...	◇ l.m.p...
Spontaneous abortion	△ male	△ female	
Relationships			
Siblings		Twins (monozygotic)	
Marriage		Twins (dizygotic)	
Divorce		Consanguinity	

Figure 2.12 Standard Symbols used in Pedigree

Table 2.3   Basic Patterns of Inheritance

Pattern and features	Representative Pedigree
Autosomal dominant *A dominant alteration on an autosome –* *non sex – chromosome* Often affected individuals in more than one generation Affects males and females Can be transmitted by either sex Affected individual has a 50 per cent risk of transmitting the condition	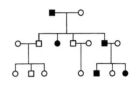
Autosomal recessive *A recessive alteration on an autosome –* *non sex – chromosome* Affected people usually have unaffected parents who are 'carriers' Risk that a sibling will be affected is 1 in 4 Affects either sex Low chance that they will transmit the disorder Consanguinity may be present	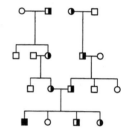
X-linked recessive *A recessive alteration on the X chromosome* Affects males (carrier females may be mildly affected) Insert table 3 (3) No male to male transmission Parents usually unaffected Mother may have affected male relatives Carrier mother has a 1 in 2 risk for male pregnancies	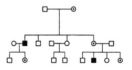
X-linked dominant *A dominant alteration on the X chromosome* Affects either sex but females more (lethality in males) Variable phenotype in females Affected male transmits only to daughters Affected females 1 in 2 offspring risk for either sex	
Y-linked *An alteration on the Y chromosome* Characters described but no known disease Only male to male transmission and all sons affected	

Common Dominantly Inherited Conditions

In general, dominant conditions are often compatible with an adult lifespan and involve structural components of the body such as muscle, collagen and fibrillin.

Neurofibromatosis Type I (NF1) is caused by mutations in the neurofibromin gene at 17q11.2, has a birth incidence of 1 in 3000 and can usually be diagnosed by five years. Around 50 per cent of cases have no family history and are therefore new mutations. NF1 is usually diagnosed in childhood by the presence of six or more café au lait patches over 1cm in diameter. Neurofibromas (small benign lumps under the skin) tend to develop from puberty onwards. Lisch nodules, benign tumours of the iris of the eye, may be present in older children. However some children will have larger and more complex neurofibromas, which may be on the face, pseudoarthrosis (a false joint) of the tibia, optic nerve tumour, scoliosis (curvature of the spine) or hemihypertrophy (one side of the body or limb larger than another). About 30 per cent have learning problems. There is a low risk of malignant tumours, particularly in the Central Nervous System. Neurofibromin has an influence on the regulation of cell division and, in tumours, changes in the second gene copy are found (see tumour suppressor genes below).

Other examples of dominantly inherited conditions include tuberous sclerosis (TS), Treacher Collins syndrome and Marfan syndrome. Mutations in other structural genes, such as those producing collagen, may give rise to problems with bone formation, as in Osteogenesis Imperfecta, or skin and ligamentous elasticity as seen in the Ehlers Danlos syndromes

Developmental genes

Human developmental genes act early in embryogenesis and are pivotal to laying down the basic structure. Embryonic patterning is segmental, with developmental genes influencing several segments determining how cells arrange themselves and develop within them. Mutations in the segmentation gene, sonic hedgehog, can cause holoprosencephaly (failure of front part of the brain to separate into two lobes), and abnormalities in differentiating right from left in heart development. Genes containing a 'paired-box' (called PAX genes) are an important group of genes vital for development of the vertebral column and nervous system. Dominant mutations in PAX3 at 2q37 cause Waardenburg syndrome, with pigmentary iris and hair anomalies and deafness. Mutations in PAX6 cause a range of developmental eye problems including dominantly inherited aniridia.

Many developmental genes are growth factors that regulate cell division, migration and differentiation. Mutations in different fibroblast growth factor receptor genes are associated with craniosynostosis syndromes (where the cranial sutures fuse too early), such as Pfeiffer, Apert and Crouzon syndromes, or skeletal dysplasias including achondroplasia.

Common Recessively Inherited Conditions

The majority of recessive conditions involve abnormalities of body chemistry such as the production of enzymes or transport molecules. For the disease to manifest, both copies of the gene need to be altered. Both parents will be 'carriers' for the condition. A carrier will have one normally functioning gene and one with altered or no function. Often half of the normal level of product is produced and this can be used to help diagnose carriers where a direct genetic test is not available. Cystic fibrosis, with a carrier frequency of 1 in 20, is the commonest recessive condition in the Caucasian population, but beta thalassaemia and sickle cell disease have similar or higher carriage rate in specific ethnic groups.

Other recessive conditions include spinal muscular atrophy (Wernig-Hoffman disease) and alpha-1-antitrypsin deficiency. Another group of disorders, the mucopolysaccharidoses, involve deficiency of a lysosomal enzyme. This reduces the cells' ability to remove waste products and the accumulation causes neurological damage, coarsens facial features and affects joint mobility. Recessive genes also account for a high proportion of severe sensorineural deafness.

Common X-linked Conditions

The X chromosome carries many genes vital for early brain development, and X-linked gene changes make a significant contribution to male learning disability, e.g. Fragile X syndrome. Some changes will just affect learning but others will have associated physical features such as facial dysmorphism, abnormality of fat distribution, spasticity, hydrocephalus or dermatological signs which may allow a specific diagnosis. Duchenne muscular dystrophy presents with progressive weakness in early childhood. Haemophilia, a blood clotting disorder, is X-linked as are various immunodeficiency syndromes.

Penetrance and Expression

For some conditions an individual may carry a genetic change but not demonstrate any problem. The phenotype is the way that the genetic inheritance is expressed in the body and the penetrance of a particular phenotype is the probability that features will be manifest in the affected individual. Occasionally even dominant conditions can appear to 'skip' a generation because of non-penetrance. Even when penetrant there can be great variability in the phenotype, even within families, and the term 'expression' is used to describe this. Dominant conditions generally show more variability than recessive ones. Anticipation is a particular pattern of expression where the phenotype becomes more severe with subsequent generations. This is particularly a feature where the basis of the mutation is an unstable repeat sequence as described earlier.

DNA in Mitochondria

Mitochondria have their own DNA with 37 genes coded. As there are no mitochondria in sperm cells any mutation in mitochondrial DNA can only be inherited maternally. A mother may have a mixture of affected and unaffected mitochondria (heteroplasmy) and therefore severity in offspring is related to the numbers of mutant mitochondria inherited and the proportion affected in susceptible tissues. Mitochondrial disease mostly presents in adult life in various ways including myopathy, seizures, strokes, optic atrophy, diabetes and deafness, but recurrent encephalitis and some myopathies presenting in childhood have been associated with mutations in mitochondrial DNA.

Multifactorial Inheritance

For many diseases the phenotype is not determined by a single gene defect but by a combination of genetic factors often influenced by the pregnancy or postnatal environment (e.g. lifestyle and inherited risk for lipid disorders or diabetes) (see Figure 2.13). These disorders recur in families more than would be expected by chance but no simple Mendelian pattern is observed. Neural tube defect, cleft lip and palate, congenital heart disease and atopy show familial clustering. The environmental element is demonstrated for neural tube defect when recurrence risk after an affected pregnancy can be reduced by a factor of five by the use of preconceptual folic acid which is an important requirement for neural tube closure.

For multifactorial conditions such as these the recurrence risk generally increases:

- with increasing severity of the condition of the affected individual (the affected individual is known as the proband);
- if more than one relative is affected;
- if the disease has an unequal sex distribution, and the proband is of the sex less commonly affected.

The risk for family members who are less than second degree relatives of the proband rapidly returns to that of the general population. Our knowledge of the risks associated with these conditions is derived from the experiences of other families with the same prior histories.

Cancer Genetics

Cancer is a genetic disease in that cancer development involves a series of changes in the genes causing loss of control of cell division. However it is important to stress that a spontaneous change in a control gene, rather than

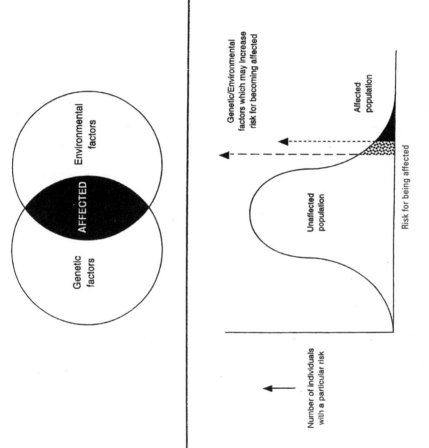

Figure 2.13 Multifactorial Inheritance – Threshold Model

an inherited change, is the trigger for cancer development in the majority of cases. Often when a predisposition to cancer is inherited, a mutation in one of the two copies of a specific tumour suppressor gene is present in all cells. If a further mutation occurs in the other copy within a cell both copies are lost and a tumour results. This was described by Knudson in his 'two hit' theory (Knudson, 1971) and the best-known paediatric example is retinoblastoma presenting with tumours at the back of the eye from birth to five years. The tumours in this pattern of inheritance are characteristically bilateral and multi-focal. In contrast sporadic retinoblastoma tends to be isolated after *both* changes have occurred in a *single* cell.

Leukaemia is one of the commonest paediatric cancers. Individuals with Down's syndrome have 20 times the general population risk of leukaemia. Leukaemia is rarely familial. About 3 per cent of childhood leukaemia is asso-ciated with a genetic disorder. Examples would be those inherited in a reces-sive pattern associated with mutations in genes that act to stabilize the DNA helix during replication and repair any mistakes made at that time. Often these can be diagnosed because the chromosomes break when cultured. One exam-ple would be Bloom syndrome, a rare recessive disorder where a sun-sensitive rash and pigmentary abnormality is associated with severe immune deficiency and a high risk of malignancy. Another example is Fanconi's anaemia, where abnormalities of the radius are associated with an increased risk of malignancy. Immunodeficiency syndromes also have an increase risk of leukaemia.

A further group of children may have an increased risk of malignancy because of the dosage of growth factors operating during development, such as in children with Beckwith-Weidermann syndrome where high birthweight and hemihypertrophy is associated with an increased risk of Wilms' tumour.

Assessment in Relation to Genetic Disorders

A Clinical Geneticist may be involved with a family prenatally if a chromoso-mal disorder or congenital malformation has been diagnosed. An older child where there are concerns regarding developmental progress with or without any unusual physical features may also need assessment.

The aim is to make an accurate diagnosis where possible, to share informa-tion as appropriate and to help parents adjust to a future that may be very different to their expectations. The risk of recurrence in future pregnancies and the role of prenatal testing need to be considered. While every situation is different, there are some key stages in a genetic assessment:

- taking a three-generation family history (pedigree);
- full pregnancy history: to include history of bleeding, fever, medication, exposure to teratogens, investigations, fetal movement and mode of delivery;
- neonatal history – measurements, resuscitation;
- developmental milestones, hearing and vision assessments;

- behavioural phenotype;
- physical examination to include assessment of any dysmorphic features (see below); and
- identify the need for further investigations, such as chromosome analysis.

Obtaining a Karyotype Analysis

The appearance of the human chromosome pattern (karyotype) is most commonly obtained from blood. In the laboratory a blood sample is cultured to encourage growth of the T lymphocytes. After 48–72 hours the cells are treated so that the chromosomes can be seen under the microscope.

Newer techniques involve fluorescently labelling known sequences of DNA which then attach to their corresponding chromosome location [FISH – fluorescence in situ hybridization]. This has made it possible to develop specific tests for known sub-microscopic deletions, and to look for losses at the tips (or telomeres) of chromosomes that are associated with learning disability. Fluorescent whole chromosome 'paints' are now available for all chromosomes and these are particularly useful in characterizing complex rearrangements.

The Dysmorphic Child

A child may have unusual facial or other physical characteristics (dysmorphism) with or without learning disability. These dysmorphic features can be described using standard terminology and taking measurements, for example around the face, which can then be compared to standards for age. Positive findings are often termed 'handles' and these can be used when searching the literature and dysmorphology databases – such as the London Dysmorphology database – to try and discern a known syndrome.

Example

A child has been born with pulmonary valve disease but is hypotonic and not feeding, and concern has been raised that there may be an underlying problem. Chromosome analysis has resulted in a normal female karyotype. Positive findings on examination include widely spaced eyes and slightly low set ears. A clinical geneticist meets the child's mother and takes a family tree. The mother is of normal stature. Her husband is 158 cm tall. Several members of his family are also short and one child has been referred for investigation of growth. A separate appointment is made to meet both parents and a request is made for the parents to bring photographs of themselves as children and of family pictures if these are available. The father also has widely spaced eyes but no other features on examination. However childhood photographs of himself and members of his family are consistent with a diagnosis of Noonan syndrome. Hypertelorism, with downturned palpebral fissures, lowset posteriorly rotated ears and neck webbing is associated with short adult stature. This is generally a benign condition but has a raised risk of congenital heart disease and feeding problems in the first year of life. Accurate diagnosis in the family can allow appropriate screening for heart disease in pregnancy as well as height prediction and preventing inappropriate investigation.

Conclusion

Our understanding of genetic disease mechanisms has increased rapidly over the last few years with promises of improvements in diagnostic strategy and treatment. Efforts have been concentrated on single gene diseases but are now looking at genetic predisposition to the major causes of adult morbidity. All advances are associated with moral dilemmas and an increased understanding of ourselves combined with increased choice both in reproduction and lifestyle will have the potential for good and bad. However for individuals and their families a great deal can be achieved by accurate diagnosis with sensitive disclosure of information.

Review Questions

1. How does DNA act as a blueprint for the design of functional proteins and how are these proteins manufactured in the cell?
2. Using the example of Down's syndrome, describe the way in which the genetic error arises.
3. What is meant by the term 'mutation?' Give two examples of mutations and analyse their impact.
4. What is meant by multifactorial inheritance? Consider how this can influence approaches to care and management.

Further Reading

Aase, J (1990) *Diagnostic Dysmorphology.* London: Plenum Medical Book Company. A detailed text in examining children for dysmorphic signs.

Clarke, A (ed.) (1994) *Genetic Counselling. Practice and Principles.* London: Routledge. A thoughtful book on difficult issues surrounding genetic information and a good insight into the specialty.

Clarke, A (1994) The Genetic testing of children. Working Party of the Clinical Genetics Society (UK). *Journal of Medical Genetics,* 31, 785–97.

Connor, JM and Ferguson-Smith, MA (1997) *Essential Medical Genetics.* Oxford, Blackwell Scientific Publications. Chapters 1–9. General basic textbook.

Dawkins, R (1989) The Selfish Gene. 2nd edn. Oxford: Oxford University Press. Interesting and thought provoking idea.

Eeles, RA, Ponder, BAJ, Easton, DF and Horwich, A (eds) (1996) *Genetic Predisposition to Cancer.* London, Chapman and Hall Medical. A good summary text for anyone interested in genetic mechanisms in cancer and cancer syndromes.

Gardner, RJM and Sutherland, GR (1996) Chromosome Abnormalities and Genetic Counselling. 2nd edn. Oxford: Oxford University Press. A useful guide for counselling families but also good explanations of cell division.

Hall, JG, Froster-Iskenius, UG and Allanson, JE (1989) *Handbook of Normal Physical Measurements.* Oxford: Oxford Medical Publishers. Useful for gaining an understanding of normal child growth patterns and proportions.

Harper, PS (1998) *Practical Genetic Counselling.* 5th edn. Oxford: Butterworth Heinemann.

Jones, KL (1997) *Smith's Recognizable Patterns of Human Malformation.* London: WB Saunders Company. A catalogue of the commonest syndromes with photographs and references.

Kingston, HM (1994) *An ABC of Clinical Genetics.* 2nd edn. London: British Medical Association. A simple first book of genetics.

Marteau, M and Richards, M (1996) *The Troubled Helix: Social and Psychological Implications of the New Genetics.* Cambridge: Cambridge University Press. If you want to delve into ethical aspects of genetics.

McKusick, VA (1994) (ed.) *Mendelian Inheritance in Man.* 11th edn. Baltimore, Johns Hopkins University Press. Also available online (OMIM – see below) – exhaustive catalogue of all known Mendelian traits.

Modell, B and Modell, M (1992) *Towards a Healthy Baby.* Parts 1–3. Oxford University Press. Well written guide to genetic counselling and community genetics.

Mueller, RF and Young, ID (2001) *Emery's Elements of Medical Genetics.* London: Churchill Livingstone. Excellent general genetics book with clear explanation of genetic principles and many paediatric examples with illustrations.

Strachan, T and Read, AP (1996) *Human Molecular Genetics.* Oxford, Bios Scientific Publishers Ltd. A comprehensive textbook for individuals who want to pursue more information about molecular mechanisms. Dip into for specific diseases.

Vogel, F and Motulsky, AG (1997) *Human Genetics, problems and approaches.* 3rd edn. Berlin: Springer-Verlag. Comprehensive textbook with good chapters on cytogenetics and cell division.

Useful websites

http://www3.ncbi.nlm.nih.gov/Omim/ *Online Mendelian Inherited in Man.*
Human Genome Organization. http://hugo.gdb.org/ Useful articles on current research and ethics.
Public Health Genetics Unit. http://www.medschl.cam.ac.uk/phgu Articles on the wider application of genetic testing.
BBC Summary of a genetics series. http://www.bbc.co.uk/health/genes Genetic summary in lay language.

References

Hall, JG (1990) *Genomic imprinting: review and relevance to human diseases. American Journal of Human Genetics,* 45, 857–73.
Knudson, AG (1971) *Mutation and cancer: a statistical study of retinoblastoma. Proceedings of the National Academy of Science USA,* 68, 820–3.
Mueller, RF and Young, ID (1998) *Emery's Elements of Medical Genetics.* Chapter 1. 10th edn. London: Churchill Livingstone.
Watson, JD and Crick, FHC (1953a) *Molecular studies of nucleic acids. Nature,* 171, 737–8.
Watson, JD and Crick, FHC (1953b) *Genetical implications of the structure of deoxyribonucleic acid. Nature,* 171, 964–7.

CHAPTER **3**

Central Nervous System Development

Sarah Neill and Lorraine Bowden

Contents

Learning Outcomes

At the end of the chapter you will be able to:

- Describe the development of the brain and central nervous system from the embryonic period through relevant stages of childhood.
- Identify positive and negative factors that influence the development of the central nervous system.
- Relate the healthy development of the brain and nervous system to normal co-ordination and control in the developing infant and child.
- Discuss the assessment of nervous system function in health.

Introduction

The nervous system consists of a network of highly complex structures that provides the body with the means to interact with the internal and external environment. Pivotal to the whole nervous system is the central nervous system, the development of which forms the focus of this chapter.

Overview of the Major Divisions of the Nervous System

A brief overview of the whole nervous system is given first to set in context the information on the development of the nervous system which is the main focus on this chapter.

The mature nervous system is divided into two parts – the central nervous system *(CNS)* and the peripheral nervous system. The CNS is composed of the brain and spinal cord, which receives, interprets or integrates stimuli and relays nerve impulses to muscles and glands. The peripheral nervous system is made up of nerves that form connections between the brain and spinal cord and those glands and muscles.

The peripheral nervous system is further sub-divided into the afferent (sensory) system, which sends information from peripheral receptors to the CNS, and the efferent (motor) system, which carries information from the CNS to muscles and glands. The efferent motor system is divided again from a functional perspective into the somatic nervous system, which transmits information from the CNS to skeletal muscles and the autonomic nervous system, which sends information from the CNS to glands, smooth muscle and cardiac muscle. The latter is also divided into the sympathetic and parasympathetic nervous systems. Further information on the detailed structure of the nervous system as a whole can be found in any good anatomy and physiology textbook.

The Central Nervous System

The central nervous system (CNS), consisting of the brain and spinal cord, therefore: 'may be thought of as the body's central control system, receiving and interpreting or integrating stimuli and relaying nerve impulses to muscles and glands, where designated actions actually take place.' (Carola *et al.*, 1992, p. 327) It receives and interprets stimuli from the internal environment (internal organs and systems such as muscles and glands), sending out nerve impulses to target organs, which stimulate responses designed to maintain homeostasis within the internal environment. The central nervous system also enables the body to receive, interpret and respond to stimuli from the external environment, for example information received by the senses: sight, hearing, taste, smell and balance. Information from both internal and external sources are analysed, compared and co-ordinated within the central nervous system, a process termed integration (Carola *et al.*, 1992). This process facilitates learning about the environment and the control of responses to the optimum effect for the survival of the individual and in the case of the child to optimize growth and development. Consequently the development of a healthy nervous system is essential for the future health and development of the child.

Prenatal Development of the Central Nervous System

The development of the central nervous system occurs very early in the embryological stage, the timing and success of which are essential as the presence of the nervous system will influence the development and organization of several other body systems. This development involves complex relationships between genetic information and specific kinds of experiences, some of which need to occur at particular periods in time.

A thorough review of the embryological development of the nervous system is beyond the scope of this book. Readers are referred to Brown *et al.* (1997) for a more detailed overview. However, the main steps in development of the central nervous system will be explored and where relevant the more common congenital problems, which occur when development does not proceed normally, will be signposted.

Early Development of the Central Nervous System from the Neural Tube

According to Moore and Persaud (1993) the development of the nervous system coincides with the first missed week of the menstrual cycle, therefore by the time the woman is aware of the pregnancy, the development of the nervous system is well under way.

The two main structures in the early embryo that contribute to the developing tissues of the nervous system are:

1. the neural tube (which forms the brain and spinal cord, along with the motor component of the peripheral nervous system); and
2. neural crest cells (which form the sensory component of the peripheral nervous system).

Week Three

Central nervous system development commences during the *third week* of gestation, originating in the thickened ectodermal layer, with the formation of the neural plate of the embryo above the notochordal process (see Figure 3.1).

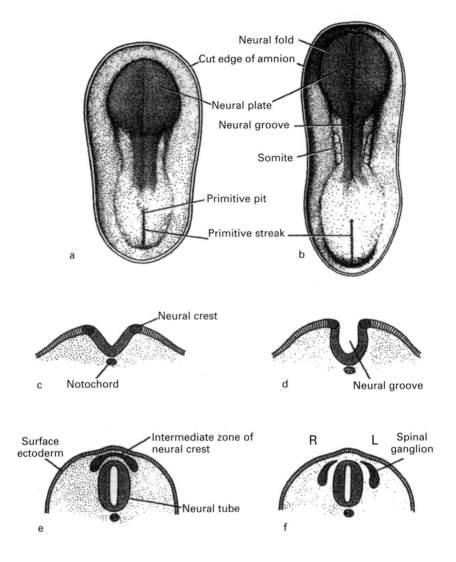

Figure 3.1 Early Development of the Neural Tube

a)   Dorsal view of an embryo at approximately 18 days.
b)   Dorsal view at approximately 20 days.
c)–f) Transverse sections showing formation of the neural groove, neural tube and neural crest.

Source: Lippincott, Williams and Wilkins from *Langman's Medical Embryology*, 8th edition, Sadler, copyright 2000.

Underlying mesodermal cells stimulate the craniocaudal (head–tail) region-alization which divides the neural plate into regions down its length before fusion of the neural tube takes place. These regions will later become specific areas within the brain and spinal cord. 'Shaping', a region-specific mechanism by which the contours of the neural plate are changed, renders the plate narrow and long.

Eighteen days post fertilization

At approximately 18 days post fertilization, a simple invagination on the dorsal portion of the ectodermal layer initiates the formation of a *neural groove* (Fitzgerald and Fitzgerald, 1994). The neural groove has raised edges known as neural folds on each side, amalgamation of which begins in the future neck region of the embryo. Differentiated cells at the edge of each neural fold escape from the line of fusion to form the neural crest cells positioned ventro-laterally on the side of the neural tube.

Around the *end of week three* to *early in week four*, before the neural tube is completely formed, two parallel areas of mesoderm undergo segmentation to form the somites (Fitzgerald and Fitzgerald, 1994; Larsen, 1998). Somites create the segmental organisation of the body, from which most of the skeleton develops, including the vertebral column. Neural crest cells migrate, clustering around each somite (see Figure 3.1).

Week 4: 22 days post fertilization

At the cranial (or head) end of the embryo the folds enlarge. These enlarged areas of the folds are the first signs of the developing brain (Fitzgerald and Fitzgerald, 1994). At about the same time the embryo bends sharply ventrally (forwards) (Larsen, 1998). The resulting mesencephalic flexure (curve) identifies the position of the future mesencephalon (midbrain). The part of the neural groove at the cranial end of the flexure will become the prosencephalon (forebrain) and the part of the future brain caudal to the flexure, the rhombencephalon (hindbrain) (Larsen, 1998). The narrower part of the groove at the caudal (tail) end of the neural groove will form the spinal cord (Fitzgerald and Fitzgerald, 1994) (see Figure 3.2).

The neural folds then increase in height and meet to fuse and form the neural tube (Fitzgerald and Fitzgerald, 1994; Larsen, 1998), which then separates from the surface ectoderm. The free edges of the ectoderm then fuse to provide the epidermis of the skin. The formation of the neural plate, neural folds and neural tube is called neurulation (Moore, 1988). The neural tube has two openings – neuropores, at the cranial and caudal ends, which usually close before the end of the fourth week of gestation.

Occasionally one or both of the neuropores may remain open resulting in serious defects to the fetus and baby. For example: Failure of the cranial neuropore to close results in the fatal condition of anencephaly – incidence ranges from 1·6/1000 births (Fitzgerald and Fitzgerald, 1994); failure of closure of the neural tube in the lumbosacral area of the spinal cord region, will result in spina bifida with a myelomeningocoele – incidence in the UK is

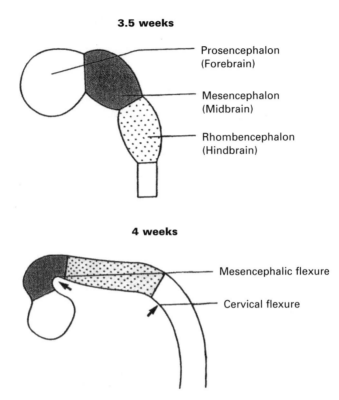

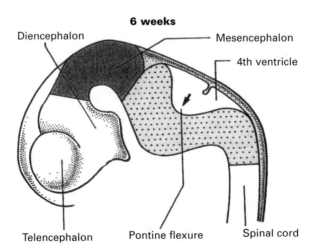

Figure 3.2 Early Development of the Brain Showing the Development of Flexures

Source: Reprinted from *Human Embryology*, Fitzgerald and Fitzgerald, copyright 1994, with permission from Elsevier.

1.7/1000 live births. This type of malformation accounts for 90 per cent of all spinal cord lesions (Campbell and Glasper, 1995).

The Development of the Brain

By the *end of the fourth week*, the enlarged cranial end of the neural tube undergoes rapid and unequal growth, giving rise to the early structures of the brain, which will sub-divide to constitute the basis for the fundamental organization of the adult brain.

As development progresses the brain forms a series of flexures producing additional vesicles. The first of these flexures, the mesencephalic flexure, contributes to the development of the three major primary fluid-filled vesicles from the neural tube as above, beginning the development of the brain.

These three vesicles undergo several further flexures resulting in subdivisions to create five secondary vesicles by *the end of the fifth week of development*. Further subdivisions promote the development of more specialized structures within the brain. Table 3.1 provides an overview of these divisions and the structures that develop from them. Cranial nerve nuclei appear in the brain stem during the *fifth week*. All of which, except the first and second, arise from nuclei located in the brain stem (Larsen, 1998). The final sub-divisions have usually occurred by the end of *the sixth week of gestation*.

Box 3.1   Brain Development before the Awareness of Pregnancy

The central nervous system begins to develop in the third week of gestation, around the time of the first missed period when the woman may not yet know she is pregnant. Pregnancy tests are not usually carried out until after the sixth week of pregnancy. The following parts of the brain will already have developed:

- Neural tube by 22 days
- Closure of neuropores before day 28
- Early development of brain vesicles during the fourth week
- All major subdivisions of the brain by the end of the sixth week.

This information should be used to support preconceptual health education, in particular advice to avoid teratogens (see later section on Factors Influencing Nervous System Development) and take folic acid supplements to reduce the likelihood of neural tube defects (see Chapter 1).

The midbrain, together with the medulla and pons, constitute the brain stem, which connects the hemispheres of the brain, cerebellum and spinal cord. The

Table 3.1 Development of Brain Structures and Cranial Nerves

Primary brain vesicles	Secondary brain vesicles	Adult brain structures	Cranial nerves	Adult neural cavities
Prosencephalon (forebrain)	Telencephalon	Cerebral hemispheres: cortex, white matter, basal nuclei.	I Olfactory	Lateral ventricles and superior part of third ventricle.
	Diencephalon	Thalamus, hypothalamus, epithalamus.	II Optic	Most of third ventricle.
Mesencephalon (midbrain)	Mesencephalon	Brain stem: midbrain.	III Oculomotor IV Trochlear	Cerebral aqueduct
Rhombencephalon (hindbrain)	Metencephalon	Brain stem: pons	V, VI, VII, VIII	Fourth ventricle
		Cerebellum		
	Myelencephalon	Brain stem: medulla oblongata	IX, X, XI, XII	
		Spinal cord		Central canal

Source: Adapted from Moore and Persaud (1998) and Marieb (1992).

brain stem also contains a collection of nuclei, which connect with the reticular formation. This network of tissue receives collateral information from afferent sensory pathways, which it filters, preventing the cortex from being flooded and overloaded with sensory stimuli. The reticular formation also governs arousal of the brain (wakefulness and level of consciousness) and some vital reflexes such as those involved with vasomotor, cardiac and respiratory function.

During the development of the brain, cavities within the vesicles – formed from the lumen of the neural tube – evolve into the ventricles of the brain and the central canal of the spinal cord. As the neural canal dilates within the cerebral hemispheres of the telencephalon, the lateral ventricles are formed following the curvature of the hemispheres created by the early folding of the prosencephalon. These then communicate with the third ventricle situated within the diencephalon. The third and fourth ventricles communicate through the aqueduct of the midbrain (cerebral aqueduct or the Aqueduct of Sylvius) (see Figure 3.3).

The prosencephalon and rhombencephalon have very thin roofs, which are penetrated by tufts of capillaries to form the choroid plexuses of the four ventricles. These plexuses secrete cerebrospinal fluid (CSF), which then circulates around the ventricular system and bathes the brain and spinal cord in later development and during life (see Figure 3. 4).

 Where the circulation of CSF is obstructed, hydrocephalus will result, as CSF builds up in the ventricles of the brain (McCance & Huether 1994).

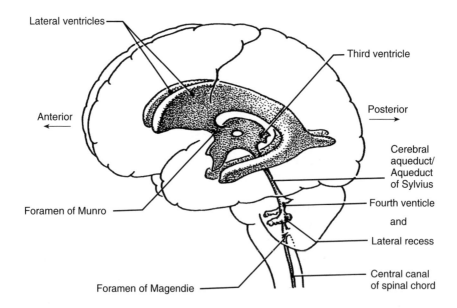

Figure 3.3 Ventricular System of the Brain

Source: Reprinted from *Physiology for Nursing Practice*, Hinchliffe S., *et al.*, copyright 1887, with permission from Elsevier.

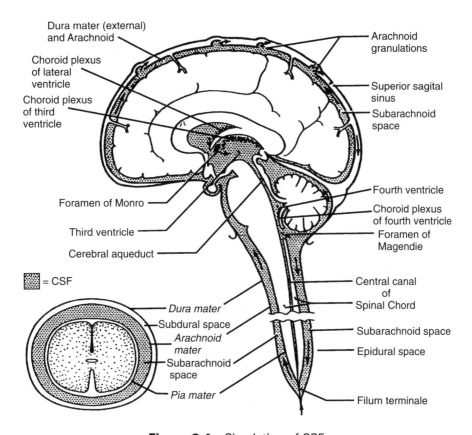

Dura mater (external) and Arachnoid

Choroid plexus of lateral ventricle

Choroid plexus of third ventricle

Arachnoid granulations

Superior sagital sinus

Subarachnoid space

Foramen of Monro

Third ventricle

Cerebral aqueduct

Fourth ventricle

Choroid plexus of fourth ventricle

Foramen of Magendie

= CSF

Dura mater

Subdural space

Arachnoid mater

Subarachnoid space

Pia mater

Central canal of Spinal Chord

Subarachnoid space

Epidural space

Filum terminale

Figure 3.4 Circulation of CSF

Source: Reprinted from *Physiology for Nursing Practice*, Hinchliffe S., *et al.*, copyright 1887, with permission from Elsevier.

Cells of the Brain

Some of the cells of the neural tube differentiate to form the two types of functional cells within the brain:

- spongioblasts or glioblasts which will produce neuroglial cells; and
- neuroblasts which will produce neurones.

Neurones: These cells are the basic anatomical and functional unit of the nervous system. They transmit impulses, and are responsible for the synthesis and transmission of neuropeptide hormones, e.g. acetylcholine in the parasympathetic nervous system, and noradrenaline in the sympathetic nervous system. In addition, neurones develop axonal and dendritic processes which form connections with other neurones and organs. The axonal process or axon is a single long process that extends from the cell body carrying nerve impulses away from it, while the dendritic processes, or *dendrites* are shorter processes from the cell body that make contact with other cells at synapses. Most of the cell bodies of the neurones in the CNS are formed between *10 and 18 weeks* of fetal life, axons and dendrites forming later in development (Tanner, 1989, p. 107).

Neuroglia: These cells or glial cells play a major support function within the nervous system. They are smaller in size but far greater in number than the neurones, occupying half the cellular volume of the brain (Tanner, 1989, p. 107) and providing a link between the neurones and blood supply. They provide structural support, nourishment and protection for the nervous system. One important function of glial cells is the provision of the myelin sheath, composed of phospholipid and protein, which insulates nerve fibres and speeds up the transmission of impulses. Glial cells begin to form from *15 weeks* gestation, with new cells continuing to form in the cerebrum up to *2 years* after birth (Tanner, 1989) (see Table 3.2).

The continuation of glial cell mitosis explains why they are a major source of primary tumours of the nervous system. These tumours are collectively termed gliomas and account for 75 per cent of childhood brain tumours, medulloblastoma being the commonest in the first decade of life (Brett, 1997).

Development of cerebral hemispheres

The cerebral hemispheres begin to develop during *week five* as bilateral bulges of the lateral walls of the prosencephalon, which then develops into the telencephalon anteriorly. These develop rapidly folding backwards to cover the diencephalon, mesencephalon and the upper part of the metencephalon (the brain stem) by *week 16*. The cerebral hemispheres then continue to grow in anterior, dorsal and inferior directions to form the frontal, temporal and occipital lobes between the *sixth and seventh months of gestation* (Larsen, 1998; Sadler, 2000). During the rest of fetal life the rapid growth of the hemispheres creates the characteristic gyri (elevated ridges of tissue) and sulci (grooves) as the hemispheres fold inwards on themselves. At birth, most of the major gyri and sulci are already present (see Figure 3.5).

Cerebral cortex development

The surface of the cerebral hemispheres forms the cerebral cortex. The mature cerebral cortex is composed of several cell layers. These develop during the migration of neuroblasts from their origins close to the ventricles of the brain outwards towards the periphery or pial surface of the cortex (outer surface of the cortex immediately below the pia mater – the inner most layer of the meninges which line the brain and spinal cord). Set patterns are followed, which result in the multilayered grey matter (the darker coloured tissues of the CNS composed mainly of cell bodies) of the brain. Radial glial cells play a key

Table 3.2 Glial Cell Type and Functions

Cell type	Function
Radial glial cells	Present in the embryonic nervous system where they act as 'guide wires' for neurone migration from the lumen of the ventricles / neural tube towards the outer surface of the brain and spinal cord.
Oligodendrocytes	Myelinate the axons of neurons in the central nervous system. A single cell is able to maintain the myelin sheaths of several axons.
Astrocytes	Star like appearance due to the presence of branching processes extending from the cell body. Found between nerve tissue and blood vessels, providing transport for nutrients and metabolites, they control chemical environment, buffer extracellular potassium ions (K+), release and recycle neurotransmitters (Marieb, 1992).
Ependyma	Line the ventricular system in the brain and spinal cord, aid production and circulation of CSF and form a fairly permeable barrier between CSF and interstitial fluid of the CNS (Guyton, 1991; Marieb 1992). This provides a route for drug therapy (intrathecal – into the subarachnoid space) which bypasses the blood–brain barrier as many drugs cannot cross from blood plasma into the CSF or the CNS.
Microglia	Minute cells with phagocytic function, removing waste products of neurone degeneration and metabolic processes.
Schwann cells	Myelinate the axons of the Peripheral Nervous System (PNS), act as phagocytes and are vital to nerve fibre regeneration.
Satellite cells	Closely associated with Schwann cells, they support neurone cell bodies within the ganglia of the Peripheral Nervous System and may regulate chemical environment in the PNS (Marieb, 1992).

process in guiding the developing neurones along lengthy processes which act as guide wires towards the outside of the cerebral cortex (Carlson, 1994; Nowakowski, 1993) (see Figure 3.6).

Cell migration in the cerebral cortex occurs by active neuronal migration. The first cells to migrate are overtaken by later migrating neurones. As a result, the first neuroblasts to migrate are positioned deeper in the cortex than later migrating cells, which occupy positions closer to the pial surface (Larsen, 1993; Nowakowski, 1993; Sadler, 2000).

The pattern of cell migration in the thalamus, hypothalamus, spinal cord, brainstem and the retina differs, as subsequent migrations of cells push the

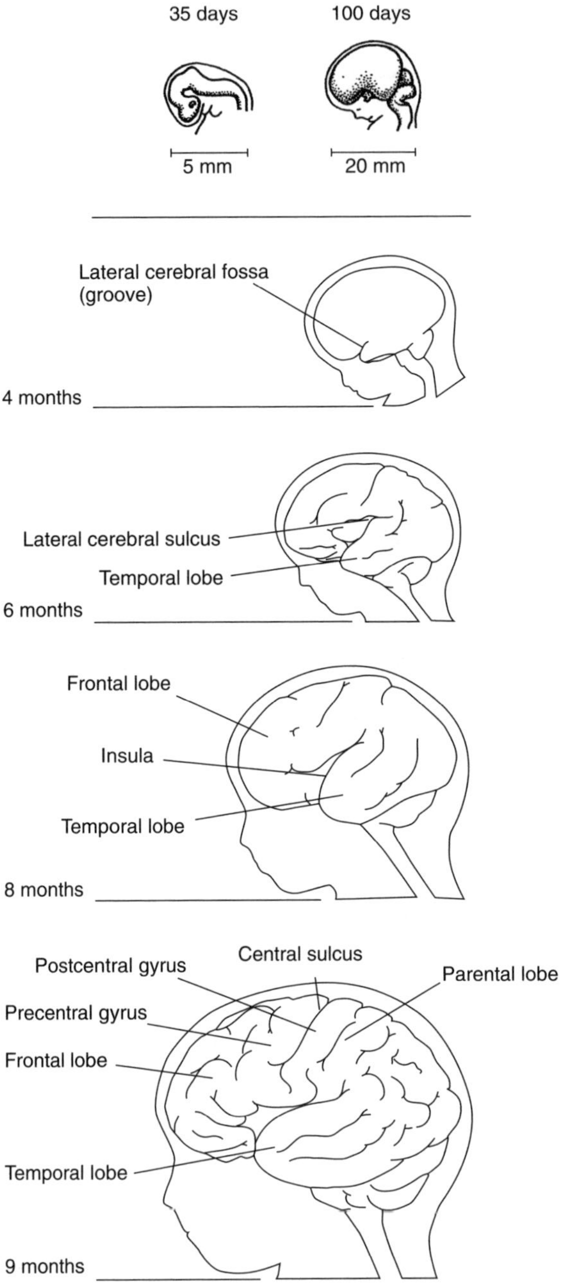

Figure 3.5   Development of the Cerebral Hemispheres

Source: Reprinted from *Physiology for Nursing Practice*, Hinchliffe S., *et al.*, copyright 1887, with permission from Elsevier.

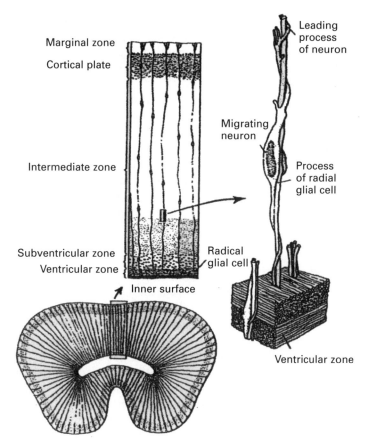

Marginal zone

Cortical plate

Intermediate zone

Subventricular zone
Ventricular zone

Inner surface

Leading
process
of neuron

Migrating
neuron

Process
of radial
glial cell

Radical
glial cell

Ventricular zone

Figure 3.6 Radial Glial Cells' Role in Neuron Migration

Source: From *Brain, Mind and Behavior* by Floyd E Bloom and Arlyne Lazerson, copyright 1985, 1988, 2001 by Educational Broadcasting Corp. Used with permission of Worth Publishers.

original ones upwards towards the pial surface. This pattern of migration is known as passive cell displacement (Nowakowski, 1993).

Once the neuroblasts reach their destination they differentiate initially into simple bipolar neurones with no axons or dendrites, which develop later. The destination of neurones is not random; those originating from the same part of the neural tube stay in the corresponding part of the brain (Carlson, 1994).

Zones of the developing cortex (see Figure 3.6):
- *Ventricular zone*, the first zone to appear immediately adjacent to the surface of the ventricle, from which cell proliferation takes place. The ventricular zone is present throughout the developing CNS (Nowakowski, 1993). Initially it produces neuroblasts, but once the cortical plate is formed this productivity ceases and the zone produces glioblasts and then ependyma, eventually becoming the ependymal layer (Larsen, 1993).

- *Intermediate zone,* develops between the ventricular zone and the marginal zone. It later becomes devoid of neuroblast cells bodies, differentiating into the white matter (paler than the grey matter, it is composed mostly of nerve fibres and therefore contains larger amounts of myelin) of the cerebral hemispheres (Larsen, 1998).
- *Subventricular zone,* adjacent to the ventricular zone, it takes over the neuroblast proliferative function of the ventricular zone once the cortical plate is formed (Larsen, 1993). It is present in the developing neocortex (Nowakowski, 1993).
- *Cortical plate,* develops between the intermediate zone and the marginal zone which later forms the different layers of the cerebral cortex, the grey matter.
- *Marginal zone,* created by the first cells to migrate from the ventricular zone, this zone remains the more peripheral zone closest to the pial surface.

Growth in brain cell number, size and structure

Two periods of rapid brain cell growth occur during the fetal period, the first increasing the number of neurones between *10 and 18 weeks* gestation, after which neurones no longer divide (Nowakowski, 1993; Tanner, 1989). The second period of growth begins at *23 weeks* gestation and continues through-out the *first year of life.* During this second period cell size increases due to an increase of cytoplasm around the nuclei of existing cells. This growth in cyto-plasm enables the development of axons and dendrites, the characteristic branching of which is termed arborization. In general, large neurones are produced first, followed by small ones and association ones. The development of motor neurones is complete before that of sensory neurones.

Developing connectivity

Dendrites and synapses first appear in the brainstem and thalamus and then in the cerebral cortex at about *23 weeks.* At approximately *32 weeks* gestation, there is a great spurt in the development and arborization of dendrites, which continue to form postnatally. Within the first three months after birth, there is a ten fold increase in dendritic growth and by *6 months post-natally* the dendrites are fully formed. The dramatic development of dendrites, commencing at about *32 weeks* when there is some over-production of neuronal connections, is asso-ciated with a period of selective cell death or 'pruning'. Since this pruning process coincides with the arrival of afferent fibres, Smith (1989) suggests these may stabilize the neurones that survive by providing synaptic junctions. Another explanation offered by Brown *et al.* (1997) is that changes in the level of fetal activity or the size of the target group of neurones (corresponding to differences in levels of trophic (nutritive) factors) could affect the extent of cell death. For a more detailed account of the complex processes involved readers are referred to Brown *et al.* (1991) or Menkes and Sarnat (2000).

These processes increase the intricacy of communications with cells within the expanding body of the growing infant. As a result increasingly complex behaviour and movement of the child is possible. Neural networks are constantly being developed and refined in response to nerve stimuli.

The Development of the Spinal Cord

The caudal part of the neural tube develops into the spinal cord, the lumen diminishing into a small cavity constituting the central canal of the spinal cord by *9 weeks gestation*. The developing spinal cord preserves its fundamental organization through most of the developmental stages. Cellular differentiation commences within the neural tube where the neuroepithelium thickens, developing into three layers. Each layer will provide a specific function later in the developmental process:

1. *Ventricular zone or ependymal layer.* As in the brain, the cells closest to the lumen initially produce neuroblasts and glioblasts. Once accomplished the ventricular zone differentiates into the ependymal layer which will line the ventricles of the brain, spinal cord, and central canal of the CNS. Neuroepithelial tumours (ependymomas) of the brain arise as a result of a mutation during the numerous mitotic divisions. These tumours account for between five and ten per cent of childhood brain tumours, the mean age at diagnosis being 5 years (Brett, 1997).
2. *Intermediate zone.* Farther away from the lumen, the intermediate zone containing cell bodies of differentiating post-mitotic neuroblasts, eventually develops into the grey matter (responsible for receiving and integrating information) of the central nervous system.
3. *Marginal zone.* On the periphery of the lumen is the third and final zone, the marginal zone, which forms shortly after the intermediate zone. This layer develops into the white matter of the spinal cord, when myelinated nerve fibres infiltrate the zone to assist with impulse conduction.

The dorsal part of the neural tube, known as the alar plate, generates sensory neurones and receives dorsal nerve roots from the spinal ganglia. In contrast, the ventral part of the neural tube, the basal plate produces neurones with a motor function and which generate ventral nerve roots. The dorsal and ventral roots are bundled together laterally to form spinal nerves (Marieb, 1992) (see Figure 3.7). Axons, which grow out of the neural tube, will innervate muscles throughout the body, forming the motor component of the peripheral nervous system. Synaptic connections between dendrites are continuously forming and degenerating. The development of more stable dendritic connections is highly dependent on the volume of electrochemical signals that pass through them, although this process remains highly plastic throughout life.

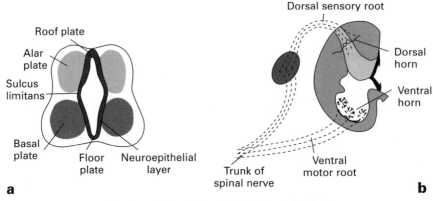

Figure 3.7   Spinal Cord Development

a) Alar & basal plates of the developing spinal cord.
b) Development of ventral motor and dorsal sensory nerve.

Source: Salder (2000).

Box 3.2   Interrelationship of Stimuli and Brain Development

- Neural networks in the brain are constantly being developed and refined in response to nerve stimuli.
- The development of more stable dendritic connections between neurones is highly dependent on the volume of electrochemical signals that pass through them.
- Therefore, repetition of movements and stimuli (the nerve impulse for which creates the electrochemical signals) enables the nervous system to make nerve pathways more permanent, seen in the child learning new knowledge and skills.
- The range of stimuli the baby and young child receives has a direct effect on the development of brain and spinal cord.

The spinal cord differs from the brain in the organization of the grey matter. In the spinal cord, the white matter, responsible for impulse conduction is situated around an inner core of grey matter, responsible for receiving and integrating information. In many parts of the brain the arrangement is reversed. The grey matter of the spinal cord is divided into three main regions, each displaying specific functional attributes:

1. *Dorsal horn* contains the nerve cell bodies for sensory pathways and the substantia gelatinosa, an area involved in the transmission of pain impulses.
2. *Lateral horn*, present in the thoracic and upper lumbar regions, contains neurones for sympathetic motor pathways for visceral organs.

3. *Ventral horn* contains nerve cell bodies for motor pathways. Poliomyelitis, an infectious disease, causes destruction of these neurones.

The white matter is divided into three pathways: ascending sensory, descending motor and commissural (transverse) pathways (Marieb, 1992).

During the first trimester the spinal cord extends the whole length of the body, with spinal nerves passing through intervertebral spaces. After *week 12*, spinal cord growth falls behind that of the vertebral column so that by birth the cord terminates at the level of the second or third lumbar vertebra (Fitzgerald and Fitzgerald, 1994). In the adult, the cord terminates at the first or second lumbar vertebrae (see Figure 3.8). As a result, ventral spinal nerve roots have to elongate to traverse the distance between their point of origin and their intervertebral space. The spinal roots which collect together here are known as the cauda equina.

Fluid can be withdrawn from beneath the cauda equina (lumbar puncture), for analysis. Although, where raised intracranial pressure (ICP) has resulted in

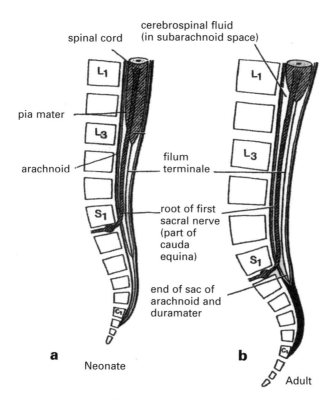

Figure 3.8 Position of the Caudal End of the Spinal Cord in (a) Neonate and (b) Adult

Source: Reprinted from *Family Centred Nursing Care of Children*, Betz, Hunsberger and Wright, copyright 1994, with permission from Elsevier.

dilated pupils, papilledema or severely depressed levels of consciousness, lumbar puncture should be delayed. When the ICP is this high this procedure may precipitate coning – the herniation of the brainstem through the foramen magnum, the aperture in the base of the skull (Aicardi, 1998).

Development of reflexes

As the spinal cord develops, the presence of primitive reflexes is demonstrated by the fetus. Between *six and eight weeks* gestation the fetus experiences tactile stimulation of the skin, spreading in a craniocaudal direction, starting from the face, indicating the development of somatosensory reflexes but not the transmission of sensory information to the thalamus or cerebral cortex (Carlson, 1994; Fitzgerald 1993). This sensitivity increases over the body except the back and top of the head. Readers are referred to the Table 4.3 for further detail on the development of neonatal reflexes.

Structural Development from Neural Crest Cells

Migration of neural crest cells occurs in a craniocaudal sequence commencing at the start of the *fourth week* (Larsen, 1998). Neural crest cells develop cell types appropriate to both the locality of their destination and the level on the craniocaudal axis from which the cells originated. Cervical neural crest cells contribute to parasympathetic nerves and thoracic neural crest cells contribute to the sympathetic nerves (McLachlan, 1994). At what point the fate of a neural crest cell is determined, continues to be a major research area (Larsen, 1998).

The neural crest separates into right and left parts (see Figure 3.1) that migrate to the dorsolateral aspects of the neural tube where they produce major components of the peripheral nervous system including: peripheral sensory neurones and associated dorsal root ganglia; and the parasympathetic and sympathetic motor neurones and associated ganglia (Larsen, 1998). Neural crest cells also contribute to the development of the ganglia of cranial nerves III (parasympathetic) V, VII & IX (parasympathetic), and X. Some neural crest cells migrate and disperse within the mesoderm to become progenitors (originators) of Schwann cells and two layers of meninges – pia mater and arachnoid mater – surrounding the brain and spinal cord (see Figure 3.4). Other crest cells will become pigment cells of the skin, chromaffin cells of the suprarenal medulla, parafollicular cells of the thyroid and many facial structures (Fitzgerald and Fitzgerald, 1994).

Myelination in the Brain and Spinal Cord

The effectiveness of the transmission of impulses depends on some degree of myelination. Although myelination is not essential to nerve transmission, it greatly speeds up conduction velocity by as much as tenfold, although this is proportional to the diameter of the nerve fibre. The sequence of myelination is thought to be predictable, according to the myelinogenetic cycles of Yakovlev and Lecours (1967), beginning in the peripheral nerves, followed by the spinal cord, brain stem, cerebellum, basal ganglia, thalamus and cerebral cortex.

In the peripheral nerves the motor nerve roots myelinate before sensory nerve roots, between the *second and fifth months* of pregnancy (Carlson, 1994), possibly reflecting the early development of protective reflexes. In the brain and spinal cord the process starts in the sensory nerves first, the opposite sequence to the peripheral nervous system (Carlson, 1994). Myelination begins in the spinal cord at about *11 weeks* gestation, following a craniocaudal pattern, while the myelination of the brain begins later in the *third trimester* of pregnancy. A very rapid period of myelination begins at *38 weeks* gestation lasting until *6 weeks postnatally*, particularly in areas of the brainstem, cerebellum and cerebral cortex. At birth, myelination of the corticospinal tracts, connecting the spinal cord to the cerebral cortex, has only progressed caudally to the level of the medulla (Carlson, 1994), although Sarnat and Menkes (2000) state that part of the pons is also myelinated at birth.

This limited myelination of the brain may explain the 'periodic breathing' of some newborn babies, as the medullary respiratory centre is myelinated at 40 weeks, while the pneumotaxic and apneustic centres in the pons may not yet have fully myelinated. In clinical practice when apnoea alarms are used with neonates, the alarm is therefore usually set for no less than 20 seconds as apnoea of up to 15 seconds is common in premature neonates and some term babies (Hunsberger and Leenan 1994).

Growth of the Central Nervous System After Birth

After birth, many aspects of the brain continue to develop, for example dendrites continue to form connections, synapses stabilize, more nerves become myelinated and association pathways mature. In addition, there is a great increase in the size of the brain, particularly during the first *4 or 5 years*, by which time it has tripled in weight. The gyri of the cerebral hemispheres, which have begun to form before birth, become more infolded and complex after birth. Frontal and temporal lobes and some of the sulci separating lobes of the cerebrum also develop postnatally.

Myleination continues rapidly in the first *6 weeks postnatally*. By *3 months* of age the cerebellum has been nearly completely myelinated. However some of the association pathways in the brain are only myelinated by the age of *16 years*. Although the first 6 weeks of life see the faster period of myelination, Sinclair and Dangerfield (1998) note that myelination continues to be fairly rapid for *a 6 month period after birth*, continuing at a slower rate thereafter into puberty and beyond with myelination of the cerebral cortex continuing into adult life (Sinclair and Dangerfield, 1998).

According to Brown *et al.* (1997) the earliest areas to myelinate are not necessarily those where function develops first. However, they do suggest that the onset of myelination is often associated with the emergence of function which may be later refined.

Therefore, all tracts and pathways in the nervous system are fully functional at birth. The continuing development can been seen in the developing child's gradual mastery of muscle control in cephalo-caudal and promixal-distal directions, reflecting the process of myelination of motor nerves moving from the head down the body and from gross limb and body movements to manual dexterity at the periphery. To read more on motor development see Chapter 4. Development within the central nervous system itself is harder to measure. However it can be seen in the development of autonomic control centres, such as those for respiration (mentioned before), thermoregulation and fluid balance, the latter two developing over the *first five and two years of life* respectively. Please refer to Chapter 9 for further detail on the development of fluid balance. The development in association areas can been seen in: the development of speech and language; the development of the limbic system in the young child's gradual mastery of his/her emotions; and the development of the higher thought centres in the cognitive development of the child.

Factors Influencing Nervous System Development

There are numerous factors that interact with each other to influence the development of the nervous system, a comprehensive review of which is beyond the scope of this chapter. However five significant areas are explored below. These are the influence of teratogens, nutrition, thyroid function, exposure to stimuli and the effect of androgens on the development of sex-typical behaviour. The influence of teratogens and nutrition is also discussed in Chapter 1.

Teratogens

A teratogen is any substance that induces the formation of abnormalities in the fetus. The period of greatest sensitivity to teratogens occurs between *3 and 8 weeks* of embryonic life (Sadler, 2000), much of it before the woman is aware of the pregnancy. Sensitivity gradually declines from this point to *birth*. The greatest period of sensitivity occurs as each organ system is undergoing its initial development.

Several factors can influence the capacity of a teratogen to produce birth factors. These include:

- Genotype of the fetus and that of the mother (where drug metabolism and resistance to infection is concerned);

- Gestation of the pregnancy (as mentioned above). Each organ system may have more than one specific period of susceptibility – termed a critical period (see section below on factors affecting nervous system development for further explanation). Although it should be noted that no stage of development is completely immune to such effects;
- Dose and duration of exposure to the teratogen;
- Mechanism through which the teratogen has its effect.

Different types of teratogens and their effects are summarized in Table 3.3.

Nutrition

A healthy diet is needed by the pregnant female (See Chapter 1) and the developing child in order to promote maturity of the nervous system. It is well known that folic acid supplementation during pregnancy reduces the incidence of neural tube defects, such as spina bifida. Less well know is the growing body of evidence that long chain polyunsaturated fatty acids (LCPUFAs) are needed for brain growth and neural development (Department of Health, 1994). LCPUFAs are rich in phospholipids, which

Table 3.3   Effects of Teratogens on the Developing Nervous System

Teratogen category	Teratogen	Congenital effect on the nervous system
Infection	Cytomegalovirus	Microcephaly, mental retardation
	Herpes simplex virus	Microcephaly
	Varicella virus	Mental retardation
	HIV	Microcephaly
	Toxoplasmosis	Hydrocephalus, cerebral calcifications
Physical agent	X-rays	Microcephaly, spina bifida
	Hyperthermia	Anencephaly
Chemicals	Warfarin	Microcephaly
	Cocaine	Microcephaly, behavioural abnormalities
	Alcohol	Fetal alcohol syndrome, mental retardation
	Lead	Neurological disorders
Maternal metabolic disorder	Diabetes mellitus	Neural tube defects.

Source: Sadler (2000).

are needed for the development of myelin. These fatty acids are synthesized in the adult and older child from the essential dietary fatty acids linoleic and linolenic acids. However in fetal life and early infancy this mechanism is immature. Consequently, the fetus is reliant on placental transfer and the infant on sourcing LCPUFAs from breastmilk (Department of Health, 1994) or from formula milks to which LCPUFAs are now added. Anderson *et al.*'s (1999) metaanalysis of research comparing cognitive function between breastfed and formula-fed babies concluded that, after adjustment for key cofactors such as maternal education and socioeconomic status, breastfeeding was associated with significantly higher scores for cognitive development than formula feeding. This enhanced development persisted throughout childhood and adolescence, with increased effect when the child was breast fed for longer. However research exploring the effect of adding LCPUFAs to formula milks has only identified an advantage for premature infants (Carlson, 1999). Clearly the conclusions to be drawn from existing research is that the promotion of breastfeeding is important for brain development, especially for myelinization, both in the premature and the term baby.

Other deficiencies within the diet also impact on the function of the nervous system. For example, iron deficiency is associated with developmental delay and behavioural disturbances (Wardley et al., 1997), presumably resulting from the reduced oxygen carrying capacity of the blood. Glucose is the brain's energy resource therefore blood glucose levels are extremely important. Consequently factors that influence the availability of glucose for the brain will affect brain metabolism.

 In clinical practice it is usual to test blood glucose levels in any children presenting with a fit or seizure of unknown cause, to exclude hypoglycaemia as the cause.

Protein is also required as the brain has a high turnover of amino acids (Tanner, 1989), which must be supplied by the diet. Consequently nutritional assessment is important when making a health appraisal.

 Some inborn errors of metabolism can also affect the developing brain. For example: in phenylketonuria the absence of the enzyme phenylalanine hydroxylase results in the inability to convert the essential amino acid phenylalanine into tyrosine. The accumulation of phenylalanine in the blood leads to brain damage (Wardley *et al.*, 1997). These children require diets low in phenylalanine, a requirement which, it is now recognized, needs to be followed throughout life.

Box 3.3   Influence of Nutrition on Brain Development

- Folic acid supplementation during pregnancy reduces the incidence of neural tube defects, such as spina bifida (see Chapter 1).
- The long chain polyunsaturated fatty acids (LCPUFAs) in breastmilk are thought to be responsible for enhanced cognitive development of

breastfed babies compared to formula-feed babies. These acids are particularly important for myelinization.

- Iron deficiency is associated with developmental delay and behavioural disturbances (Wardley *et al.*, 1997), presumably resulting from the reduced oxygen carrying capacity of the blood.
- Glucose is the brain's energy resource, therefore, blood glucose levels are extremely important. Consequently factors that influence the availability of glucose for the brain will affect brain metabolism.
- Protein is required as the brain has a high turnover of amino acids (Tanner, 1989), which must be supplied by the diet.

These factors highlight the importance of maternal and infant nutrition for brain development. A key area for health promotion.

Thyroid Function

Thyroid hormone is also necessary for a healthy nervous system as it regulates the various processes involved in the final stage of brain differentiation. These include the development of axons, dendrites and synapses, neuronal migration and myelination. The brain's responsiveness to thyroid hormones is greatest during the last stages of brain development (Menkes *et al.*, 2000). As nerve tissue is unable to manufacture new cells once the growth period has ended, any correction necessary must be made within the growth period to avoid a permanent deficit in the number of neuronal cells. Consequently it is important to treat any deficiencies early in postnatal life while the brain is still within a peak period of growth and development.

Children with congenital hypothyroidism have insufficient thyroid hormone production. They need to be identified soon after birth to prevent the permanent deficits in brain development referred to above. These children will require supplementation with thyroxine throughout life, with increasing doses at times of rapid growth (Ruble and Charron-Prochownik, 1994).

Exposure to Stimuli

Children require exposure to a wide range of diverse stimuli to facilitate the development and stabilization of dendritic connections. Initially, at the peak of synaptic development a plethora of transient dendritic connections are formed (Sadler, 2000). These become more stable connections where they are repeatedly stimulated. Conversely where these connections are not used the synapses deteriorate and are eventually lost (Rutishauser, 1994).

One example given in Rutishauser (1994) is that of visual development, where early visual deprivation leads to permanent visual disability.

This flexibility in the development of dendritic connections is termed plasticity and persists throughout life although it is greatest in the *first 5 years* of childhood during the peak of brain growth. This early period of high plasticity is often referred to as a critical period, which is probably related to the presence of the excess of dendrites from which the adult pattern is created (Brown *et al.*, 1991).

Essentially, this is the basis for learning. Consequently the more stimuli the child receives the more learning will take place. During the critical period the opportunity for such learning is greater than at any other time in life, highlighting the importance of the young child's environment with regard to appropriate stimuli for development.

Effect of Androgens

It is gradually beginning to be accepted that the behavioural differences between girls and boys may not all be attributed to social learning. Increasingly, research is demonstrating the role of androgens in the development of differing behavioural patterns between boys and girls. This research has focused on exploring the differences in sex-typical behaviour in girls with congenital adrenal hyperplasia compared to controls, as they are known to have been exposed to higher than normal levels of androgens in fetal life (Berenbaum *et al.*, 2000; Hines and Kaufman, 1994), differences in behaviour are therefore attributed to this exposure. In their literature review, Berenbaum *et al.* (2000) found that these girls engage in more male-typical play, have more male-typical interests in adolescence, greater spatial ability and are less interested in infants, marriage, motherhood and feminine appearance. They conclude from their own research that the critical period for androgen effects on behaviour occurs early in prenatal development, probably between *weeks 8 and 24* of gestation when the levels of gonadal hormones are greatest, producing permanent changes in the structure of the brain. Clearly socialization has a lesser effect than has been commonly perceived on the development of sex-typical behaviours.

Conclusions on CNS development

The development of the central nervous system is an extremely complex process that can be affected by a wide range of interrelating factors. What has been presented here is an overview of the key stages in this developmental process with the intention of enabling the reader to develop an understanding of the basic processes and how these may affect the long-term functioning of the individual. Some of the key stages at which abnormalities may occur have also been highlighted to illustrate why these may occur.

The following section of the chapter focuses on the assessment of central nervous system function to enable the reader to make the links between the underlying developmental anatomy and physiology and observation of the child growing and developing.

Assessment of Neurological Function in Health

Introduction

There are various ways in which the functioning of the central nervous system can be assessed during childhood, from the assessment of gross structural development to tests of specific nerve pathways and assessment of integrated functioning of the CNS. Generally a comprehensive assessment would include all three approaches. There are a number of different methods available for each approach, some of which will be outlined here both for the neonate and the child. Whatever method is used, it is important to begin the assessment with information gathering in the form of history taking from the child (where of sufficient age and understanding) and their parents or carers. They will be able to detect subtle changes in the child long before they are detectable by health care professionals who do not know the child as well. The principles of such history taking are well described elsewhere and will therefore not be covered again here.

Gross Structural Development

The brain normally weighs 340g at birth. By *4 years of age* this has increased to 1340g, largely due to myelination, the formation of dendrites and association pathways (Campbell and McIntosh, 1992). Assessment of overall growth of the CNS can be monitored through assessments of the size and shape of the head and spine, although it must be recognized that this is a relatively insensitive test as it is restricted to the observable or measurable external signs of growth and therefore does not provide any information on functioning of the system. Whenever measurements of size are made on children, parental norms should always be taken into account.

Head circumference (HC), around the frontal and occipital bones – the largest circumference, is routinely measured at birth and at 6–8 weeks of age (Hall and Elliman, 2003). It may also be carried out utilizing ultrasonography antenatally. Larger than normal HC for age may indicate hydrocephalus, although this would be accompanied by other signs and symptoms. Small HC might indicate microcephaly or very rarely total craniostenosis (premature fusion of sutures), both of which would also have other symptoms.

Head shape assessment includes assessment of symmetry, separation or premature fusion of cranial sutures and presence and tension of fontanelles. In a neonate two fontanelles are palpable: anterior and posterior fontanelles. The posterior fontanelle closes *shortly after birth*, at the latest by *6 weeks of age*, while the anterior fontanelle remains open, closing by about *18 months of age* (see Figure 3.9).

 Assymmetry may indicate partial craniostenosis when accompanied by premature fusion of some sutures, or in the neonate the presence of cephalohaematoma

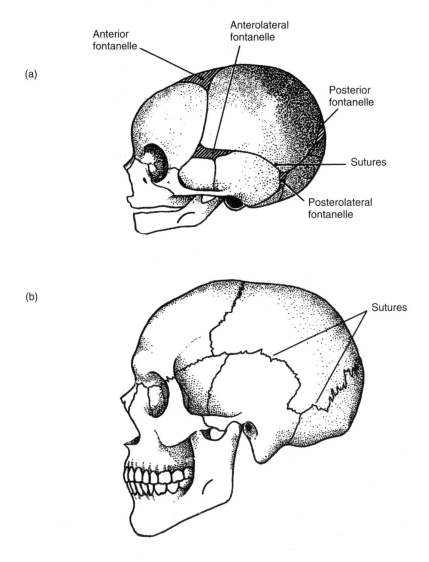

Figure 3.9 Fontanelles and Sutures in (a) an Infant Compared with (b) an Adult

Source: From Sinclair and Dangerfield, 1998, by permission.

or caput succedaneum as a result of birth trauma. Separation of sutures may indicate hydrocephalus or other pathology increasing brain volume. Tense fontanelles also indicate increasing brain volume which may be due to over-hydration or pathologically raised intracranial pressure. Sunken fontanelles are most commonly associated with dehydration.

Spine shape is usually assessed at birth for symmetry, signs of pits, hairy patches or cystic swellings (Baston and Durward, 2001). Later during child-hood growth spurts, particularly at adolescence, the spine will again be assessed for symmetry.

Pits, hairy patches and cystic swellings are all indicators of Spina bifida (Delahoussaye, 1994). Asymmetry in the neonate may indicate congenital scoliosis, while later development of asymmetry, often detected in adolescence, indicates idiopathic scoliosis (Mason and Wright, 1994).

Box 3.4 Assessment of Gross Structural Development

The following can be assessed:

- Head circumference
- Head shape – symmetry, separation or premature fusion of cranial sutures and presence and tension of fontanelles.
- Spine shape – at birth for symmetry, signs of pits, hairy patches or cystic swellings and later during childhood growth spurts, particularly at adolescence, for symmetry.

These are relatively insensitive tests as they do not provide any information on functioning of the system.

Specific Nerve Pathways

Specific nerve pathways are most commonly tested at birth in the elicitation of neonatal reflexes, in childhood through testing normal 'adult' deep tendon reflexes and through the assessment of cranial nerve function in the very sick child. Neonatal reflexes disappear at different ages and stages of development (see Table 4.3). Enduring primitive reflexes, loss of reflexes, or hyperactivity of deep tendon reflexes indicate cerebral insult or dysfunction. Hypotonia and lack of ability to pass developmental milestones also indicate possible neuro-logical maldevelopment or dysfunction. Cranial nerve testing enables the location and severity of a specific CNS disease or injury to be determined. Hazinski (1992, pp. 527–9) provides a comprehensive overview of the function and assessment of each cranial nerve.

Integrated Functioning of the CNS – Global Functional and Cognitive Development

A wide range of tools is available to assess integrated functioning of the CNS in children. For a comprehensive list of tools available, see Betz *et al.* (1994, pp. 956–7). In research studies measuring cognitive function and intelligence, the following Anderson *et al.* (1999) found to be the more commonly used:

- Bayley Mental Development Index (the Motor component is given in the following chapter)
- Peabody Picture Vocabulary Test
- General Cognitive Index of the McCarthy Scales of Children's Abilities
- Wechsler Child Intelligence Scale
- Stanford-Binet Intelligence Scale.

However, in community clinical practice, more global developmental assessment tools are used such as the Denver Developmental Screening Test (Revised) or Sheridan's charts of developmental progress. Hall & Elliman (2003) recommend that children's development is assessed at birth, 6–8 weeks, 8 months, 4–5 years and at school entry at 5 years of age.

In the hospital setting, more specific assessment of neurological functioning may be undertaken, either at birth or once concerns about the child's neurological functioning have been raised or when there are known to be potential effects of a specific disease process. This assessment may include general integrated features such as arousal and awareness, and some specific nerve pathways through testing sensation and motor responses. Stephenson *et al.* (2000) provide a succinct overview of neonate neurological assessment which includes the Dubowitz gestational neurological assessment, while Ferguson-Clark and Williams (1998) provide a good overview of the neurological assessment of children using scales adapted for (such as the Glasgow Coma Scale) or specific to children (such as the Adelaide scale). There is as yet no consensus on the most effective tool for use with children across the age groups (Warren, 2000).

Conclusions on the Assessment of CNS Function

The assessment of the nervous system is complex, as all human function is controlled by neurological impulses. Results of the tests will be somewhat determined by the developmental age and stage of the child. The accuracy of some of the tests may be hindered or complicated by the inability of the child to localize and articulate. In addition, the effectiveness of any form of neurological assessment is reliant on the skill and accuracy of the examiner. Consequently it is important that all those involved are adequately prepared to carry out the particular assessment. Much valuable information can be gleaned from the tools and approaches outlined above, however these should always be considered as just one part of the overall assessment, which should always include the child (where old enough to contribute) and his/her carers. A very careful and exact history of previous and current medical circumstances must always be obtained to place findings in context.

Conclusion

The central nervous system is composed of the brain and spinal cord, which receives, interprets or integrates stimuli and relays nerve impulses to all the muscles and glands in the body. Consequently it is involved in virtually every biological function of the body. The development of this system begins in the very early stages of embryonic life with the formation of the neural plate in the third week of gestation, usually before the mother is aware of the pregnancy. As a consequence, there is a critical period of increased vulnerability for the influence of teratogens. Most of the cell bodies of the neurones in the CNS are formed between 10 and 18 weeks of fetal life, while the glial cells continue to form until 2 years after birth with myelination peaking in the first year of life but continuing into adulthood. The brain remains a highly plastic structure throughout life enabling the continuation of learning. The major structures of the brain are present by the fourth month of gestation, although the brain has further development to complete before and after birth. Much of postnatal development is highly dependent on the stimuli and diet received by the developing child.

Assessment of neurological function in the developing child is inevitably complex. As a result, a wide range of tools and approaches exist to assess the child's neurological function. However in health, beyond the assessment of reflexes during neonatal assessment, the assessment of the child's central nervous system function is embedded within the general developmental assessments conducted by community health care services.

Review Questions

1. From which structure within the developing embryo does the nervous system originate?
2. At what stage is the developing embryo most vulnerable to the effects of teratogens and why?
3. Explain the meaning of 'plasticity' in relation to the developing human brain.
4. Discuss the implications of the development of myelination for the child during the first year of life.
5. Describe the three main approaches to neurological assessment, giving examples of tools or methods used in each.

Further Reading

Fitzgerald, MJT and Fitzgerald, M (1994) *Human Embryology*. London: Ballière Tindall.

Carlson, BM (1994) *Human Embryology and Developmental Biology*. London: Mosby.

Both of the above texts provide a good, easy to read, overview of the development of the central nervous system in utero.

Larsen, WJ (1998) *Essentials of Human Embryology*. New York: Churchill Livingstone.

This is the latest of Larsen's detailed books on the subject, which includes a detailed section of the development of the brain and spinal cord. If you would like to add greater depth to your understanding of central nervous system development in utero, this is the book for you.

Brown, MC, Hopkins WG and Keynes, RJ (1991) *Essentials of Neural Development*. Cambridge: Cambridge University Press.

Menkes, JH and Sarnat, HB (eds) (2000) *Child Neurology*. 6th edn. Philadephia: Lippincott Williams & Wilkins.

Brown, M, Keynes, R and Lumsden, A (2001) *The Developing Brain*. Oxford: Oxford University Press.

All three of the above books will provide readers with a comprehensive overview with much greater detail than has been possible within the scope of this book. The latter text is a comprehensive review of the latest research concerning brain development, much of which is from animal studies.

Aicardi, J (1998) *Diseases of the Nervous System in Childhood*. 2nd edn. Cambridge: Cambridge University Press.

Brett, EM (1997) *Paediatric Neurology*. 3rd edn. New York: Churchill Livingstone.

Both Aicardi and Brett are extensive medical texts on diseases of the nervous system, ideal for readers who wish to learn more about the range of disorders that may affect this body system during childhood.

References

Aicardi, J (1998) *Diseases of the Nervous System in Childhood*. 2nd edn. Cambridge: Cambridge University Press.

Anderson, JW, Johnstone, BM and Remley, DT (1999) Breast-feeding and cognitive development: a meta-analysis. *Am. J. Clin. Nutr*, 70, 525–35.

Baston, H and Durward, H (2001) *Examination of the Newborn. A Practical Guide*. London: Routledge.

Berenbaum, SA, Duck, SC and Bryk, K (2000) Behavioural effects of prenatal versus postnatal androgen excess in children with 21-hydroxylase-deficient congential adrenal hyperplasia. *J. Clin. Endocrinol. Metab.*, Feb. 85(2), 727–33.

Betz, CL, Hunsberger, M and Wright, S (eds) (1994) *Family-Centered Nursing Care of Children*. 2nd edn. Philadelphia: WB Saunders.

Brett, EM (1997) *Paediatric Neurology*. 3rd edn. New York: Churchill Livingstone.

Brown, JK, Omar, T and O'Regan, M (1997) Brain development and the development of tone and movement. In KJ Connoly and H Forssberg (eds) *Neurophysiology and Neuropsychology of Motor Development. Clinics in Developmental Medicine,* 143/144, 319–45.

Brown, MC, Hopkins, WG and Keynes, RJ (1991) *Essentials of Neural Development.* Cambridge: Cambridge University Press.

Campbell, AGM and McIntosh, N (eds) (1992) *Forfar and Arneil's Textbook of Paediatrics.* Edinburgh: Churchill Livingstone.

Campbell, S and Glasper, EA (eds) (1995) *Whaley and Wong's Children's Nursing.* London: Mosby

Carlson, BM (1994) *Human Embryology and Developmental Biology.* London: Mosby.

Carlson, SE (1999) Long-chain polyunsaturated fatty acids and development of human infants. *Acta Paediatr. Suppl.*, Aug, 88(430), 72–7.

Carola, R, Harley, JP and Noback, CR (1992) *Human Anatomy & Physiology.* 2nd edn. New York: McGraw-Hill.

Carter, B (1994) *Child and Infant Pain. Principles of Nursing Care and Management.* London: Chapman & Hall.

Delahoussaye, CP (1994) Families with neonates. In CL Betz, M Hunsberger and S Wright(eds) *Family-Centered Nursing Care of Children.* 2nd edn. Philadelphia: WB Saunders.

Department of Health (1994) *Report on Health & Social Subjects 45. Weaning and the Weaning Diet.* Report of the Working Group on the Weaning Diet of the Committee on Medical Aspects of Food Policy. London: HMSO.

Ferguson-Clark, L and Williams, C (1998) Neurological Assessment in Children. *Paediatric Nursing*, 10(4), 29–35.

Fitzgerald, M (1993) *Sensory Physiology.* In PD Gluckman and MA Heymann (eds) *Perinatal and Pediatric Pathophysiology. A Clinical Perspective.* London: Edward Arnold.

Fitzgerald, MJT and Fitzgerald, M (1994) *Human Embryology.* London: Ballière Tindall.

Gluckman, PD and Heymann, MA (eds) (1993) *Perinatal and Pediatric Pathophysiology. A Clinical Perspective.* London: Edward Arnold.

Guyton, AC (1991) *Textbook of Medical Physiology.* 8th edn. Philadelphia. WB Saunders.

Hall, DMB and Elliman D (ed.) (2003) *Health for All Children.* 4th edn. Oxford: Oxford University Press.

Hazinski, MF (1992) *Nursing Care of the Critically Ill Child.* 2nd edn. St Louis: Mosby Year Book.

Hines, M and Kaufman, FR (1994) Androgen and the development of human sex-typical behaviour in rough-and-tumble play and sex of preferred playmates in children with congenital adrenal hyperplasia. *Child. Dev.*, Aug. 65(4), 1042–53.

Hunsberger, M and Leenan, L(1994) Altered respiratory function. In CL Betz, M Hunsberger and S Wright (eds) *Family-Centered Nursing Care of Children.* 2nd edn. Philadelphia: WB Saunders.

Larsen, WJ (1993) *Human Embryology.* New York: Churchill Livingstone.

Larsen, WJ (1998) *Essentials of Human Embryology.* New York: Churchill Livingstone.

Marieb, EN (1992) *Human Anatomy and Physiology.* 2nd edn. Redwood City, CA: Benjamin Cummings.

Mason, KJ and Wright, S (1994) Altered musculoskeletal function. In CL Betz, M Hunsberger and S Wright (eds) *Family-Centered Nursing Care of Children.* 2nd edn. Philadelphia: WB Saunders.

McCance, KL and Huether, SE (1994) *Pathophysiology: The Biologic Basis for Disease in Adults and Children*. St Louis: Mosby.

McLachlan, J (1994) *Medical Embryology*. Wokingham: Addison-Wesley.

Menkes, JH and Sarnat, HB (2000) *Child Neurology*. 6th edn. Philadelphia: Lippincott Williams & Wilkins.

Menkes, JH, Fink, BW, Hurvitz, CGH, Hyman, CB, Jordan, SC and Wantabe, F (2000) Neurologic manifestations of systemic disease. In JH Menkes and HB Sarnat (eds) *Child Neurology*. 6th edn. Philadephia: Lippincott Williams & Wilkins.

Moore, KL (1988) *Essentials of Human Embryology*. Ontario. Decker.

Moore, K and Persaud, T (1993) *The Developing Human: Clinically Oriented Embryology*. 5th edn. London: W.B. Saunders.

Nowakowski, RS (1993) Development of the CNS. In PD Gluckman and MA Heymann (eds) *Perinatal and Pediatric Pathophysiology. A Clinical Perspective*. London: Edward Arnold.

Royal College of Nursing Institute (RCNI) (1999) *Clinical Guidelines for the Recognition and Assessment of Acute Pain in Children*. London: RCN.

Royal College of Paediatrics and Child Health (RCPCH) (1997) *Prevention and Control of Pain in Children. A Manual for Health Care Professionals*. London: BMJ Publishing.

Ruble, JA and Charron-Prochownik, D (1994) Altered endocrine function. In CL Betz, M Hunsberger and S Wright (eds) *Family-Centered Nursing Care of Children*. 2nd edn. Philadelphia: WB Saunders.

Rutishauser, S (1994) *Physiology and Anatomy. A Basis for Nursing and Health Care*. Edinburgh: Churchill Livingstone.

Sadler, TW (2000) *Langham's Medical Embryology*. 8th edn. Philadelphia: Lippincott Williams & Wilkins.

Sarnat, HB and Menkes, JH (2000) The new neuroembryology. In JH Menkes and HB Sarnat (eds) *Child Neurology*. 6th edn. Philadephia: Lippincott Williams & Wilkins.

Sinclair, D and Dangerfield, P (1998) *Human Growth After Birth*. Oxford: Oxford University Press.

Smith, CUM (1989) *Elements of Molecular Neurobiology*. New York: John Wiley & Sons.

Stephenson, T, Marlow, N, Watkin, S and Grant, J (2000) *Pocket Neonatology*. Edinburgh: Churchill Livingstone.

Tanner, JM (1989) *Foetus into Man*. 2nd edn,Castlemead: Ware.

Twycross, A, Moriarty, A and Betts, T (eds) (1998) *Paediatric Pain Management. A Multi-disciplinary Approach*. Oxford: Radcliffe Medical Press.

Wall, PD and Melzack, R (1989) *Textbook of Pain*. London: Churchill Livingstone.

Wardley, BL, Puntis, JWL and Taitz, LS (1997) *Handbook of child nutrition*. 2nd edn. Oxford: Oxford University Press.

Warren, A (2000) Paediatric coma scoring researched and benchmarked. *Paediatric Nursing*, 12(3). 14–18.

Yakovlev, PI and Lecours, AR (1967) The myelogenetic cycles of regional maturation of the brain. In A Minowski (ed.), *Regional Development of the Brain in Early Life*. Philadelphia: F.A. Davis.

CHAPTER 4

The Development of Movement

Sandy Oldfield

Contents

- Somatic Nervous System and Musculoskeletal System Development, Linked to the Development of Purposeful Movement
- Assessment of Motor Development in Health
- Review Questions
- Further Reading
- References

Learning Outcomes

At the end of the chapter, you should be able to:

- Define motor development and describe how motor activities are often classified.
- Explain how pre- and postnatal motor development is related to the maturing, plastic nervous system, and bone and muscle development.
- Describe the role of primitive reflexes, postural reflexes and stereotypic movements in early motor development.
- Discuss environmental influences on motor development, for example in relation to massage or stroking of preterm infants and practice opportunities postnatally.
- Describe the sequence of fundamental motor skills development during childhood and how these skills are assessed.
- Outline early and more recent theoretical perspectives that attempt to explain motor development.
- Discuss the assessment and promotion of normal motor development.

Introduction

There are few areas of development that are not expressed through motor behaviour, particularly during infancy. This emphasizes the importance of understanding what underlies this area of development. Children's neuromotor function can be a useful indicator of progress in the development of nervous and musculoskeletal system function, as well as highlighting possible deficits in their environment. This assessment is important when considering clinical interventions.

The purpose of this chapter is to map the development of early motor function, while at the same time indicating the contribution of experience, nervous system, bone and muscle development to this process. The significance of the interplay between experience and biological development is discussed with reference to dynamic systems theory. It is hoped that this chapter will inform and inspire curiosity about this important and interesting aspect of development.

Somatic Nervous System and Musculoskeletal System Development, Linked to the Development of Purposeful Movement

Defining Motor Development, Motor Patterns and Motor Skills

Motor development is the attainment of patterns and skills of movement that results from neuromuscular maturation, growth and experience. The term motor pattern is used to describe a general kind of action (such as reaching, walking and hopping) but not the quality of that action. For example, a *toddler's* way of walking is very different from that of *a five year old* but the pattern is still described as walking. Motor skills, on the other hand, refer to the degree of proficiency, accuracy and efficiency of a particular movement.

Classification of Motor Patterns and Skills

One way of classifying motor patterns is as either gross motor (involving the whole or major part of the body) or fine motor (involving manual dexterity) activities. In practice, it is common for both gross and fine motor patterns to be expressed together in motor tasks. For example, writing requires fine motor movement when forming letters but also gross motor movement of the arm and torso.

Developmental assessment forms often differentiate between gross and fine motor movements, as there is a tendency for the latter to develop later. For example, reaching and grasping movements increase in efficiency and precision with age – from the early stiff, swatting movements of the whole arm in *early infancy* to more flexible arm movements with precise pincer movements of *the toddler.*

Another form of classification is in relation to the type of fundamental motor patterns. These are elementary forms of movement described as loco-motion (e.g. walking, jumping), non-locomotion (e.g. bending, pulling, pushing) and manipulation or prehension (e.g. grasping, throwing). Skills from these areas are often used in combination with each other to make up complex motor activities.

Aspects of Biological Development and Experience Affecting Motor Development

Early movement patterns can be detected in utero from as early as *8 weeks gestation* and development proceeds in a relatively predictable fashion well into childhood. The predictability of this development is related to genetic regulation of neuromuscular maturation that both constrains and enables developing motor abilities. However, a number of other factors influence motor function, including:

- opportunities for and motivation to practice,
- prior motor experiences,
- muscle tone and posture,
- environmental conditions in which an action is carried out; and
- the child's size.

These factors are discussed in the sections that follow.

Box 4.1 Factors that Influence the Development of Motor Function

- genetic regulation of neuromuscular maturation;
- opportunities for and motivation to practice;
- prior motor experiences;
- muscle tone and posture;
- environmental conditions in which an action is carried out; and
- the child's size.

Nervous System Development

The classification of the nervous system – related to movement

Before outlining the course of nervous system development, it may be helpful to recall the parts of the nervous system and their relationship to movement.

An overview of nervous system structure can be found in the preceding chapter. Those aspects related to movement are reviewed below and are summarized in Table 4.1.

The central nervous system (CNS) is composed of the brain and spinal cord, and this is where sensory impulses are interpreted. With regard to movement, important information about proprioception, the awareness of the position, balance and movement of the body or any of its parts, is conveyed to the brain. The CNS is also the origin of most nerve impulses that stimulate muscles to contract. The peripheral nervous system (PNS) forms connections between the brain and spinal cord and the muscles that are innervated (and also to glands).

The peripheral nervous system is divided into the afferent (sensory) system, which sends information from peripheral receptors to the CNS, and the efferent (motor) system that carries information from the CNS to muscles. The efferent motor system is divided again into the somatic nervous system, which transmits information from the motor cortex in the CNS to skeletal muscles, although not all originate from there. The sensory cortex relays sensory information to the motor cortex and the cerebellum and basal ganglia transmit information via the thalamus to the motor cortex. The autonomic nervous system in contrast, sends information from the CNS to glands, smooth muscle and cardiac muscle.

Therefore, when considering the nervous system in relation to the control of movement, we must recognize the role of the CNS and the PNS (including the afferent, efferent and somatic nervous systems). Afferent or sensory neurones convey proprioceptive information from muscles, tendons and the labyrinth to the brain to enable information to be perceived about posture, balance and results of movement. Efferent or motor neurones carry impulses to muscles to enable movement. In skeletal muscle, a single motor neurone may innervate hundreds of muscle fibres. This combination of a motor neurone and the muscle it stimulates is termed a motor unit.

Prenatal development of the nervous system

The preceding chapter has provided an overview of the prenatal development of the nervous system. A thorough review of the embryological development of the nervous system is beyond the scope of this book. Readers are referred to Brown *et al.* (1997) for a more detailed overview. However, the main steps in development and relationship to development of movement will be outlined in brief.

The neural crest is the precursor of all peripheral autonomic nerve fibres, sensory nerve fibres and Schwann cells. The latter two are clearly important in the development of motor function. The neural tube is the origin of many of the other structures of the nervous system which are important in human movement. For example, the cerebellum, necessary for postural control and coordination, grows out of the metencephalon. However, the most important

Table 4.1 An Overview of Aspects of the Nervous System Involved in Motor Function

Name of part of CNS	Neural connections relating to motor function and or balance	Role in relation to motor function and/or balance
Brainstem	• *From* cerebral cortex • *To and from* spinal cord	• Posture and balance control • Coordination of head and eye movements
Cerebral (motor) cortex 1. Prefrontal 2. Primary motor 3. Premotor 4. Supplementary motor	(Connections from or to one or more of the four areas of cerebral cortex) • *From* thalamus (and basal ganglia, spinal cord via thalamus) and association areas • *To* brainstem, spinal cord directly and via brainstem, and to posterior parietal cortex	• Initiates planned movement/planning of motor task • Regulates rate of force required to move • Stabilizes muscles relating to planning movement • Involved in coordination of posture and voluntary movements
Cerebellum • Anterior lobe • Posterior lobe	• *From* motor/premotor cortex, spinal motoneurones, spinal interneurones • *To* brainstem regions, proximal/distal limb muscles, via thalamus to motor and premotor cortex	• Monitors cortical and brainstem activity, comparing against sensory feedback • Alters function based on learning from experience • Regulates muscle tone, balance and coordination of movements/time of movements
Basal ganglia (Five paired nuclei)	• *From* cerebral cortex and directly from thalamus • *To* thalamus and all parts of motor cortex plus areas of cortex relating to memory and behaviour	• Involved in control of voluntary and involuntary movement

Source: Davis *et al.*, in Gluckman and Heymann (1996).

structures that will relate to sensation, perception, and motor patterns arise from the telencephalon, from which the cerebrum, with its two cerebral hemispheres, is formed. It is in the cerebrum that sensory information is collated and analysed.

Development of motoneurones

Cells that will later become motoneurones migrate from the ventricular zone. As the first cells are pushed outwards by later ones, a continuous column of cells form in the cephalocaudal (head-to-tail) axis of the developing spinal cord. This column later divides as the newly differentiated motoneurones reach muscle masses in limb buds. Later migrating cells form different regions of the spinal cord. When migration is complete, there are six main clusters of motoneurones corresponding to muscle groups in each of the limb buds.

Even before migration is complete, the neurones are attaining their differentiated form. The axons grow in length and dendrites form and arborize (develop a characteristic branching structure). The development of motoneurones is complete before that of sensory neurones, with glial cells being the last to differentiate.

Initially an over-abundance of dendritic branches develop, the purpose of which is uncertain. One possibility suggested by Brown *et al.* (1997) is that they may be needed to obtain the right number of muscle fibres. It is known that the number of motoneurones innervating the muscle regulates production of muscle fibres. Therefore, an over-abundance of motoneurones could ensure that sufficient muscle fibres are produced.

Establishing connections in the CNS and with developing muscle

Outside the brain and spinal cord, motoneurone axons find their way to the belly of developing muscle, guided by chemical guidance factors and later by growth cones on the tips of the axons. Growth cones enable contact with muscle fibres to form neuromuscular junctions in the same regions. As a result of influences from the developing muscle, the growth cone differentiates into a presynaptic terminal. In turn, this influences the differentiation of the muscle fibre. Neuromuscular junctions appear and other changes take place in the muscle to enable motor and sensory impulses to be transmitted. As the muscle fibres continue to be innervated, an excess number of axons come to innervate the same muscle fibres. These excess neurones are pruned out before birth and die. This is a similar process to selective pruning in the CNS (see preceding chapter).

Myelination

The next stage of development is the myelination of neurones in the central and peripheral nervous systems by glial cells. While this is not essential to nerve transmission, it greatly speeds up conduction velocity by as much as tenfold, although this is proportional to the diameter of the nerve fibre. The process of myelination is discussed in more detail in the preceding chapter. *At birth*, much of the cerebral cortex has not yet been myelinated, although the nerves relating to the leg and vision are furthest advanced. There is also myelination of part of the brainstem, thalamus and cerebellum.

Box 4.2 Myelination

Myelination of neurones in the central and peripheral nervous systems, by glial cells, is not essential to nerve transmission, but it greatly speeds up conduction velocity by as much as tenfold, although this is proportional to the diameter of the nerve fibre.

Growth of the nervous system after birth in relation to movement

In the context of motor development, the postnatal development of the cerebral cortex and cerebellum are of particular interest. The cerebral cortex becomes somewhat thicker with age (it doubles between birth and adulthood). Maturation is in three areas, and in this order – the primary areas (related to sensori-motor function), the association areas (related to vision, hearing, speech and writing) and the terminal zones (relating to establishing connections between the thalamus and parts of the frontal lobe first through long association fibres and then short association fibres).

At birth, the cerebellum still retains an external granular layer of cells until one year, when these redundant cells are removed. As mentioned in the preceding chapter, myelination within the cerebellum mostly occurs postnatally, particularly during the *first two months*.

Skeletal Muscle Development

Skeletal muscles are the type of muscle that produce body movements. As muscles contract or relax, tendons (attached to bones and usually crossing joints) exert some force on the joint. The place where the muscle is attached to stationary bone is the origin, and the moveable joint, the insertion. The lever–fulcrum principle can explain how movement occurs. The bones act as fixed and rigid levers, and the joints as fulcrums for the levers. In the lever–fulcrum principle, effort (muscle contraction) is balanced by resistance (force or weight, including weight of the limb). Muscles, usually opposing pairs, work in groups to coordinate movement, as in flexing the arm. In this example, the biceps brachii is the flexor muscle, which is the agonist, or prime mover. The triceps brachii is the extensor muscle, which is the antagonist, or relaxing muscle. Other muscles, synergists, steady movements and fixators, a type of synergistic muscle, stabilize the origin of the agonist muscle. The remaining parts of this section will provide an overview of embryonic and postnatal development of muscle.

Prenatal muscle development

Muscle tissue arises from embryonic mesoderm. Following gastrulation, a portion of the dorsal mesoderm from which skeletal muscle will eventually arise, divides, forming blocks of tissue known as somites. Some of the somites are responsible for formation of the vertebral column, ribs and dermis, while others form the limb bud and muscle masses. The instruction to the somites to form muscle rather than other tissue is provided by myogenic master regulatory genes or homeobox genes in the mesodermal cells.

Formation of skeletal muscle fibres

The cells that will form muscle fibres originate from mesoderm, and are known as myoblasts (early muscle-forming cells), which, after a proliferative stage, fuse together to become myotubes. The first myotubes are formed at about *7 weeks gestation*. Myotubes will eventually become muscle fibres (see Figure 4.1).

The following sequence of events occurs in the formation of muscle fibres. (Please see the left side of Figure 4.1). The description excludes details about induction and regulatory mechanisms.

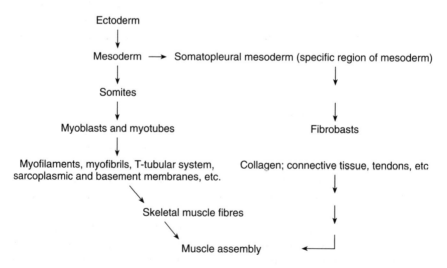

Figure 4.1 Development of Skeletal Muscle

a. *Massive proliferation of cells* starts in somites, and then among myoblasts.

b. *Motility and exploration*: Myoblasts divide rapidly, become mobile and their cytoplasmic processes explore other nearby myoblasts and previously formed myotubes.

c. *Alignment*: Myoblasts line up against and adhere to other nearby myoblasts and myotubes.

d. *Development of electrodense structures; myotube formation*: After the myoblasts have adhered to each other, structures similar to gap junctions are then formed. (A gap junction is a tubular structure though which a nerve impulse passes from one cell to another.) Next, during transient depolarisation of myoblasts, calcium ions (Ca^{2+}) are enabled to enter the cells, which promote fusion of myoblasts with each other. As more and more myoblasts fuse together into a chain, myotubes are formed.

e. *Protein synthesis; formation of myofilaments, myofibrils, etc*: After this, myosin and actin (proteins found in myofilaments) are formed, myofilaments group into bundles and become thicker to form myofibrils. The 'slow' myosin is evident at *8–10 weeks*, with 'fast' myosin appearing in myotubes at *14–15 weeks* (Draeger *et al.*, in McComas, 1996). Additionally, a basic form of the T-system (transverse tubules), sarcoplasmic reticulum and basement membrane of the myotube are formed. The plasma membrane on the surface of the myotube is called the plasmalemma. (The plasmalemma and basement membrane make up the sarcolemma of the mature skeletal muscle fibre.) The plasmalemma is beginning to develop important properties of excitability, enabling action potentials to be fired and it now contains acetylcholine receptors (AChRs). Twitching of myotubules can now be seen in culture. These receptors are important for muscle stimulation, as acetylcholine is the neurotransmitter that diffuses across the sarcolemma. As it combines with AChRs, the permeability of the sarcolemma to sodium and potassium ions is altered, ultimately resulting in development of muscle action potential and muscle contraction.

f. *Formation of muscle fibres*: The final transition of the myotube to become a muscle fibre occurs with the enlargement of the myotube, addition of more myofilaments, better differentiation of the sarcoplasmic and T-system, and the movement of the nuclei to the area under the plasmalemma. Proliferation of myotubes and muscle fibres continues until approximately *25 weeks gestation*; then it slows or stops. However, myotubes are still acquiring myosin until *31 to 34 weeks gestation*. Muscle fibres continue to grow in number and become more closely packed together as *term* approaches.

On the right side of Figure 4.1, it may be seen that the muscle masses (dorsal and ventral) are beginning to develop from somites. These masses of muscle divide, eventually forming individual muscles. Connective tissue, arising from fibroblasts, originating from the somatopleural mesoderm, supports and envelopes each muscle belly, groups muscle fibres into bundles, and defines the tendons at the ends of the muscles.

From *20 weeks gestation*, some muscle fibres are beginning to differentiate into different types – large Type I fibres appear first (between *20 and 30 weeks*), with normally-sized Type I fibres appearing at *30 weeks*. The large Type I fibres are usually not present any more *at birth*, but the normal-sized ones increase in number, constituting 40 per cent of the muscle fibres *at birth*. Type II fibres also appear at *30 weeks*, and about 45 per cent of the muscle fibres *at birth* are of this type. The remaining 15 per cent of muscle fibres are undifferentiated. Type I fibres are also known as slow twitch fibres as contraction velocity is slow, although resistant to fatigue. Type II (a and b) fibres are sometimes called fast twitch fibres; their contraction velocity is fast, but they are not as resistant to fatigue. The proportion of Type I fibres *at birth* is lower than it is at *1 year post-natally* (when the distribution is about the same as in an adult).

Postnatal muscle development

The number of muscle fibres increases until about *4 months postnatally*. Their size increases during *childhood*, with adult diameters being reached during *adolescence*. However, variations in the contractile and metabolic features of muscle fibres and the extent of increase in size are influenced by the degree of muscle activity. The girth of muscles increases *after birth*, due to the continued growth of muscle fibres.

The size of muscle fibres is related to increases in the number of nuclei in muscle cells. Boys show a 14-fold increase in number of nuclei in muscle cells between *birth* and *adolescence*, while girls have a 10-fold increase. The increase of muscle length, which occurs at the muscle–tendon junction, is related to increases in the length and numbers of sarcomeres. In addition, as the skeleton grows, so do the lengths of corresponding muscle fibres. This probably results from the range of movement required of a joint. The stimulus for increasing length of the tendon is also thought to be related to tension.

It should be recognized that regular physical activity is very significant for muscle function. The percentage of certain types of muscle fibre and their size may vary with exercise or other factors.

For example, children who walk late, at about *19 months* have been found to have reduced muscle fibre size (especially type 11) (Lundberg *et al.*, 1979a in Malina, 1986).

Nutritional factors also appear to have some influence:

Lundberg *et al.* (1979b) also reported that a sample of children with coeliac disease had poor gross motor development associated with a reduced percentage of type 1 fibres, but this number and their diameter increased when the nutritional deficiency was corrected.

It is known that training can greatly increase the area and size of muscle fibres.

For example, high resistance weight training in children as well as adults is associated with hypertrophy of relevant muscles and changes in the ratio of type 1 to type 11 fibre areas (Malina, 1986). Endurance training in children and adolescents, in contrast, has less of an effect on muscle size, although Eriksson (1972) has reported chemical changes. Marked changes were observed in oxidative potential of muscle (as measured by 30 per cent increase in succinate dehydrogenase (SDH) activity) and glycolytic potential (as measured by 8 per cent increase in phosphofructokinase (PFK) activity) in 11 year old boys after six months of training. In adult males, after the same amount of training, the PFK activity was higher but SDH activity was lower. This suggests that although both adults and children can benefit from training, the type and degree of response will vary with age.

Bone Development and Growth

Bones and cartilage form the framework of the skeletal system. In addition to facilitating movement, functions of the skeletal system include protection of internal organs, support of soft tissues and muscles at their points of attachment, and storage of minerals, haemopoetic cells and lipids. One of the main types of bone is the long bone (examples being the femur and humerus). The shaft of the long bone is called the diaphysis, within which is the medullary cavity, lined by the endosteum. The ends of the bone are the epiphyses and the place where the diaphysis meets the epiphysis is the metaphysis. In a *child*, the metaphysis is the place where the epiphyseal plate is located, the importance of which will be discussed later. On the epiphysis, there is a thin layer of articular cartilage, where the bone forms a joint. The bone is covered elsewhere by periosteum, which is involved in bone growth and repair.

This section of the chapter will provide an overview of the origins of bone tissue and the process of development of bones, or ossification. Two types of bone are formed in the skeletal system, spongy bone and compact bone. Compact bone, found below the periosteum, is densely packed, and, unlike spongy bone, has Haversian systems or osteons. These have central Haversian canals surrounded by concentric rings called lamellae, canaliculi or small canals connecting lacunae (spaces) and osteocytes. Blood vessels, nerves and lymphatic vessels travel through Haversian canals. In contrast, spongy bone is made up of thin plates of bone, known as trabeculae, forming an irregular latticework pattern. It is not densely packed as in compact bone, and the spaces (lacunae) may be filled with red marrow, where blood-forming cells develop.

Histological origins of bone tissue and mechanisms of bone formation

As noted in the section on muscle development, bone also arises from embryonic mesoderm. A loosely organized embryonic connective tissue known as mesenchyme develops from mesodermal cells. The mesenchyme can differentiate into many types of cells, including chondroblasts (involved in cartilage formation), osteoblasts (involved in bone formation) or fibroblasts (involved in connective tissue formation). Bone is formed through either of two processes of bone formation, intramembranous ossification, where bones are formed directly from osteoblasts, or through endochondral ossification, where cartilage is formed first from chondroblasts, and later is transformed from cartilage to bone. Some bones, such as the cranium and clavicles, are mostly formed by intramembranous ossification. Other bones, such as long bones, are formed by endochondral ossification. In summary, both forms of ossification start with mesenchyme, but in intramembranous ossification, bone is formed without going though a stage of first being cartilage.

Box 4.3   Types of Ossification

Bone is formed through either of two processes of bone formation:

1. *Intramembranous ossification*, where bones are formed directly from osteoblasts, for example the cranium and clavicles; or
2. *Endochondral ossification*, where cartilage is formed first from chondroblasts, and later is transformed from cartilage to bone, for example the long bones.

Both forms develop from a loosely organised embryonic connective tissue known as mesenchyme which itself develops from mesodermal cell

---

The timing of ossification varies with different bones. At about *6 weeks* of embryonic life (see Figure 4.2a), some mesenchymal cells become closely packed, or condensed, forming a model or template of a bone. Some of these cells form a membrane around the model, called the perichondrium. The inner layer of cells of the perichondrium do not differentiate as yet, but the outer layer becomes fibroblasts, roughly defining the shape of the eventual bone. At this point, the development differs in long bones (where endochondral ossification occurs) and some other bones (where intramembranous ossification occurs). Therefore, these two types of ossification will be discussed separately.

Prenatal development of long bones (eg femur)

The model begins to enlarge mainly through a process called apposition. This is a form of growth characterized by surface depositing of material, where the original tissue mass does not itself expand. Enlargement also occurs though interstitial growth, which is the uniform growth throughout a tissue mass during early development of bones. The apposition involved in this case is the depositing of newly formed cartilage cells called chondrocytes, which originate from previously undifferentiated cells of the perichondrium. The newly forming cells are

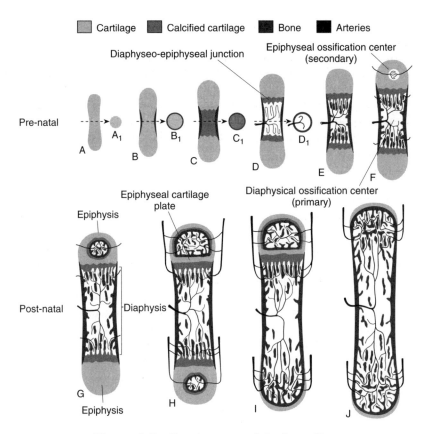

Figure 4.2 Development of the Long Bones

Source: Reprinted from *The Developing Human: Clinically Orientated Embryology*, 4th edition, with permission from WB Saunders.

deposited near the top and bottom ends of the model. As more chondrocytes and intercellular material of collagenous and/or elastic fibres are deposited, these areas become more densely packed, forming hypertrophied cartilage. This causes an increase in length and width (especially at the ends) of the model.

Between *7 and 12 weeks*, the cells closer to the centre of the model begin to disintegrate, resulting in cartilage being most dense to the top and bottom of the central area. Older chondrocytes in these areas of hypertrophied cartilage begin to secrete alkaline phosphatase, an enzyme that enables the intercellular material around the chondrocytes to become calcified.

After these areas become calcified, ossification in the diaphysis area of the model begins. Osteoid tissue (uncalcified bone matrix) is formed directly from within the perichondrium membrane. A collar of this osteoid tissue forms on the inner aspect of the membrane in the central area of the model, and soon becomes calcified when calcium phosphate is deposited in the osteoid tissue (see Figure 4.2b, c). Osteoblasts (bone forming cells) become trapped in the matrix and develop into osteocytes (bone cells), so enabling periosteal bone to be formed. The outside aspect of the membrane becomes the periosteum following the appearance of osteoblasts.

Blood vessels, which carry osteoclasts (cells that remove bone) and undifferentiated cells, extend from the periosteum to the central area of the model. The osteoclasts remove cartilage cells from the central area, and the blood supply extends further along the model. Some undifferentiated cells become osteoblasts, which will form bone around calcified cartilage (see Figure 4.2d). Others become haemopoetic cells.

By *12 weeks*, endochondral ossification occurs within the central area of the model. This is termed the primary centre of ossification. Osteoblasts cluster around remaining calcified cartilage, forming trabeculae as osteoblasts become trapped in lacunae and develop into osteocytes. Successive layers of trabeculae fuse together, forming the latticework pattern typical of spongy bone. Later, more central trabeculae are absorbed by osteoclasts, forming a marrow cavity. Meanwhile, trabeculae continue to widen on the edges of the marrow cavity and become incorporated into the cortex (see Figure 4.2e).

Sub-periosteal bone, which is compact, is also being formed by this time. In addition, towards either end of the model, there is emerging a narrow zone of calcified cartilage next to a zone of hypertrophied chondrocytes nearest the ends of the model. The model becomes longer and wider as chondrocytes continue to divide and intercellular substance increases (see Figure 4.2f). From this point and *throughout life*, remodelling of bone occurs. The growth in the size of the marrow cavity through resorption (diameter is increased by osteoclast activity) is balanced with growth of the model mainly through apposition, but also through interstitial growth. Interstitial growth occurs in cartilage matrix until it becomes too impliable for growth to continue in this way.

The model at this stage therefore has compact bone around most of its external aspect (periosteum), which surrounds either spongy bone composed of trabeculae or cartilage (the latter being concentrated at the extreme ends). There is a marrow cavity, and zones of cartilage and hypertrophied chondrocytes lie towards either end of the model. These areas later become the locations of the epiphyseal plates/discs, which will be responsible for the lengthwise growth of bones.

Prenatal development of other types of bones

As mentioned previously, a few bones (the clavicle, cranium) develop through intramembranous ossification. After a period of appositional growth, blood vessels carrying osteoblasts and osteoclasts enter the primary ossification centre. A matrix is formed by collagen fibres that are deposited by the osteoblasts, and then the matrix becomes calcified after calcium and other inorganic salts are deposited.

In irregularly shaped short bones such as the carpals and tarsals, the process is essentially the same as in long bones, except that instead of a cavity developing in the middle, they occur at sites of future joints. After the shapes of the models are evident, each bone then articulates with neighbouring bones and they are covered by perichondrium. Blood vessels invade cartilage from the perichondrium, and thereafter ossification occurs from ossification centres (mainly *postnatally*) in a similar way to long bones. There may be more than one ossification centre. However, in these bones, with the exception of the calcaneum (heel bone), there are no epiphyseal plates. Figure 4.3 shows the extent of ossification of the skeleton *at birth*.

Postnatal bone growth

In long bones, secondary centres of ossification develop (see Figure 4.2f–i), initially at one epiphysis and then at the other (see Figure 2g, h). In some bones, several centres develop, which later fuse together. Although these centres exist, some are not active until *adolescence*. Between the epiphysis and diaphysis is the epiphyseal plate or disc. Here chondrocytes lie in columns along the axis of the bone, in parallel with calcified cartilage strips. Above the chondrocytes lies a layer of resting cartilage. The chondrocytes divide and mature, and interstitial growth within the plate occurs lengthwise.

After a time, many of chondrocytes die and are resorbed, while the smaller resting cartilage layer remains. Ossification occurs on this layer of cartilage on the part facing the diaphysis, enabling the shaft to lengthen. The epiphyseal plate remains a similar thickness throughout childhood – as new chondrocytes are formed within it, which would deepen the cartilage layer, cartilage closer to the diaphysis is replaced by bone, so keeping its thickness constant.

In all types of bones, ossification continues to proceed outwards from the centres of ossification. Remodelling, including of the Haversian system, continues during *childhood*. Towards *late adolescence* (*16–18 in females* or *18–21 in males*), the bone growth within the diaphysis of long bones overtakes the interstitial growth in the cartilaginous, epiphyseal plate, and it is converted to bone. There is then continuous bone between diaphysis and epiphysis. Bones can no longer grow when the epiphyseal plate is converted to bone. In addition to the lengthwise growth of bones just described, the width increases by apposition and resorption. Apposition exceeds resorption, so the cortex of the diaphysis does increase in thickness until *adolescence*. Finally, there is some adjustment in moveable joints with increased range of motion.

The predictable sequence of bone development is used in clinical practice to measure bone age in children with growth problems by comparing ossification visible on X-ray with published standards.

Movements and Reflexes in the Prenatal and Early Postnatal Period

It is well known that both spontaneous and elicited movements can be detected as early as *7.5 weeks gestation* (deVries, 1982, cited in Brown *et al.*,

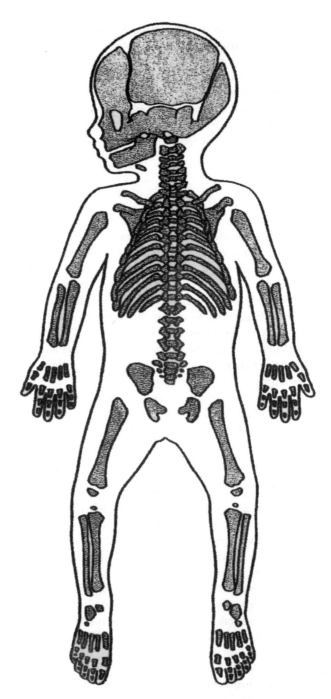

Figure 4.3   Ossification of the Skeleton at Birth

Source: From Sinclair and Dangerfield, 1998, by permission.

1997). Preyer (1885, cited in Brown *et al.*, 1997) was the first to observe that spontaneous, 'impulsive' movements occur several days before reflexes can be invoked through sensory stimuli. This suggested that motor systems begin to function prior to sensory ones. The movements have been described as having rhythmic and sometimes writhing quality. It is evident that there are links between sensory input and motor function in the *fetus*, although *after birth* exposure to the external environment and maturation of nervous and muscle tissue, enables these patterns to become more coordinated.

Box 4.4   First Prenatal Movements

Both spontaneous and elicited movements can be detected as early as *7.5 weeks gestation* (deVries, 1982, cited in Brown *et al.*, 1997), around the time pregnancy is first confirmed.

Brown *et al.* (1997) report findings concerning muscle tone and reflexes in the prenatal period, based on observational studies by Hooker (1952) and Humphrey (1964). These are summarized in Table 4.2. Note that although movements are evident from the first flexor stage, the characteristics change over time, and it is only from *6 months of age* that movement is more flexible and less reliant on environmental cues such as contact with a surface and position of the head and neck. This relates to improved muscle tone, loss of primitive reflexes that could interfere with voluntary movement, better balance and maturation of the nervous system.

Function of primitive reflexes, postural reflexes and stereotypic movements in early motor development

Primitive and postural reflexes. Primitive reflexes are thought to be remnants from our evolutionary past, and some retain a useful function (for example, rooting, sucking). Most authors view them to be sub-cortical in origin, suggesting that as the *infant's* higher mental functions develop, they are inhibited. However, they can reappear, for example in brain injury.

Children with neurological deficits (for example, with cerebral palsy) retain some of these reflexes past *infancy*.

A description of these reflexes, how they are elicited and their relevance to motor development can be found in the Table 4.3. Figure 4.4 shows that some of these reflexes are evident *in utero*, and they persist for different lengths of time in *early infancy*.

Most authors view primitive reflexes as an impediment to mature motor function, requiring inhibition for smooth voluntary motor actions to be possible (eg, Fiorentino, 1973; Blasco, 1994; Capute *et al.*'s, (1978) description of the primitive reflex profile is well known).

Table 4.2   Stages in the Development of Muscle Tone and Reflexes

Name of Stage	Age range	Features of this state
First flexor stage	9–17 weeks gestation	Predominant flexor tone Possible to elicit limb flexor reflexes Myoclonic jerks – Spontaneous movements (jerking/jumping) of all limbs (8–16 weeks) Rhythmic movements, e.g. movements of individual limbs, pronation and supination of hands (by 10–12 weeks) *Rooting reflex*, grasp reflex Pursing of lips elicited by perioral stimulation
First extensor stage	18–30 weeks gestation	Strong flexor tone is lost Spontaneous rhythmic movements involving flexion and extension, eg, cycling, boxing, grasping, increase in variety and speed (up to 20 weeks) EEG waves appear (indicating brainstem oscillatory circuits starting to operate) Asymmetric tonic neck reflex (ATNR) (by 18 weeks) *Moro reflex* (by 22 weeks) Fine mouth and tongue, 'crying' and yawning movements (by 22 weeks) Sucking and swallowing reflexes, but poor coordination (12–30 weeks)
Second flexor stage	30–44 weeks gestation	Flexor tone returning, especially after 35 weeks Synchronous, rhythmic reciprocal patterns of movement capable of propelling foetus in utero (swimming, hatching behaviour) (from 30 weeks) – probably organized at level of red nucleus in mid-brain Legs tend to be flexed and abducted Arms flex (35 weeks) and recoil when extended (38 weeks) Hips will not abduct more than 45° (40 weeks) Adduction of limbs (from 35 weeks) Vestibular apparatus activated (from 33 weeks) – i.e. if born, posture adopted relative to gravity
Second extensor stage	Birth–6 months	Inhibition of flexor tone in arms (4 weeks postnatal) – so infant lies with arms extended and legs flexed Active leg extension when lying suprine (6–8 weeks postnatal) When prone, legs extended at the hip, chest lifted off ground and head vertical (16 weeks) When prone, fully extended arms support weight (6 months) Re-emergence of extensor reflexes after birth (ATNR, trunk incurvation, Moro reflexes), disappearing again by 5–6 months Early posture adopted related to infant's position in space, neck reflexes and contact with a surface Flexion/extension less dependent on position (4–6 months) When pulled to sitting, head raised in anticipation, and later can voluntarily pull up (4 months) Infant does not fall over when sitting if leans to side (5 months) Improved balance and limb righting enables independent sitting and standing with support (6 months) Protective parachute response develops from 5 months
Cortical stage	From 6 months	Posture no longer dependent on position of head, neck, trunk or surface contact. As able to freely flex one part of limb and extend other, capable of standing balance and movement (requiring functioning of one cerebral hemisphere and basal ganglia). Manual and postural skills developing

Table 4.3 Primitive Reflexes

Name of Primitive reflex	Mode of elicitation	Description	Significance for motor development
Moro	Sit child upright, allow head to fall back 20° OR lower baby quickly OR make a loud noise	Back straightens, arms extend outwards, with hands open, then arms move to midline, hands clenched.	If persists, may interfere with sitting. Persistence may indicate neurological deficit
Palmar	Place finger in palm of hand	Baby grips finger	Persistence could interfere with voluntary handling of objects/signal neurological deficit
Plantar	Place finger across ball of foot near toes	Toes appear to 'grip' finger	Persistence could signal neurological deficit
Asymmetrical tonic neck reflex (ATNR)	Infant placed supine, with legs and arms extended, turn head to side	Arm extends on side where infant is facing, and other arm flexes at elbow (like fencing or stance).	Continued presence may inhibit ability to roll over (arm is in the way), balance, visual tracking unilaterality of brain function.
Spinal Galant/trunk incurvation	Stroke infant's back along spine	Hips move towards side stimulated.	Persistence could interfere with balance.
Rooting/sucking	Stroke/touch cheek (rooting). Object/teat in mouth (sucking)	Infant will turn towards finger touching cheek, and suck when found	Persistence may indicate neurological deficit
Tonic Labyrinthe Reflex (TLR) TLS = supine, TLP = prone	Two positions: Place infant *supine* on palm, let head drop back below midline; then raise head above midline. Place infant *prone*	Supine: Extensor thrust of limbs with back arch when head drops, mild tongue thrust; legs flex, adopts foetal position when head raised. Prone: Flexes limbs	Tongue-thrust action can interfere with sucking and swallowing (as in cerebral palsy), or with speech. Persistence could affect balance
Babinski	Stroke sole of foot from outside edge of heel, up length of foot on that side, and across ball of foot towards big toe	Large toe dorsiflexes, and toes fan out	Persistence may indicate neurological deficit
Symmetrical Tonic Neck Reflex (STNR)	Place supine, move head to the side.	Flexion of arms, extension of legs	Enables rolling over to occur as no longer ATNR
Landau	Place infant prone, holding under chest	Head and then torso lift up	Importance for learning to crawl and for development of muscle tone
Heading righting reflex (HRR)	Infant sitting; body leans to one side	Head moves to upright position even if body isn't	Helps with stability in sitting
Amphibian	Frequently elicited in supine position or in times of excitement	Contralateral arms and legs move alternately	Relevant for learning to crawl
Segmental Rolling reflex/body righting	Rotate infants hips towards midline	Rest of torso follows direction of hips	Helps with skill of rolling over.
Transformed Tonic Neck Reflex (TTNR)	Place infant supine, turn head to side	Arm and leg on side where face directed, flexes, other side extends	Relevant for positioning in skills such as throwing ball

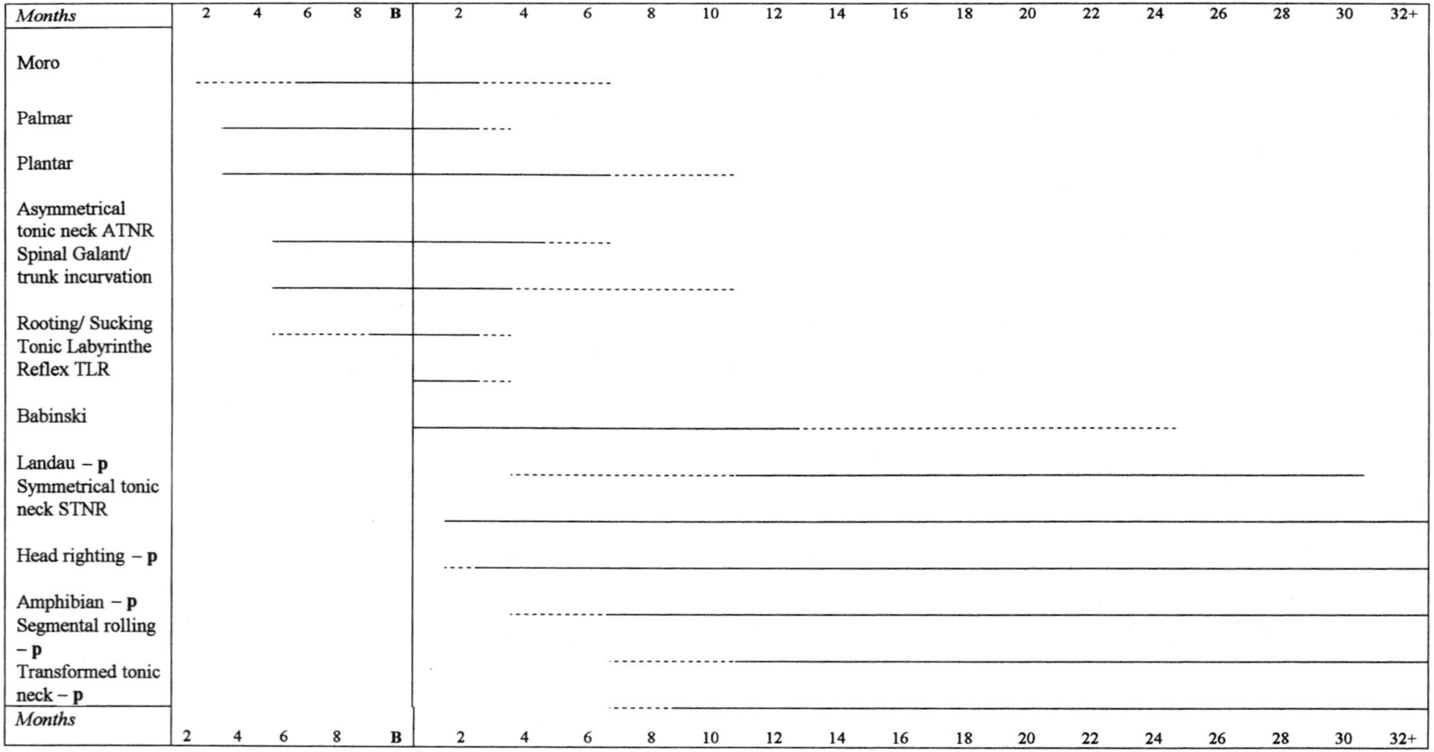

Months	2	4	6	8	B	2	4	6	8	10	12	14	16	18	20	22	24	26	28	30	32+

Moro

Palmar

Plantar

Asymmetrical tonic neck ATNR
Spinal Galant/ trunk incurvation

Rooting/ Sucking
Tonic Labyrinthe Reflex TLR

Babinski

Landau – **p**
Symmetrical tonic neck STNR

Head righting – **p**

Amphibian – **p**
Segmental rolling – **p**
Transformed tonic neck – **p**

| Months | 2 | 4 | 6 | 8 | B | 2 | 4 | 6 | 8 | 10 | 12 | 14 | 16 | 18 | 20 | 22 | 24 | 26 | 28 | 30 | 32+ |

Key: Primitive reflex present ———— Reflex possibly present - - - - - -
p = Postural reflex

Figure 4.4 Profile of Emergence and Disappearance of Primitive Reflexes and Appearance of Postural Reflexes

Source: Adapted from Beuret LJ (1985), in Goddard S (1990) *A Developmental Basis for Learning Difficulties and Language Disorders*, Goddard SA, INPP Monograph Series 1/90, copyright 1990, with permission from Sally Goddard Blythe, at the Institute for Neuro-Physiological Psychology.

This is why some physiotherapy interventions, for example of children with cerebral palsy, attempt to inhibit these reflexes to facilitate righting and equilibrium reactions (Bobath, 1980).

Some evidence for the importance of reduction of primitive reflexes is found in a study by Marquis *et al.* (1984), who found that in very low birth-weight *infants*, there was an association between the strength of retained primitive reflexes and incidence of later motor delays. Others suggest that certain primitive reflexes may be incorporated into mature motor actions (eg, Thelen and Cooke, 1987; Zelazo *et al.*, 1993). Interestingly, some recent studies have questioned whether there is any relationship between primitive reflexes and motor development (Bartlett, 1997; Pimentel, 1996). These suggest that the spontaneous, rhythmical, stereotypical movements seen in *infancy* may be more important. This is discussed further in the next section.

The inhibition of primitive reflexes precedes emergence of postural reflexes (see Figure 4.3). Postural reflexes, found in most adults, facilitate general motor activities.

For example, when the *infant* is learning to roll, they usually start by rolling their hips towards the mid-line. The segmental rolling reflex is then elicited, and this helps the rest of the body to follow.

Other examples are seen in Table 4.3. The emerging postural reflexes appear as primitive reflexes decline, and often parallel the time of acquisition of definitive motor actions.

Stereotypical movements: It will be recalled from the previous section that there are many characteristic movements of the *fetus, embryo* and *young infant.* These include stereotypic movements (or stereotypies), which are rhythmical, repetitive and intrinsically generated movement patterns. These are thought by some researchers to be important precursors of related mature motor actions. This view was initially proposed by Thelen (1979) and has been researched extensively, mainly by this author.

This view has significant implications for child-rearing practices. In particular, it would be considered beneficial to maximize opportunities for stereotypic movements in *early infancy* that would provide practice, for example, in stepping movements that are later incorporated into walking.

Common practices such as use of baby walkers may reduce stereotypy normally displayed prior to walking (such as alternate leg kicking).

Environmental Influences on Motor Development

As pointed out in the previous chapter, the nervous system continues to have plasticity *postnatally*. This means that it is capable of change as a result of experience. It was noted that *prior to birth*, there is remodelling in neural development, including 'pruning' of excess connections. Greenough *et al.* (1987) indicate that this continues into *infancy*, often during what is commonly termed as sensitive periods (ie, windows in time when an organism is more responsive to particular kinds of experience). They report findings show that in *early post-natal development*, synapses are over-produced in a chaotic manner in the nervous system and skeletal muscle (as well as in oculomotor system). As development progresses, some of these synapses are selectively pruned, leaving a well-defined and organized system, for example at neuromuscular junctions.

Greenough *et al.* (1987) suggest that it is helpful to recognize that there are probably two different sorts of plasticity relating to storing of environmental experience. The first results from the kinds of experiences that would be expected during the normal course of *infancy*, coined 'experience expectant', resulting in retention of synapses and storing of information reflecting this species-specific experience. They suggest this may underlie the well-known sensitive period phenomenon. However, they also propose a second form of plasticity, coined 'experience dependent', which relates to specific individual experience. It is this latter form of plasticity that may be of particular interest when considering possible beneficial effects of tactile stimulation on neuromotor development. Stimulation may result in over-production of neuronal synapses that would not have occurred in the absence of this experience. This could finally result in a better-organized system, possibly affecting motor development.

There has been some support for this view, in relation to effects of tactile or vestibular stimulation/rocking, stroking and/or massage of *preterm infants* on their early neuromotor development in recent years, although the evidence does not consistently support these benefits. Although only one study has apparently been undertaken in this area with *term infants*, no similar effects were found (Koniak-Griffin *et al.*, 1995). On the other hand, passive tactile stimulation has been shown to have a beneficial effect on muscle tone of hypotonic, *developmentally delayed young children* (Linkous and Stutts, 1990). Most research, however, has focused on benefits for *preterm infants.*

A number of studies have supported the benefits of early stimulation for neuromotor development. Barnard and Bee (1983) conducted one of the earliest studies in this area, showing benefits of temporally patterned stimuli in this age group. Field *et al.* (1986) showed that tactile/kinaesthetic stimulation given to *preterm neonates* involving stroking and passive movements resulted, among other benefits, in more mature motor responses as measured on the Brazelton NBAS scale (1973). Clark *et al.* (1989) found that motion stimulation (rocking) accelerated motor development and weight gain in *premature infants.* After thrice daily rocking on the longitudinal axis for 15-minute periods for 2 weeks, neuromuscular maturation was significantly greater in all treatment (versus control) infants. Passive muscle tone and active motility showed improvement as well as auditory and visual orientation, alertness and defensive reactions. There were no significant differences in weight gain, although the larger infants in the treatment group showed marked increases in weight gain. More recently, de Roiste and Bushnell (1996) have shown similar benefits of tactile stimulation in this age group.

Practice can also affect the speed and quality of motor skills in *infancy* and *later childhood.* Cross-cultural research illustrates effects of restrictions or enhancement opportunities for particular motor milestones. For example, through use of cross-cultural comparisons, deVries (1999) showed how nutrition, culture and maternal health in pregnancy could affect motor development. In comparing genetically similar tribal groups in rural Kenya, he reported variations in beliefs and practices about infancy and child-rearing, which appeared to be related to neuromotor development.

For example, Digo people value child autonomy and independence and believe that *infants* can learn from birth. The early child autonomy enables the mother to attend to other tasks required of her. This tribe also sees the infant as robust. These factors lead to cultural practices of early training in motor skills and encouragement of independence. These children reach milestones such as sitting, standing, walking and vocalization earlier than other tribal groups. In the Kikuyu tribe, the *infant* is more often seen as vulnerable and the view that infants are capable of learning from birth is less common. For example, the women do not carry infants on their backs as early as in other tribes. These infants have later motor milestones than Digo infants.

These brief examples illustrate how cultural and child-rearing practices may enhance or delay motor development.

Other studies have shown that practice in *early infancy* can accelerate motor development.

For example, Zelazo *et al.* (1993) showed that practice in stepping and sitting for *infants under the age of 6 months* improved their ability to sit for long periods and to step at a faster rate.

However, it is unclear if such advantages would be maintained, or if this would produce only a temporary acceleration of development.

Theoretical Explanations of Motor Development and Functioning

Early description and explanations of motor functioning

Much of the early research in motor development involved painstaking and detailed longitudinal study and descriptions of children's motor milestones. Gessell (1928), Bayley (1935) and others undertook this valuable work. Many contemporary assessment scales are based on their descriptions. The largely invariant sequence of development was explained according to neural changes and general rules governing the order of change. An example of a rule was that development progressed in a cephalocaudal and proximodistal manner. Unfortunately, this early work did not describe the underlying processes, assuming instead that such development was predetermined due to 'hard-wiring' of the nervous system for motor skills.

This view limited research in this area. Consequently, very little research was carried out in this area until the 1970s, when interest was aroused with new theories concerning motor functioning, such as information-processing explanations of motor development, including the 'Closed Loop Model' (Adams, 1971) and the 'Open Loop Model' (Keele, 1982). These attempted to explain how motor actions were executed and stored in memory for future use. The former suggested motor behaviour depended largely on peripheral feedback systems and memory storage of motor sequences, while the latter postulated the existence of predetermined motor programmes that could account for the speed and accuracy of human movement.

There is some physiological evidence for the existence of very early sub-cortical motor programmes, although similar evidence for mature motor programmes is lacking. These early motor programmes have been described by physiologists including Grillner (1975) as neural oscillators or central pattern generators (CPGs), and are postulated to be responsible for the early rhythmical patterned movement seen in animals and humans, such as the stereotypical *infant* movements described earlier in this chapter.

However, information-processing models have not been able to explain the variability and flexibility of complex motor skills, or to provide an adequate explanation of the neuroanatomical basis of mature motor actions.

Recent explanations of motor functioning

Neuronal group-selection theory: More satisfactory explanations of motor func-tioning have been proposed and developed in recent years and these have gone some way to addressing problems of models discussed earlier. One of the most influential of these is the neuronal group-selection model, first proposed by Edelman (1978). Unlike other models, this not only provided a developmen-tal perspective but also a proposed account of how the brain may be involved in more flexible motor actions and higher brain functions. This view is quite complex and only an overview can be provided. Interested readers should refer to Edelman (1978) or Sporns and Edelman (1993) for further details.

The model is based on both empirical evidence and theoretical propositions based on the evidence. It is known that in the brain, neurones are grouped in modules or groups. It is also known that cortical cells are organized in columns in sensory projection areas (Hubel and Wiesel, 1974; Mountcastle, 1967). It is likely that different neuronal groups are organized within such columns. Edelman proposes that local circuit neurones (LCNs) provide interconnections within these modules (intrinsic connections) and extrinsic connections exist between these neuronal groups. Most of the variability of interconnections is thought to be in these intrinsic rather than extrinsic connections. This latter point is proposed based on the appreciation that in order for motor responses to be flexible, there must be more than one set of connections within a neuronal group able to recognize and initiate responses to the same signals. However, with repeated experience, some may be selected over others, result-ing in more committed patterns of recognition and response. This accounts for one of the main features of this model, that the brain is a selective system.

Unlike other theories, Edelman's approach explicitly differentiates between responses in early development and those evident later on. It was mentioned in the previous paragraph that diverse collections of neuronal groups are necessary for recognition and response to perceptual stimuli. These collections of neuronal groups are called *repertoires*. In *infancy and early development*, these repertoires are believed to have pre-determined functions (not dependent on particular experience), where they can respond to a particular signal configuration with a limited range of output. He calls this the primary repertoire. This would account in part for the more limited and less variable movements seen in *early infancy*. As the child matures and gains experience, the secondary repertoire dominates. Edelman (1978, p. 65) suggests that the secondary repertoire, defined as 'collections of different higher order neuronal groups whose internal or external synaptic function has been altered by selection and commitment during experience', enables the *older child* to respond to stimuli in a much more varied way.

Dynamic systems theory: The dynamic systems perspective has been developed by psychologists, although the neuronal group-selection theory is consistent with this view. In common with neuronal group-selection theory, it also attempts to explain the diversity in human motor performance on the basis of not just neural but also dynamic and contextual factors. Ulrich (1997) provides a very readable and comprehensive overview of this approach from a developmental perspective and readers are referred to this source for further details.

Dynamic systems theory originated in ideas from Bernstein (1967), who suggested that motor functioning cannot be described by one-to-one mapping of neuronal impulses and particular movements. He argued that a theory was needed that was able to account for the contribution of contextual factors in movement. A neural explanation was not sufficient, partly because there are so many muscles and bones involved in motor actions that it is impossible to adequately explain variability of movement. For example, Ulrich (1997) notes that over 700 muscles and 100 joints are used in walking. Imagine the number of nerve connections that would be needed for the variety of movements shown in walking alone. A key question posed by this was what Bernstein called 'the degrees of freedom problem', how the brain can control and coordinate movement with so much potential variation.

A further limitation of previous theories was that the role of context in variability was not adequately considered. Forces such as inertia and gravity influence movement. Furthermore, contexts for actions are rarely the same, as they are defined by ever-changing active and passive forces. Bernstein (1967, cited in Turvey *et al.*, 1982) recognized this problem and defined three sources of this context-conditioned variability: anatomical (eg, function of muscles is specified by angles of their pull), mechanical (eg, initial state of a muscle affects the movement possibilities) and physiological variability. In the latter, because of the influence of interneurones from different parts of the spinal cord, cortical and spinal neural transmissions function cooperatively to execute action, rather than resulting from direct cortical control.

Summary

The major part of this section of the chapter has provided an overview of pre- and post-natal development of muscle, bone and the nervous system as relevant to purposeful movement. Although these have been presented as separate systems, they are highly interdependent during development. For example, it will be recalled that muscle fibre production *prenatally* is regulated by the number of motoneurones innervating the muscle. Similarly, *postnatal* muscle fibre and tendon lengthening is associated with bone growth and the increasing range of movement.

Dynamic systems theory helps us to appreciate that while the integration of these systems is important, the nature and quality of movements is also dependent upon the environmental context in which the motor actions are occurring. Factors such as a child's weight or other anatomical factors, the initial state of the muscles to be used in a motor task, or physical limitations of the environment are recognized as significant in explaining the variability of motor actions. Neuronal group-selection theory helps us to understand why early motor activity is more limited in variability, and emphasizes the importance of experience for both neurological and motor development.

There are many points raised in the preceding section of this chapter that are relevant to the practice of health care professionals, including the important area of health promotion. The healthy development of systems involved in motor actions is influenced both *pre- and post-natally* by environmental factors such as nutrition and sensory experience. Health care professionals are in good positions to promote parents' or prospective parents' understanding and influence interventions to promote normal development.

Other aspects of the preceding discussion have more direct significance for the nature of practice by some health care professionals. For example, the importance of early kinaesthetic and tactile experience for neuromotor and other areas of development is relevant to health care professionals working with *premature infants* in Neonatal/Special Care Baby Units.

As our knowledge and understanding of the influences on developing systems increases, it is our responsibility to continue to review standard practices to ensure that they are underpinned by evidence. The next section, focusing on assessment of motor development, raises the issue that in the light of emerging theories of motor development, we perhaps need to review some aspects of our approach to the practice of assessing children's motor development.

Assessment of Motor Development in Health

The choice of approach will vary to some extent depending on the purpose of the assessment. Most health care professionals working with children will be familiar with some of the standard screening assessment tools that focus on achievement of milestones, particularly in *infancy* and *early childhood*. These measures originate from traditional, neural or maturation-based approaches and therefore do not provide information about underlying mechanisms of motor development. However, they can be useful screening tools in the general population. Most of these measure milestones relating to locomotion, posture and manipulation (prehension). An example of such a test is the motor items within the Bayley Scales of Infant Development (1969), a selection of which is reproduced in Table 4.4. Although these or similar scales may be used in screening by, for example, Occupational Therapists, many health visitors in the UK do not consider their use to be necessary or cost-effective, and rely on parent report of concern about developmental delay. On the other hand, tests of some primitive reflexes (previously discussed) may form part of the neurological examination of a *neonate*.

If motor difficulties have been noticed before *school age*, children in the older age groups may need to be assessed using a battery of tests. This is because the nature of a motor difficulty may reflect one or more of a range of problems, including neurological dysfunction, perceptual-motor difficulties or visual-motor integration (Jongmans *et al.*, 1997). Such tests may be used to detect or assess the extent of motor difficulties, for example in clumsiness (Developmental Co-ordination Disorder, formerly called Dyspraxia). Some assessment tools are specifically designed for assessment of children with recognized motor dysfunctions such as cerebral palsy. For example, Ketelaar *et al.* (1998) reviewed 17 assessment measures used with these children, where the purpose was either to discriminate between children with or without particular motor functions or characteristics and/or to evaluate the degree of change in motor function over time. These authors noted that in the case of measures used to assess cerebral palsy, there were no identified predictive measures, i.e. those that predict future function based on current function.

A test of neurological dysfunction for *older children* is the Touwen's Examination of the Child with Minor Neurological Dysfunction (Touwen, 1979). This includes a number of items relating to sensorimotor apparatus, posture, balance of the trunk, coordination of extremities, fine manipulative skills, dyskinesia/kinesia, gross motor function, quality of motility, associated movements and visual system. Perceptual-motor competence can be assessed through the Movement Assessment Battery for Children (Movement ABC) (Henderson and Sugden, 1992). This test measures fine and gross motor coordination, by sampling manual dexterity, static and dynamic balance and ball skills (see Table 4.5). Visual-motor integration can be tested using the Developmental Test of Visual-Motor Integration (VMI) (Beery, 1989). The child is asked to copy various geometric shapes of increasing difficulty and these are assessed for accuracy.

The use of such measures is based on the view that motor development is largely 'hard-wired', as the order of emergence of motor skills and balance appears in a fairly predictable sequence. (On the other hand, dynamic systems

Table 4.4 Selection of Items from Bayley Scale of Infant Development

Test item	Age at which 50% of children pass (months)	Ages at which 95% of children pass (months)
Head erect – vertical	0.8	3.0
Head erect and steady	1.6	4.0
Turns from side to back	1.8	5.0
Sits with support	2.3	5.0
Sits with slight support	3.8	6.0
Sits alone momentarily	5.3	8.0
Pulls to sitting position	5.3	8.0
Rolls from back to front	6.4	10.0
Sits alone, good coordination	6.9	10.0
Pulls to standing position	8.1	12.0
Raises self to sitting position	8.3	11.0
Stands by furniture	8.6	12.0
Stepping movements	8.8	12.0
Walks with help	9.6	12.0
Sits down	9.6	14.0
Stands alone	11.0	16.0
Walks alone	11.7	17.0
Walks up stairs with help	16.1	23.0
Walks up stairs alone, both feet on each step	25.1	30+

theorists would suggest this is not all due to 'hard-wiring' in the nervous system.) It is therefore assumed that delay in attaining motor milestones or difficulty in performing motor tasks may reflect an underlying neurological cause. Although assessors generally appreciate that environmental deprivation may contribute to such problems, there is an assumption that healthy children would be expected to perform well, given normal practice opportunities.

A limitation to this approach to assessment from the dynamic systems theory viewpoint is that neural factors are only a part of the explanation for how children develop their motor skills. Various other individual factors, including weight, strength or endurance, and environmental constraints such as weight or shape of objects to be manipulated could be important. Mathiowetz and Haugen (1994) note that paradigm changes relating to motor behaviour theory is beginning to affect occupational and physiotherapy practice, with a greater recognition of the need to assess these other aspects of motor behaviour and to encourage clients to find their own best opportunities and solutions to functional problems.

Although not commonly undertaken by health care professionals, motor development researchers have observed changes in the quality/level of skill in motor skills with age (eg. stages as described in Malina and Bouchard

Table 4.5 Examples of Items from the Movement Assessment Battery for Children (Movement ABC)

ABC test	Age band (years)	Items, scored 0–5 on each	ABC checklist	12 Questions in each section, scored 0–3
Manual dexterity	4–6	Posting coins Threading beads	Section 1	Child stationary/environment stable
	7–8	Tracing a bicycle trail Placing pegs	Section 2	Child moving/environment stable
		Threading lace Tracing a flower trail	Section 3	Child stationary/environment changing
	9–10	Shifting pegs by rows Threading nuts on bolt Tracing a flower trail	Section 4	Child moving/environment changing
			Total motor score	Total scores from Sections 1–4, classifies child as OK, at risk (AR), or movement problem (MP)
Ball skills	4–6	Catching a bean bag Rolling a ball into goal	Cut-off points	OK AR MP
	7–8	One-hand bounce and catch Throwing bean bag into goal	age 6	<60 60+ 90+
	9–10	Two-hand catch Throwing bean bag into goal	age 7	<50 50+ 75+
			age 8	<35 35+ 55+
			age 9	<35 35+ 50+
Static and dynamic balance	4–6	One-leg balance Jumping over cord Walking, heels raised		
	7–8	Stork balance Jumping in squares Heel-to-toe walking	Section 5	Behavioural problems related to motor difficulties
	9–10	One-board balance Hopping in squares Ball balance		
Total motor	Cut-off same for all ages	<10 = OK >10 = motor impairment >14 = serious motor impairment		

Source: Henderson and Sugden (1992).

(1991) in selected motor skills). Maturity of motor skills is characterized by features of the movement, such as stiffness or clumsiness, range of motion or coordination with other movements, and also with outcomes such as the distance a ball is thrown or time taken to complete a movement. Malina and Bouchard notice that often there appears to be regression in maturity of movements for short periods. This often occurs at times of transition, when the child is attempting to adapt a movement to new contexts – for example throwing a ball from a stationary position versus doing this while running. These findings are consistent with the dynamic systems approach to motor learning, as there is an emphasis on the nature of the task and context.

Summary

This final section of the chapter revealed that although screening tests exist for assessment of motor skills, they are not routinely used except in the case of children with identified motor dysfunction or for those at high risk of motor developmental delay. Parental report is a typical mechanism in identifying abnormalities in motor developmental delay or dysfunction. The expense of widespread use of developmental screening and the uncertain reliability of some tests means that assessment of motor development tends to be restricted to children with recognized neuromotor problems. Finally, it was argued that there is a need to review the range and nature of current motor developmental assessment tools in keeping with changes in motor development theory.

Review Questions

1. Map the broad sequence of events of neuronal development that occur prenatally and immediately postnatally.
2. Map the broad sequence of events that occur in the development of muscle fibres prenatally.
3. What further changes occur in muscle fibres postnatally, and how does experience affect these?
4. Identify and define the two forms of ossification by which bones are formed.
5. Briefly outline the process of bone growth and development postnatally until the end of adolescence.
6. Why do movements become more flexible and less reliant on environmental cues after six months of age?
7. What are 'experience expectant' and 'experience dependent' learning and why are these processes helpful in understanding individual differences in early motor development?

8. What is the evidence for benefits of tactile stimulation for neuromotor functioning in childhood and for which groups of children?

Further Reading

Brown, JK, Omar, T and O'Regan, M (1997) Brain development and the development of tone and movement. In K J Connoly and H Forssberg (eds), *Neurophysiology and Neuropsychology of Motor Development. Clinics in Developmental Medicine*, no. 143/144, pp. 319–45. These authors provide a thorough review of the embryological development of the nervous system.

Thelen, E (1996) Chapter 2. Motor development: A new synthesis. *Annual Progress in Child Psychiatry and Child Development*. New York: Bunner/Mazel. This chapter is also available from American Psychologist, 1995, 50(2), 79–95, from which it is a reprint. Thelen, one of the leaders of developmental research in the dynamic systems tradition, provides an overview of dynamic systems theory, shows how this relates to development of motor skills, their stability and change, and points to some challenges for research. Towards the end of the chapter, neuronal group selection theory is explained simply, and discussed as a plausible neural mechanism for the acquisition of perceptual-motor skills.

Guyton, AC and Hall, JE (1996) *Textbook of Medical Physiology*. Philadelphia: W.B. Saunders Company. The following chapters are particularly useful: Chapter 54: Motor Function of the Spinal Cord: The Cord Reflexes; Chapter 55: Cortical and Brainstem Control of Motor Function; and Chapter 56: The Cerebellum, Basal Ganglia and Overall Motor Control. The book is easy to understand and terms are defined. Unlike many anatomy and physiology textbooks, the authors organize the content from the perspective of function and then relate it to structure, rather than the other way around. This means that the chapters are organized into sections such as 'supporting the body against gravity' and 'maintaining equilibrium', relating these to the structure and function of parts of the nervous system involved. This is helpful when reading this from a practice perspective. The authors also make reference to dysfunction to facilitate understanding of normal anatomy and physiology.

Gallahue, DL and Ozmun, JC (1995) *Understanding Motor Development: Infants, Children, Adolescents and Adults* (3rd edn). Madison: WCB Brown and Benchmark Publishers. This book was written for students as an introduction to motor development across the life span. In addition to material that is very specific to motor development, it also includes content on general growth and development of children and some psychological aspects of development related to physical activity. It includes chapters on areas referred to in this chapter, such as infant reflexes and stereotypies, and motor assessment.

Haywood, KM and Getchell, N (2001) *Life Span Motor Development* (3rd edn). Champaign, IL: Human Kinetics. This simply written book provides an overview of a range of aspects of motor development through the life span, rather than an in-depth review of these areas. It includes an introduction to growth, the development of different aspects of motor function and constraints on motor-development.

Nowakaowski, RS and Hayes, NL (2002) Principles of CNS Development. In MH Johnson, Y Munakata and RO Gilmore, *Brain Development and Cognition: A Reader* (2nd edn). Oxford: Blackwell Publishing Ltd. The recommended chapter provides a succinct overview of CNS development. Although some of the language is quite technical, terms are defined clearly.

References

Adams, JA (1971) A closed-loop theory of motor learning. *Journal of Motor Behavior*, 3, 111–49.

Barnard, K and Bee, H (1983) The impact of temporally patterned stimulation on the development of preterm infants. *Child Development*, Oct., 54(5), 1156–67.

Bartlett, D (1997) Primitive reflexes and early motor development. *Journal of Developmental and Behavioral Pediatrics*, June, 18(3), 151–7.

Bayley, N (1935) The development of motor abilities during the first three years. *Society for Research in Child Development Monographs*, 1(1), 1–26.

Bayley, N (1969) *The Bayley Scales of Infant Development*. Copyright © by the Psychological Corporation.

Beery, KE (1989) *The VMI: Developmental Test of Visual-Motor Integration* (3rd revision). Cleveland, OH: Modem Curriculum Press.

Behrman, RE and Kliegman, RM (eds) (1992) *Nelson Essentials of Pediatrics* (2nd edn). Philadelphia: W.B. Saunders Co.

Bernstein, N (1967) *The Co-ordination and Regulation of Movements*. Oxford: Pergamon Press.

Beuret, LJ (1985) American Institute for Neurophysiological Psychology. In S Goddard (1990) A developmental basis for learning difficulties and language disorders. *INNP Monograph Series 1*. Chester: Institute for Neurophysiological Psychology. Paper presented at the 2nd European conference of Neurodevelopmental Delay in Children with Specific Learning Difficulties, held in Chester on 2nd, 3rd and 4th March 1990.

Blasco, PA (1994) Primitive reflexes: Their contribution to the early detection of cerebral palsy. *Clinical Pediatrics*, 33, 388–97.

Bobath, K (1980) A Neurophysiological Basis for the Treatment of Cerebral Palsy (2nd edn). *Clinics in Developmental Medicine*, 75, 77–87.

Brazelton, TB (1973) *Neonatal Behavioral Assessment Scale. Clinics in Developmental Medicine* no. 50. Spastics International Medical Publications. London: William Heinemann Medical Books Ltd.

Brown, JK, Omar, T and O'Regan, M (1997) Brain development and the development of tone and movement. In KJ Connoly and H Forssberg (eds), *Neurophysiology and Neuropsychology of Motor Development. Clinics in Developmental Medicine*, 143/144, 319–45.

Capute, AJ, Accardo, PJ, Vining, EPG, Robenstein, JE and Harryman, S (1978) *Primitive Reflex Profile*. Baltimore: University Park Press.

Clark, DL, Cordero, L, Goss, KC and Manos, D (1989) Effects of rocking on neuromuscular development in the premature. *Biology of the Neonate*, Dec., 56(6), 306–14.

Davis, SL, Farssberg, H, Lennerstrand, G and Ygge, J (1996) Motar Systems. In PD Gluckman and MA Heymann (eds) *Pediatric Perinatology. The Scientific Basis* (2nd edn) London: Edward Arnold.

de Roiste, A and Bushnell, IWR (1996) Tactile stimulation: Short and long-term benefits for pre-term infants. *British Journal of Developmental Psychology*, March 14(1), 41–53.

deVries, JIP, Visser, GHA and Prechtl, HFR (1982) The emergence of fetal behavior 1: Qualitative aspects. *Early Human Development*, 7, 301–22. In JK Brown, T Omar and M O'Regan (1997) Brain development and the development of tone and movement. In KJ Connoly and H Forssberg (eds) *Neurophysiology and Neuropsychology of Motor Development, Clinics in Developmental Medicine*, 143/144, 319–45.

deVries, MW (1999) Babies, brains and culture: optimizing neurodevelopment on the savanna. *Acta Paediatrica*, Supplement 429: 43–8.

Draeger, A, Weeds, AG and Fitzsimons, RB (1987) Primary, secondary and tertiatry myotubes in developing skeletal muscle: A new approach to the analysis of human myogenesis. *Journal of the Neurological Sciences*, 81, 19–43. In AJ McComas (1996) *Skeletal Muscle: Form and Function*. Champaign, IL: Human Kinetics.

Edelman, GM (1978) Group selection and phasic reentrant signalling; A theory of higher brain function. In GM Edelman and VB Mountcastle (1978) (eds), *The Mindful Brain: Cortical Organisation and the Group-Selective Theory of Higher Brain Function*. Cambridge: MIT Press.

Eriksson, BO (1972) Physical training, oxygen supply and muscle metabolism in 11–13 year old boys. *Acta Physiol. Scand. (Suppl.)*, 384. In RM Malina (1986) Growth of muscle tissue and muscle mass (Chapter 4). In F Faulkner and JM Tanner (1986) (eds), *Human Growth: A Comprehensive Treatise* (2nd edn), vol 2, *Postnatal Growth and Neurobiology*. New York: Plenum Press.

Field, TM, Schanberg, SM, Scafidi, F, Bauer, CR, Vega-Lahr, N, Garcia, R, Nystrom, J and Kuhn, CM (1986) Tactile/kinesthetic stimulation effects on preterm neonates. *Pediatrics*, 77(5), May, 654–9.

Fiorentino, MA (1973) *Reflex Testing Methods for Evaluating CNS Development* (2nd edn). Springfield, IL: Charles C. Thomas. In V Mathiowetz and JB Haugen (1994) Motor behavior research: Implications for therapeutic approaches to central nervous system dysfunction. *The American Journal of Occupational Therapy*, 48(8), 733–45.

Gessell, A (1928) *Infancy and Human Growth*. New York: Macmillan.

Gluckman, P and Heymann, M (1996) *Paediatric and perinatology: The Scientific Basis*. London: Arnold.

Goddard, S (1990) A developmental basis for learning difficulties and language disorders. *INNP Monograph Series 1*. Chester: Institute for Neurophysiological Psychology. Paper presented at the 2nd European Conference of Neurodevelopmental Delay in Children with Specific Learning Difficulties, held in Chester on 2nd, 3rd and 4th March 1990.

Greenough, WT, Black, JE, Wallace, CS (1987) Experience and brain development. *Child Development*, 58, 539–59.

Grillner, S (1975) Locomotion in vertebrates: Central mechanisms and reflex interaction. *Physiological Review*, 55, 247–304.

Henderson, SE and Sugden, DA (1992) *Movement Assessment Battery for Children.* London: The Psychological Corporation, Harcourt Brace Jovanovich.

Hooker, D (1952) *The Prenatal Origin of Behavior.* Lawrence, KA: University of Kansas Press. In JK Brown, T Omar and M O'Regan, M (1997) Brain development and the development of tone and movement. In KJ Connoly and H Forssberg (eds), *Neurophysiology and Neuropsychology of Motor Development. Clinics in Developmental Medicine.* 143/144, pp. 319–45.

Hubel, DH and Wiesel, TN (1974) Sequence regularity and geometry of orientation columns in the monkey striate cortex. *Journal of Comparative Neurology,* 158, 267–94.

Humphrey, T (1964) Some correlations between the appearance of human fetal reflexes and the development of the nervous system. *Progress in Brain Research,* 4, 93–135.

Jongmans, M, Mercuri, E, deVries, L, Dubowitz, L and Henderson, SE (1997) Minor neurological signs and perceptual-motor difficulties in prematurely born children. *Archives of Disease in Childhood,* 76, F9–F14.

Keele, SW (1982) Learning and control of coordinated motor patterns: The programming perspective. In JAS Kelso *Human Motor Behavior: An Introduction.* Hillsdale, NJ: Lawrence Erlbaum.

Kelso, JAS (1982) *Human Motor Behavior: An Introduction.* Hillsdale, NJ: Lawrence Erlbaum.

Koniak-Griffin, D, Ludington-Hoe, S and Verzemnieks, I (1994) Longitudinal effects of unimodal and multimodal stimulation on development and interaction of healthy infants. *Research in Nursing and Health,* Feb., 18(1), 27–38.

Linkous, LW and Stutts, RM (1990) Passive tactile stimulation effects on the muscle tone of hypotonic, developmentally delayed young children. *Perceptual and Motor Skills,* 7, 951–4.

Lundberg, A, Eriksson, BO and Mallgren, G (1979a) Metabolic substrates, muscle fibre composition and fibre size in late walking and normal children. *European Journal of Pediatrics,* 130, 79. In RM Malina (1986) Chapter 4. Growth of muscle tissue and muscle mass. In F Faulkner and JM Tanner (eds) (1986) *Human Growth: A Comprehensive Treatise* (2nd edn), vol 2, Postnatal Growth and Neurobiology, New York: Plenum Press.

Lundberg, A, Eriksson, BO and Jansson, G (1979b) Muscle abnormalities in coeliac disease: Studies on gross motor development and muscle fibre composition, size and metabolic substrates. *European Journal of Pediatrics,* 130, 93. In RM Malina (1986) Chapter 4. Growth of muscle tissue and muscle mass. In F Faulkner and JM Tanner (1986) (eds) *Human Growth: A Comprehensive Treatise* (2nd edn), vol 2, *Postnatal Growth and Neurobiology,* New York: Plenum Press.

McComas, AJ (1996) *Skeletal Muscle: Form and Function.* Champaign, IL: Human Kinetics.

Malina, RM (1986) Chapter 4. Growth of muscle tissue and muscle mass. In F Faulkner and JM Tanner (eds) (1986) *Human Growth: A Comprehensive Treatise* (2nd edn.) vol 2, *Postnatal Growth and Neurobiology,* New York: Plenum Press.

Malina, RM and Bouchard, C (1991) Chapter 11. Motor development during infancy and childhood. In: *Growth, Maturation and Physical Activity.* Champaign, IL: Human Kinetics Publications Inc.

Marquis, PJ, Ruiz, NA, Lundy, MS and Dillard, RG (1984) Retention of primitive reflexes and delayed motor development in very low birth weight infants. *Journal of Developmental and Behavioral Pediatrics,* Jun., 5(3), 124–6.

Mathiowetz, V and Haugen, JB (1994) Motor behavior research: Implications for therapeutic approaches to central nervous system dysfunction. *The American Journal of Occupational Therapy*, 48(8), 733–45.

Mountcastle, VB (1967) The problems of sensing and the neural coding of sensory events. In GC Quarton, T Melnechuk and FO Schmitt (eds), *The Neurosciences: A Study Program*, New York: The Rockerfeller University Press, pp. 393–408. In GM Edelman and VB Mountcastle (eds) (1978) *The Mindful Brain: Cortical Organisation and the Group -Selective Theory of Higher Brain Function.* Cambridge: MIT Press.

Pimentel, ED (1996) The disappearing reflex: A reevaluation of its role in normal and abnormal development. *Physical and Occupational Therapy in Pediatrics*, 16(4), 19–41.

Preyer, W (1885) *Specielle Physiologie des Embryo.* Leipzig: Grieben's Verlag. In JK Brown, T Omar and M O'Regan (1997) Brain development and the development of tone and movement. In KJ Connoly and H Forssberg (eds), *Neurophysiology and Neuropsychology of Motor Development. Clinics in Developmental Medicine.* 143/144, pp. 319–45.

Roche, AF (1983) Chapter 2. Bone growth and maturation. In F Faulkner and JM Tanner (eds) (1986) *Human Growth: A Comprehensive Treatise* (2nd edn), vol 2, *Postnatal Growth and Neurobiology*, New York: Plenum Press.

Sinclair, D and Dangerfield, P (1998) *Human Growth after Birth.* Oxford: Oxford University Press.

Smith, CUM (1989) *Elements of Molecular Neurobiology.* New York: John Wiley & Sons.

Sporns, O and Edelman GM (1993) Solving Bernstein's problem: A proposal for the development of movement by selection. *Child Development*, 64, 960–81.

Thelen, E (1979) Rhythmical stereotypies in normal human infants. *Animal Behaviour*, 27, 699–715.

Thelen, E and Cooke, DW (1987) Relationship between newborn stepping and later walking: A new interpretation. *Developmental Medicine and Child Neurology*, Jun., 29(3), 380–93.

Touwen, BCL (1979) Examination of the child with minor neurological dysfunction. *Clinics in Developmental Medicine*, 71, London: William Heinemann Medical Books.

Turvey, MT. Fitch, HL and Tuller, B (1982) The Bernstein perspective I: The problems of degrees of freedom and context-conditioned variability. In JAS Kelso (ed), *Human Motor Behavior: An Introduction.* Hillsdale, NJ: Lawrence Erlbaum.

Ulrich, BD (1997) Dynamic systems theory and skill development in infants and children in neurophysiology and neuropsychology of motor development. In JK Connoly and H Forssberg (eds), *Neurophysiology and Neuropsychology of Motor Development. Clinics in Developmental Medicine.* 143/144, pp. 319–45.

Yakovlev, PI and Lecours, AR (1967) The myelogenetic cycles of regional maturation of the brain. In A Minowski (ed), *Regional Development of the Brain in Early Life.* Philadelphia: FA Davis.

Zelazo, NA, Zelazo, PR, Cohen, KM and Zelazo PD (1993) Specificity of practice effects on elementary neuromotor patterns. *Developmental Psychology*, 29(4), 686–91.

CHAPTER 5

The Respiratory System in Infancy and Early Childhood

Ah-Fong Hoo

Contents

- Development of the Respiratory System
- Assessment and Monitoring of Respiratory function
- Review Questions
- Further Reading
- References

Learning Outcomes

At the end of this chapter you will be able to:

- Describe the characteristics and function of the respiratory system.
- Outline the normal growth and development of this system during postnatal life and early childhood.
- Discuss how the cyclical rhythm of respiration is generated and relate this phenomenon to changes in intrapleural pressure.
- Describe the gas exchange process in the lungs and how respiratory disorders may affect this function.
- Compare the major differences in terms of respiratory physiology in a young child with that in an adolescent or adult.
- Describe how the differences between the respiratory physiology of the young child and an adolescent or adult may predispose the young child to respiratory illnesses.
- Describe the process of evaluating a child's respiratory status, taking into account the normal function of the respiratory system.

Introduction

In its simplest form, breathing can be thought of as the automated and rhythmic mechanism by which air passes through the lungs to allow the acquisition of oxygen (O_2) and the removal of carbon dioxide (CO_2) and other gaseous waste products from the venous blood. The contraction and relaxation of the skeletal muscles of the abdomen, rib cage and diaphragm enable gases to move in and out of the pulmonary terminal air sacs (alveoli) via the branching airway system. Respiration, which includes breathing, is the overall process by which body cells utilize O_2, produce CO_2 and exchange these gases between the blood circulation and the atmosphere.

Although the lungs have several important functions, including the synthesis of complex compounds such as pulmonary surfactant and other proteins (eg, building collagen and elastin to form the structural framework of the lung), their principle function, however, is gas exchange by diffusion (that is, gas molecules moving from an area of high to another of low tension or partial pressure). For this process to occur efficiently, the lungs must be supplied with adequate quantities of air (ventilation) matched appropriately in proportion with pulmonary circulation (perfusion) to optimize exchange of gases. The rate and depth of breathing, according to the body requirements, must also be carefully regulated by the respiratory control centre.

In this chapter the early development of the respiratory system is explored. The implications of developmental characteristics of the system at significant stages for the health of the child are identified, followed by an overview of the assessment of the respiratory system in the infant and young child. However, to set this development in context a brief overview is first provided into the basics of respiratory anatomy and physiology, including, where known some of the characteristic differences in the infant and young child.

Development of the Respiratory System

Introduction

The production of energy by tissue cells requires a continuous supply of oxygen (O_2) for various metabolic reactions. As a result of these reactions, cells also release quantities of carbon dioxide (CO_2) which must be eliminated rapidly and efficiently, since an excess of CO_2 produces acid conditions that are harmful to cells. The two systems that supply O_2 and CO_2 are the circulatory and respiratory systems. The circulatory system transports the gases in the blood between the cells and the lungs. The respiratory system consists of the nose, pharynx, larynx, trachea, bronchi and lungs. The term upper respiratory tract refers to the nose, throat and associated structures, whereas the lower respiratory tract refers to the remainder of the branching system.

Respiration is the overall exchange of gases between the atmosphere, blood and cells. This is accomplished by a well-coordinated interaction of the lungs with the respiratory oscillator (formed by a group of respiratory neurons which drives the respiratory muscles), the diaphragm, chest wall musculature, and the circulatory system.

Principal Function of the Lung

The lung is designed to provide an adequate supply of inspired air and pulmonary blood flow to allow O_2 and CO_2 exchange between the alveolar gas and pulmonary capillaries. In humans, the basic processes involved are: pulmonary ventilation (or breathing) which constitutes inspiration (inflow) and expiration (outflow) of air between the atmosphere and the lungs, and the exchange of gases within the body. The gas exchange between the lungs and blood is referred to as external respiration, and that between the blood and the cells is known as internal respiration.

Prenatal Lung Development

Structure and development history of the lung

Lung growth and development occurs mostly during fetal life, a time when the lung is not required to fulfil its extra-uterine function, since the placenta is the site for gas exchange for the fetus. Although the pattern of growth may be genetically determined (Hislop, 1995), several intra-uterine environmental factors have been recognized as important modulating influences, such as the volume of fetal lung liquid, its rate of secretion and absorption (Walters, 1994). The fetal lungs are sustained in an expanded state by lung fluid which is continuously secreted by the alveolar cells. The pattern of fetal breathing movements with respect to changes in thoracic dimensions (ie, the degree of stretch) during development is an important determinant of its growth and structural maturation (Harding, 1994).

 In the presence of oligohydramnious (reduced amniotic fluid volume), for example in Potter's syndrome, fetal lung growth and development are retarded. A congenital diaphragmatic hernia occurs due to the failure of the tissues, from which the diaphragm develops, to fuse during the embryonic period, and commonly allows part of the bowel to herniate through the left pleuroperitoneal canal into the thoracic cavity. Babies born with this condition have hypoplastic lungs, in which airway and/or alveolar numbers are reduced depending on the time of the onset of the insult. This condition could produce an acute emergency *at birth* as the lungs may not expand adequately.

Other factors such as maternal smoking and nutrition during pregnancy, low birthweight for gestational age and factors associated with premature

delivery, are likely to have adverse effects on not only *fetal* lung development, they may also be associated with the increased risk of respiratory
morbidity and mortality during *infancy, childhood* and *late life* (Aubard
and Magne, 2000; Barker, 1994; Barker *et al.*, 1991; Brooke *et al.*, 1989;
Chan *et al.*, 1989; Collins *et al.*, 1985; Dezateux *et al.*, 2001; Haglund
and Cnattingius, 1990; Hoo *et al.*, 1998; Lum *et al.*, 2001; Wadsworth and
Kuh, 1997).

Box 5.1   Factors Affecting Early Lung Development

- Volume of lung liquid *in utero*
- Maternal smoking during pregnancy
- Maternal nutrition during pregnancy
- Low birth weight for gestational age
- Premature delivery

Development stages

Human fetal lung development is a complex process which continues for the
first 3 years following birth (Burri, 1994; Hislop, 1995). During the *embryonic
period (0–7 weeks' gestation)*, the lung begins as a simple ventral diverticulum
from the primitive foregut at approximately *4 weeks' gestation*. The lining of
the whole respiratory system derives from this endodermal bud. As it separates
from the foregut, the bud continues to grow in and develops into a midline
tubular structure forming the trachea and two lateral lung buds. This process
usually completes by *28 days*. The lung buds continue to grow and penetrate
the surrounding mesoderm in a caudolateral direction. Following the embryonic period, four overlapping stages of lung development have been described
based on the appearance of the lung tissue (Jeffery and Hislop 1995). The
timing of the stages varies between individuals and species.

Pseudoglandular phase (6–17 weeks gestation)

Further branching of the duct system establishes the conducting portion of
the respiratory airway (the pre-acinus) from the trachea up to the level of the
terminal bronchioles. The most rapid phase of branching is from the *tenth to
fourteenth weeks of gestation*. From about *10 weeks gestation*, cartilage plates
appear in the trachea; smooth muscle cells become present in the trachea and
lobar bronchi; and epithelial lining cells differentiate into ciliated and goblet
cells. During this stage, the future airways are narrow with little lumens, and
by the *sixteenth week*, all the pre-acinus airway branching is complete (Hislop,
1995). These branches may increase in size with subsequent lung growth but
no further new branches are formed.

Canalicular phase (16–26 weeks gestation)

This period involves maturation of the airways and the extensive angiogenisis within the thinning mesenchyme, which surrounds the more distal sections of the fetal respiratory system, to form a dense vascular network. The diameter of the airways increases and the peripheral airways continue to divide forming prospective respiratory bronchioles and alveolar ducts. Proliferations of the capillaries become closely associated with, and gradually protrude into, the airway epithelium, in particular with the respiratory bronchioles and alveolar ducts. The lungs are thus being prepared for their future role in gas exchange. By the *twenty-fourth week of gestation*, the cartilage and submucosal glands extend as far down the airway as the adult level.

Saccular/alveolar phase (24 weeks–term gestation)

The terminal bronchioles undergo further differentiation into respiratory bronchioles and alveolar ducts, which then give off subdivisions or alveolar saccules. These saccules appear as shallow indentations in the walls of the distal air spaces at around *weeks 28 and 29*. Each of the distal respiratory portions of the lung (respiratory unit or acinus) comprises a single terminal bronchiole and its subsequent divisions of respiratory bronchioles, alveolar ducts and saccules. Two epithelial cell types are present in the saccular alveolar walls: a) pneumocyte type I, a very thin squamous cell type, covers more than 95 per cent of the alveolar surface and functions in gas exchange; b) the larger and rounded pneumocyte type II cells function to secrete low levels of pulmonary surfactant. With advancing gestation, the pneumocyte type I cells become thinner and flatten out to increase the epithelial surface area by dilation of the saccules, giving rise to immature alveoli. The distribution of the arterial and venous blood vessels continue to divide into numerous smaller vessels, which follow closely the distribution of the branching bronchial tree ending with the capillaries protruding into the alveolar spaces. By *26 weeks gestation*, a functional though inefficient blood/gas barrier has formed. Maturation of the alveoli continues by further enlargement of the terminal sacs and deposition of elastin. The appearance of fully mature alveoli begins approximately at *36 weeks* and by *term gestation*, between 50 and 150 million alveoli are reported to be present (Dunnill, 1962; Hislop *et al.*, 1986; Seatta and Turato, 1999).

Box 5.2   Timing of Key Stages in Prenatal Lung Development

- *4 weeks gestation*: Lung development begins and the tubular structure forming the trachea and two lateral lung buds is usually complete by 28 days, often before pregnancy is confirmed.
- *6–17 weeks gestation*: The pseudoglandular phase, when the duct system branches to form the conducting airways. Cartilage plates

appear in the trachea and smooth muscle cells in the trachea and lobar bronchi from about 10 weeks' gestation.

- *16–26 weeks gestation*: The canalicular phase, when the vascular network begins to form and the peripheral airways divide producing respiratory bronchioles and alveola ducts. A functional, albeit inefficient, blood/gas barrier is formed by around 26 weeks gestation.
- *24 weeks to term gestation*: The saccular/alveolar phase, when terminal bronchioles differentiate into respiratory bronchioles and alveolar ducts, which then develop subdivisions or alveolar saccules at around weeks 28–29.
- *36 weeks gestation*: Fully mature alveoli appear.

The Structure and Function of the Respiratory System

The lung and the thoracic cavity

The lungs are conical in shape and made of highly elastic, spongy tissue. They are two in number, each placed on either side within the thorax, and are separated from each other by the heart and the contents of the mediastinum (see Figure 5.1). They are attached to the thoracic cage by serous membranes called the pleurae; the visceral pleura covers the outer surface of each lung and is continuous with the parietal pleura that is closely attached to the inner surface of the thoracic cage, including that of the diaphragm, which forms the floor of the thoracic cavity. These membranes are separated by a thin (almost virtual) layer of pleural fluid so that each lung is enclosed within its own fluid-filled, double-walled sac. There is no communication between the intrapleural fluid surrounding each of the lungs. The left lung is divided into two lobes by an interlobular fissure, whereas the right lung is divided into three lobes by two interlobular fissures.

Intrapleural pressure

The pleural fluid seal prevents the lung from separating from the thorax. A negative pressure, relative to that of the atmosphere, is created inside the intrapleural 'space' by the opposing pulling forces resulting from the natural tendency of the thorax to spring out (outward recoil) and that of the lung to collapse (inward recoil). Intrapleural pressure is sometimes referred to as intrathoracic pressure since it is transmitted to all structures in the thorax including the heart. This negative pressure facilitates venous return by exerting a slight 'sucking' force, and is the driving force for 'pulling' air into the lung. During exercise, this force is increased since deeper breathing is accompanied by greater negative intrathoracic pressure.

Venous return may be impaired in some patients during mechanical ventilation as a result of the applied positive pressure which is transmitted not only down the airways but also around all the thoracic blood vessels.

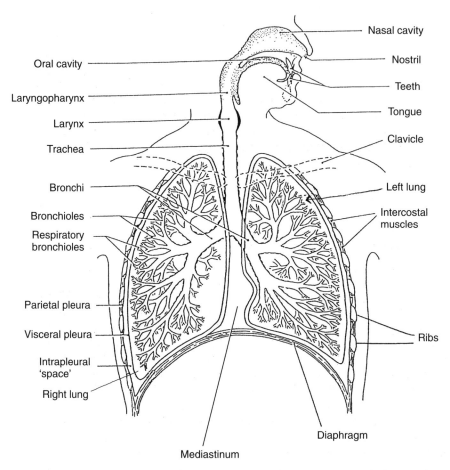

Figure 5.1   Anatomy of an Adult Respiratory System

Source: Adapted from Hinchliffe and Montague (1988).

Inspiration and expiration

During inspiration, the dome-shaped diaphragm provides the dominant muscle force. When the diaphragm contracts during inspiration, it flattens and presses down on the abdominal contents, lifting the rib cage forward and outward, therefore expanding the thoracic cage and lungs, both from top to bottom and from front to back (see Figure 5.2). Since the air in the lungs now occupies a larger volume, the alveolar pressure falls temporarily below that of the atmosphere, causing air to be drawn into the lungs by bulk flow until alveolar pressure again equals atmospheric pressure at the end of inspiration. By contrast, intrapleural pressure becomes increasingly more negative throughout inspiration, partly due to the increase in the elastic recoil of the lung and partly due to the fall in alveolar pressure. During quiet breathing, expiration

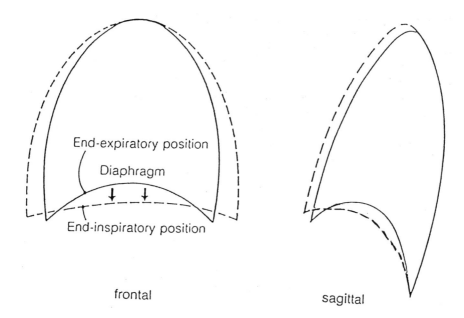

Figure 5.2　Diaphragmatic Movement During Respiration (Frontal and Sagittal Views)

Note: The piston-like movements of the adult diaphragm during ventilation are depicted by the broken (inspiration) and solid (expiration) lines. During inspiration, the diaphragm contracts and flattens, forcing the abdominal contents downwards and lifting the rib cage, thereby increasing the thoracic volume. At the end of expiration, the diaphragm and rib cage resume their resting position.

is a passive process requiring no active muscle contraction. At end-expiration, the respiratory muscles relax allowing the elastic lung and thorax to recoil to their original resting volume (functional residual capacity). The decreased volume compresses the air in the lungs such that alveolar pressure temporarily exceeds atmospheric, providing the necessary driving force to expel air out of the lungs. Expiratory flow ends when alveolar pressure again equals that of atmospheric pressure. During expiration, intrapleural pressure becomes progressively less negative. This is partly due to the increasing reduction in elastic recoil of the lung as it returns to its resting position and partly due to the positive pressure during expiration.

Gas exchange

For gas exchange to occur in the lungs or tissues, gases have to cross the cellular membranes. The pulmonary artery, which brings venous blood to the lungs for gas exchange, branches and subdivides into millions of thin-walled capillaries, forming a dense network of blood vessels covering each alveolus. The small blood vessels continue to multiply in the *initial 18 months of life*, with preferential growth of single-layered capillary network areas up to *3 years of age*, roughly parallel with alveolar multiplication and growth. Terminal respiratory (gas exchanging) unit consists of structures distal to the terminal bronchioles such as the respiratory bronchiole, alveolar ducts and alveoli. This unit is known as an acinus and has thin enough surface to allow rapid diffusion of gases. The extremely thin surfaces are known as the pulmonary, or alveolar-capillary, membranes. Travelling through the network of capillaries covering the alveoli, blood is brought into close proximity with the alveolar air, enabling gas diffusion to occur. The subdivision of the lungs into millions of alveoli vastly increases the surface area available for diffusion.

Diffusion of gases

In a gas mixture, each gas exerts its own pressure as if it were completely filling any available volume. The total pressure of a gas mixture is the sum of all the individual (or partial) pressures (Dalton's law of partial pressures). Bulk flow can only occur in the presence of a difference in total pressure between two areas. However, in the absence of a total pressure gradient, net movement of individual gases in a gas mixture (as in air) can occur by diffusion, as long as a partial pressure gradient for that particular gas exists. In the lungs and at cellular level, a perpetual partial pressure gradient for O_2 and CO_2 is maintained because of the continual renewal of alveolar gas during ventilation, and the constant consumption of O_2 and production of CO_2 by the tissue cells. This enables passive gas diffusion to occur, with O_2 diffusing into the blood for transportation to the tissue and CO_2 diffusing out of the blood into the air to be expelled during expiration.

The upper respiratory tract

The nasal cavity, pharynx, larynx, trachea and bronchi are collectively known as the conducting airways. As they do not participate in gas exchange, their portion of each breath is wasted. This is known as the anatomical dead space which, in an adult, has a volume of approximately 150 ml. The conducting airways have an important role in protecting delicate respiratory tissues in the alveoli. As air enters the upper respiratory tract, it is filtered, warmed and moistened by the mucus membranes in the nose and/or the mouth before passing through the trachea into the lungs.

The nasal cavity is relatively large and divided by a septum. Ciliated epithelium lines the cavity which ensures that air is warmed, filtered and moistened as it passes through the nose.

When a tracheostomy or endo-tracheal tube is introduced, the inspired air bypasses the nose and consequently the lower respiratory mucosa becomes dry. The ciliary activity rapidly ceases which predisposes to infection. It is therefore important to ensure that inspired gases are moistened using a humidifier when an artificial airway is in place.

The pharynx (throat) is a common passage for air and food and a resonating chamber for speech sounds. It starts from the internal nasal passages and extends to the level of the cricoid cartilage (see Figure 5.3). Its wall is composed of skeletal muscles and lined with mucous membrane. The nasopharynx (uppermost portion of the pharynx) has two openings from the internal nasal passages and two from the Eustachian (auditory) tubes. The pharyngeal tonsil (adenoid) is situated on the posterior wall. The oropharynx (middle portion of the pharynx) has the palatine and lingual tonsils. The laryngopharynx (lower portion of the pharynx) becomes continuous with the oesophagus posteriorly, through which food passes into the stomach; and the larynx anteriorly, through which air flows down to the trachea, bronchi, bronchioles and alveoli.

The larynx (or the voice box; see Figures 5.3 and 5.4) is lined with mucous membrane that is continuous with that of the pharynx and trachea. It is supported by pieces of cartilage, connected by ligaments and moved by various muscles, and has elastic vocal cords which function in sound production. The space between the vocal cords, through which air passes, is known as the glottis. The thyroid cartilage or the Adam's apple (which is more prominent following puberty in men than in women) gives the larynx its triangular shape.

The epiglottis is a leaf-shaped elastic cartilage lying above the larynx (see Figure 5.3) with one end attached to the thyroid cartilage. During the act of swallowing, it closes over the glottis so that food and liquids are routed into the oesophagus and not the respiratory tract. When anything else apart from air enters the larynx, the cough reflex is elicited to expel it.

The lower respiratory tract

The trachea: At birth, the trachea (windpipe) is funnel-shaped with the upper end wider than the lower end (Merkus *et al.*, 1996). It becomes cylindrical with increasing age and approximately 10 to 12 cm long and 2.5 cm in diameter in an adult (see Figures 5.1 and 5.3). The trachea is lined with ciliated epithelium which filters and warms inspired air. It consists of smooth muscle, elastic connective tissue and incomplete rings of cartilage shaped like a series of letter C's. The cartilages are held together by fibrous tissue and trachaelis muscle and provide rigidity to the trachea preventing it from collapsing and obstructing the flow of air during inspiration, when airway pressure becomes negative. As the open part of the of the C-shaped cartilages faces the oesophagus, the latter can expand into the trachea during swallowing.

Should the trachea become obstructed, a tracheostomy may be performed. Intubation is another method of opening air passages, in which a tube is passed into the mouth, down through the larynx and the trachea.

A child with tracheobronchomalacia, a condition due to softening or degeneration of the airway walls, is liable to stridor (noise on inspiration) due to airway obstruction.

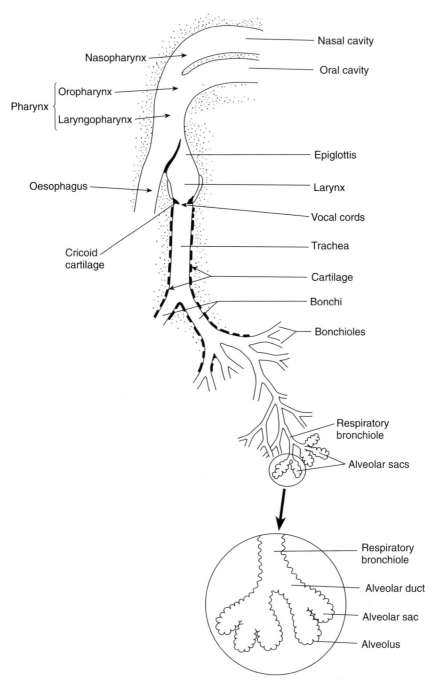

Figure 5.3   Structure and Divisions of the Airways

Source: Reprinted from *Physiology for Nursing Practice*, Hinchliffe S., *et al.*, copyright 1887, with permission from Elsevier.

a   b

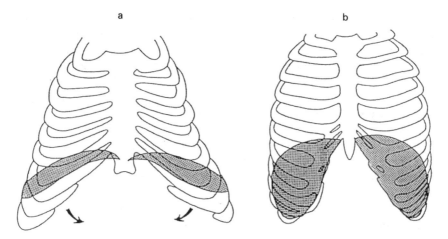

Figure 5.4 Schematic Diagram Illustrating the Differences in the Configuration of the Rib Cage and Diaphragm from Birth (a) to Adulthood (b)

Source: Professor Hugo Devlieger from his thesis, 'The Chest Wall in the Preterm Infant' copyright 1987.

The cricoid cartilage (see Figure 5.3) is the ring of cartilage forming the inferior portion of the larynx and is attached to the first ring of the tracheal cartilage. The trachea, lined with ciliated epithelium which protects against dust, bifurcates at its inferior end into the right and left primary bronchi. At the bifurcation is a sensitive cartilaginous ridge known as the carina, which represents a receptor for the cough reflex. Particles falling on the carina initiate a forceful expulsion as part of a cough. In *infants*, the trachea extends from the larynx to the level of the fourth thoracic vertebra (Ellis *et al.*, 1994).

The shorter trachea and symmetrical carinal angles, in *infants under 6 months* of age, readily allow foreign bodies to enter either primary bronchus, in contrast to preferentially entering the more vertical right primary bronchus as is the case in older children and adults (Mok, 1999).

The primary bronchi enter the right and left lungs at the hilum (recess on the medial surfaces where vessels enter the lungs). The right main bronchus divides into the right upper, middle and lower bronchi to supply the three lobes of the right lung, while the left main bronchus divides into the left upper and lower lobe bronchi (see Figure 5.1). Each lobar (or secondary) bronchus further subdivides into segmental (or tertiary) divisions. The lower airways, down to the smallest divisions supported by cartilage, are known as bronchi which divide into bronchioles (see Figures 5.1 and 5.3). This entire branching structure from the trachea is commonly referred to as the bronchiole tree.

The bronchi are lined by a pseudostratified columnar epithelium which rests on spiral bands of smooth muscle. Among many other cell types within the epithelium, there are a large number of cells with cilia, whose rhythmic beating in a thin liquid layer propels the surface film of mucus and inhaled particles effectively out of the lung through the trachea and upper respiratory tract. The diameter and length of the bronchi decrease progressively with each successive branching (generation) but the sum of the cross-sectional areas of the two dividing bronchi is greater than that of the previous generation. Their cartilage support gradually disappears, such that the cartilage no longer exists in airways less than 2 mm in diameter, which are usually referred to as bronchioles.

The bronchioles have a simple cuboidal epithelium. An important functional difference exists between the bronchioles and bronchi: that is, the bronchioles are embedded directly into the connective tissues of the lung so that their diameter depends on lung volume. For example, when the lung is fully inflated, the pulmonary distending pressure 'pulls and widens' the calibre of these small airways. The reverse happens when the lung is deflated. In older children and adults, collateral ventilation (movement of gas from one acinus to another) occurs through inter-alveolar openings (pores of Kohn) and channels between bronchioles and adjacent alveoli (canals of Lambert) to bypass an obstructed airway. However, although these structures may be found in the infant lung, they are probably not sufficiently large to allow air passage (Wohl, 1998).

Infants and younger children, in contrast to older individuals, are unlikely to ventilate beyond obstructed bronchioles or respiratory units, making them more vulnerable to atelectasis (blocked alveoli which fill with fluid or collapse), hyperinflation associated with infection and ventilation/perfusion mismatching.

Up to *5 years* of age, the peripheral conductance is relatively low with peripheral airway resistance approximately four times greater than that of the older child/adult (Hogg, 1970). Together with the late development of channels of collateral ventilation, this probably explains the high incidence of lower obstructive airway disease in young children.

From the trachea, there are approximately 8–13 divisions to the smallest bronchi, with a further 3–4 divisions of the bronchioles before reaching the terminal bronchioles. Each terminal bronchiole may contain up to 50 respiratory bronchioles which are lined with thin respiratory epithelium across which gas exchange can occur (see Figure 5.3). Similar to those of the larger airways, the walls of the bronchioles consist of smooth muscle, but unlike the trachea and bronchi, the bronchioles do not have cartilage in their walls to maintain rigidity.

The alveoli: Branching off the terminal respiratory bronchioles are fine alveolar ducts lined with squamous epithelium (see Figure 5.3). As the epithelial lining of the airways approaches the alveolar ducts, it becomes progressively less ciliated. Alveoli are hollow cup-shaped thin walled structures which open into the terminus of the alveoli ducts. Three types of cells are found in the alveolar epithelium, namely thin squamous epithelial cells covering most of the alveolar surface; large (type II) cuboidal epithelial cells, which are responsible for epithelial cell renewal and synthesis of surfactant (a phospholipid which reduces surface tension forces in the lung preventing alveolar collapse) and alveolar macrophages which are active phagocytic cells. Since there are no ciliated or mucus-producing cells in the alveolar epithelium, these macrophages are the principle defence mechanism against any bacteria or debris that enters the alveoli, by engulfing and removing them – mainly in the sputum.

In the *newborn* human lung, the number of alveoli has been estimated at approximately 50–150 million at birth, with an alveolar surface area of around 4 m² (Dunnill, 1962; Hislop *et al.*, 1986; Saetta and Turato, 1999). The average diameter of an alveolus at *2 months* of age is 150–180 μm as compared to 250–300 μm in an adult (Dunnill, 1962).

The smaller alveolar size in infants predisposes them to alveolar collapse.

The process of alveolization (production of new alveoli) starts *in utero* but occurs predominantly after birth particularly during the first *18 months to 3 years* of life. During this period, small blood vessels continue to multiply and there is a preferential growth of single-layered capillary network and remodelling of the parenchymal septa. Thereafter, all components grow proportionately until adulthood. Up to *3 years* of life, lung size increases due to alveolar multiplication, there being little change in alveolar size. The adult equivalent of about 300–400 million alveoli is reached by approximately *3-4 years* of age (Hislop *et al.*, 1986; Jeffery and Hislop, 1995), thereafter, the alveoli continue to increase in size and number up to *7 years* of age. From *8 years*, the alveoli increase in size only until the adult lung volume of approximately 3000 ml and surface area of 75 m² are reached in adolescence when the chest wall stops growing. The large expansion in alveolar number and size, hence alveolar surface area, from *birth to 8 years* of age increases the diffusing capacity of oxygen and other gases across the alveolar–capillary membrane.

Until *5 years* of age, the distal airway growth lags behind that of the proximal airways, leading to relatively higher peripheral (small) airway resistance in *infants and young children*.

The smaller diameter of the peripheral airways (<2mm) renders *infants and young children* more prone to intrathoracic or lower airway obstruction in the presence of inflammation and oedema, resulting in an increase in hyperinflation and the work of breathing (Saetta and Turato, 1999).

In contrast, as mentioned previously, mature anatomical collateral ventilatory channels in older children and adults enable ventilation distal to an obstructed airway by collateral 'flow'.

Surfactant

Pulmonary surfactant, a highly surface active substance, is synthesized by alveolar epithelial (pneumocyte) type II cells and composed of approximately 80 per cent phospholipids, 10 per cent proteins and 10 per cent neutral lipids. Surfactant production begins from about *22–24 weeks gestation* but it is not secreted in mature concentrations until about *32–34 weeks' gestation*.

Surface tension is a force that exists at the interface between fluid and air, where the force of attraction between molecules is not equal. The greatest force is in a downward and horizontal direction which contracts the surface area. In the alveoli where such an interface is present, in the absence of surfactant, the net effect is to pull the alveolar walls in towards each other, leading to alveolar collapse, resulting in areas of atelectasis. Consequently, greater effort has to be exerted by the infant in order to expand the lungs with each inspiration. This rapidly leads to exhaustion. By contrast, in the presence of surfactant, the surface tension in the lungs is reduced thereby promoting alveolar expansion and preventing their complete collapse on expiration. In addition, surfactant is also present in small airways and promotes their patency (Enhorning *et al.*, 1995).

 Respiratory distress syndrome (RDS, or hyaline membrane disease) is a condition associated with a deficiency in surfactant and occurs primarily in premature babies. Prevention of neonatal RDS may be achieved by administering antenatal glucocorticoids, which stimulates production of (fetal) surfactant, to women at risk of preterm delivery, and prophylactic treatment with surfactant soon after delivery to infants at risk of developing RDS (Kirkpatrick and Mueller, 1998; Robertson, 1993).

Box 5.3   Surfactant

Reduces surface tension in the alveoli preventing collapse on expiration.

* *22–24 weeks gestation*: production begins.
* *32–34 weeks gestation*: mature concentrations present.

Premature babies may develop respiratory distress syndrome due to surfactant insufficiency.

Postnatal Respiratory Development

Major differences exist between the infant and adult respiratory systems. The lung is only partially formed *at birth* and postnatal lung growth is characterized by multiplication of alveoli, maturation and enlargement of lung structures. Under *6 months of age*, infants are obligatory nose breathers and rarely breathe through their mouths except when crying (or in the presence of a nasal obstruction). This is because the tongue is positioned wholly within the mouth, obstructing air flow through the mouth unless it is opened wide as it is when crying. In later development, the tongue becomes a partially pharyngeal organ reducing the bulk within the mouth. As infants have relatively narrow nasal passages, and since even a small reduction in the lumen of the nasal passage will significantly increase respiratory resistance, and hence the work of breathing, it is important therefore to keep their nasal passages clear.

For example, when nasal gastric tube feeding is required, an appropriate size tube should be selected so as not to obstruct the whole nostril, thereby avoid- ing possible consequence of an increase in the work of breathing and fatigue.

At *birth* and during *early infancy*, the chest wall is highly compliant (floppy), since the ribs are more cartilaginous and therefore less rigid than they will be when fully ossified. As a result of this, the chest wall and lungs have reduced outward recoil, resulting in a relatively low resting lung volume in young infants. In addition, the high level of compliance within the tracheo-bronchial tree is likely to put the infant at risk of dynamic airway compression.

This contributes to the rapid deterioration in infants and young children with acute airway obstruction. To counteract the possible risk associated with a low lung volume, young infants often adopt the strategy of using both their larynx and post-inspiratory diaphragmatic activity to modulate (or brake) expiratory flow in an attempt to prolong expiratory time in order to maintain an adequate resting lung volume (Kosch and Stark, 1984; Stark *et al.*, 1987). This maybe heard as soft *grunting* – the sound created by the opening of the glottis. This results in a dynamically elevated resting lung volume which is above that which would be passively determined by the balance between the outward recoil of the chest wall and inward recoil of the lung. This process enables an adequate lung volume to be sustained, which in turn optimizes gas exchange.

Total resistance to airflow is high at *birth* but decreases rapidly as breathing is established. In a *term* infant, lung volume doubles by *6 months* and triples by *1 year*, and lung compliance shows a similar increase, following the general pattern of growth for the body as a whole. Transition to a more relaxed breathing pattern occurs between *6–12 months* of age with the adoption from a predominantly supine to an upright posture (Papastamelos *et al.*, 1995).

At birth, the ribs are relatively horizontal at rest thus reducing the potential contribution of the rib cage in relation to increasing the thoracic cavity cross-sectionally during tidal breathing (Openshaw *et al.*, 1984). Young infants, therefore, are predominantly diaphragmatic breathers. This is seen in the greater movement of the abdomen than the chest with each breath, as the contracting diaphragm displaces abdominal contents downwards.

Some types of apnoea alarm are designed to detect abdominal, rather than chest, movement in young infants, with the sensor placed on the abdomen.

However, the configuration of the ribs changes significantly when young children adopt the upright position which alters the forces acting on the ribcage. The action of gravity on the ribs, as well as the pull of the muscles inserted on the ribs, causes the ribs to slope caudally. This leads to relative lengthening of the thoracic cavity and the ribcage begins to acquire the ovoid adult pattern (Openshaw *et al.*, 1984). The chest wall gradually stiffens while undergoing ossification and changes in its shape during the first *2 years* of life (Papastamelos *et al.*, 1995).

The diaphragm is dome-shaped in *older children and adults*, in contrast to the relatively flattened shape in *young infants* (see Figure 5.4). During inspiration, the contraction of the flattened diaphragm (which has a larger radius) generates less pressure, resulting in less expansion of the lungs. Together with the floppy chest wall that may further predispose to inward movement (retraction) of the rib cage during inspiration, the mechanical efficiency of the respiratory system is compromised. Both normal preterm and newborn term infants have been observed to exhibit a degree of asynchronous chest wall and abdominal movements during active (rapid eye movement) sleep.

Asynchrony is also seen in infants with wheezy illness and those with acute upper airway obstruction.

Young infants have reduced high oxidative skeletal muscle fibres which are liable to fatigue more easily, thus any extra load to the respiratory muscle will potentially increase the risk of developing respiratory fatigue or failure.

Box 5.4   Timing of Postnatal Lung Development

Upper respiratory tract:

- *Up to 6 months of age* infants are obligatory nose breathers, except when crying. It should be noted that prolonged crying is exhausting for the baby.

Thoracic cavity:

- *In early infancy* the ribs are still partly cartilaginous contributing to a highly compliant chest wall, reducing outward recoil and a low lung volume. Acute airway obstruction may lead to rapid deterioration.
- Ribs are more horizontal *at birth*, consequently *young infants* are diaphragmatic breathers, observed in abdominal movements with each breath.
- Ribs change in shape during the first *2 years* of life.
- Diaphragm is flatter in shape in *infancy* compared to the dome shape of adults.

All of which increase vulnerability to retractions of the rib cage during inspiration when respiratory function is compromised.

Lung growth:

- Lung volumes double by *6 months* and treble by *1 year* of age, resulting in corresponding increases in absolute lung compliance.
- Up to *3 years* of age, the capillary network continues to develop and

the number of alveoli increases. The latter largely being responsible for the increase in lung size.

- From *3 to 7 years* of age, alveoli increase in size and number. Up to *5 years* of age, peripheral conductance is relatively low with resistance being approximately four times greater than that of adults.
- From *8 years* of age to adulthood, alveoli increase in size only. Resistance is now equivalent to adults.

Control of Breathing (Respiratory Cycles)

Nerve impulses pass from the respiratory control centre in the medulla of the brain, down the phrenic and intercostal nerves to the diaphragm and intercostal muscles, respectively, in a cyclical fashion forming the basic rhythm of respiration. Cyclical excitation of these respiratory muscles causes alternate expansion and relaxation of the chest wall and diaphragm, which in turn results in air being drawn into (inspiration) and expelled from (expiration) the lungs (for further details, see section on 'Inspiration and expiration'). Normal respirations of *newborn* and *young infants* are irregular and abdominal, with a relatively rapid rate. Resting respiratory rate is higher in children due to their relatively higher metabolic rate and oxygen consumption, and gradually reduces with age to the adult level (see Table 5.1). Breathing pattern may be observed by watching the abdominal movements associated with respiratory cycles. Apnoea is the absence of breathing for more than 15 seconds (Wong, 1999). Periods of apnoea lasting less than 15 seconds are commonly observed particularly in those born premature.

The respiratory pattern of infants who are at increased risk of developing prolonged episodes of apnoea (>15 seconds) may be monitored by using apnoea sensors, which are attached to the abdomen to detect absence of breathing movements.

Table 5.1 Normal Ranges for Respiratory Rates

Age	Respiratory rate (breaths/min)
Newborn	30–40
<12 months	25–35
1–5 years	20–30
5–12 years	20–25
>12 years	15–25
Adult	15–20

Source: Modified from Chaudry and Harvey (2001).

Vulnerability to Respiratory Infections

The newborn infant is immunologically incompetent, and as such is dependent on the immunity provided by maternal antibodies (mainly of the IgG type), which crossed the placenta in the last trimester of pregnancy. The level of maternal antibodies against infections progressively declines during the *first 6 months* of life, and since the infant's own antibody production is slow to mature, s/he is therefore more vulnerable to serious infections. As such, *infants* and *young children* who are breastfed continue to acquire maternal antibodies via the breast milk and are thus better protected against infections (Cushing *et al.*, 1998; Howie *et al.*, 1990), while those who are bottlefed (Watkins *et al.*, 1979), and those exposed to environmental tobacco smoke are more susceptible to respiratory infections (Couriel, 1994; Harsten *et al.*, 1990). Other environmental factors that increase the likelihood of acquiring respiratory infections include attendance at childcare facilities, siblings of school age, lower social class and overcrowded living conditions (Segedin, 1999).

Box 5.5   Factors that Increase the Risk of Respiratory Infection

- Bottle/formula feeding in infancy
- Exposure to tobacco smoke
- Attendance at child care facilities
- School aged siblings
- Lower socioeconomic status
- Overcrowded living conditions
- Immaturity of the respiratory system under 7–8 years of age.

Effect of Premature Delivery on Airway Development

In premature lungs, a relative increase of bronchial smooth muscle, an increased proportion of submucosal glands, and more viscous mucus have been observed. These changes are exaggerated in *preterm infants* who require mechanical ventilation (Hislop and Haworth, 1989). The increased incidence of respiratory expression of diseases in infants born prematurely is in part related to the altered structure and size of the airways. Furthermore, these infants tend to have fewer alveoli and an increase amount of interstitial collagen and elastin in their lung tissue (Cherukupalli *et al.*, 1996). Throughout childhood, the lungs of children who had been ventilated during the neonatal period have fewer alveoli and reduced surface area than expected for lung volume. Diminished lung and airway function has been observed in *infants* (Hjalmarson and Sandberg, 2002) and *young children* (Baraldi *et al.*, 1997) and in *school age children* (Coates *et al.*, 1997; Galdes-Sebaldt *et al.*, 1989; Gross *et al.*, 1998) of *preterm birth,* irrespective of whether they had experienced respiratory distress syndrome in the neonatal period, suggesting damaged or altered airway development due to factors associated with prematurity and/or mechanical ventilation.

Conclusion

Respiration is essential for life, yet it is a complex system that develops only gradually during infancy and early childhood. The majority of the lung and airway development has been accomplished by the age of around *seven to eight years* of age when all the alveoli have formed. Further development reflects an increase in size of alveoli and system as a whole, rather than an increase in number of the structures involved. Consequently vulnerability to respiratory disease is greater in early childhood.

Respiratory disorders constitute a high proportion of childhood illnesses, particularly in the *birth to five year* age group. Such illnesses account for the largest proportion of general practice consultations and a significant proportion of childhood admissions to hospital. Therefore it is important for those caring for children to have an understanding of the development of the respiratory system in early childhood and the assessment of respiratory function in this age group. The preceding section of this chapter has provided an overview of the development of the respiratory system, including some indicators of possible sources of respiratory difficulty. The following section explores assessment of children's respiratory function.

Assessment and Monitoring of Respiratory Function

Visual and auditory assessment of a child can provide enough information for formulation of a diagnosis and initiation of therapy. A child's level of activity and comfort is both affected by respiratory and non-respiratory conditions. It can be difficult to assess the respiratory status of a child who is extremely anxious or in pain. Respiratory comfort is evaluated by observing the child's body position, respiratory rate and pattern, and work of breathing (see Table 5.2).

Visual assessment of Respiratory Status

It is important to recognize that the assumed position of *infants* in the first year of life is often dependent on caregivers, and may not reflect their preference. Children with respiratory distress independently adopt the position of most comfort, for example, the child with upper airway obstruction will sit forward in the sniffing position. Respiratory rates and patterns in early life

Table 5.2 Assessment of Respiratory Status in Infants and Young Children

Signs and symptoms associated with respiratory infections	Respiratory patterns associated with respiratory infections
Nasal blockage • nasal discharge frequently accompanies respiratory infections; may be thin and watery (rhinorrhea) or thick and purulent • infant's nasal passages are easily blocked by mucosal swelling and exudation, resulting in interference with respiration and feeding. May contribute to development of otitis media and sinusitis *Pyrexia* • may be absent in newborn infants; frequent in young children between *6 months and 3 years*; often appears as first sign of infection; high temperature (39.5 to 40.5°C) may occur with mild infections, and may precede febrile seizures *Sore throat* • a frequent complaint of *older children; young children* are often unable to describe symptoms, even though the throat is highly inflamed; children often refuse to take oral fluids or solids *Loss of appetite* • frequently the initial sign of illness and affects virtually all small children with acute infections; often persists throughout febrile stage of illness and into convalescence	*Respirations* Rate – normal, slow or rapid (tachypnoea) Depth – estimate from amplitude of thoracic and abdomen excursion to determine whether normal depth, shallow (hypopnoea) or too deep (hyperpnoea) Ease – effortless, discomfort in breathing (termed *orthopnoea* when it prevents the child from lying down), flaring nares, head bobbing with inspiration (use of accessory muscles of respiration) Laboured breathing (dyspnoea) – sudden onset, intermittent or continuous; gradually becoming worse, accompanied by wheezing, grunting. In older children: at rest or associated with exercise or pain *Respiration sounds* Hoarseness – from laryngeal inflammation Grunting – due to closure of the glottis to increase pressure in the airways to prevent collapse of bronchioles and alveoli, and to prolong expiratory time to optimize gas exchange process Stridor – noise on inspiration due to upper airway obstruction Wheezing – noise more frequently on expiration due to lower airway obstruction Cough – to clear debris from airways *On auscultation* Wheezing – as above Rhonchi – course rale, a noise produced by air passage through partially obstructed bronchioles Absence of sound – indicates no air entry

Continued on next page

Table 5.2 (Cont.)

Signs and symptoms associated with respiratory infections	Respiratory patterns associated with respiratory infections
Vomiting • present at onset of illness and may persist for several hours; *small children* vomit readily with illness. In *infants*, this may be aggravated by air trapping which depresses the diaphragm thus reducing stomach capacity *Diarrhoea* • often present in association with respiratory illness, particularly viral infections; usually mild and transient but could become severe, causing dehydration	*Other observations* Posture of *older children* – discomfort, restlessness Chest pain in *older children* – may be localised, generalised or referred to base of neck or abdomen or to shoulder tip; its association with inspiration or grunting. Cyanosis – reduced oxygenation of the blood resulting in reduced saturation of haemoglobin. Not always present in *infants*; note distribution: facial or peripheral, degree, duration; may be indirectly manifested through tachypnoea and laboured breathing. Hyperinflation of chest cavity – due to air trapping in small airways. Retractions of soft thoracic tissues – which are drawn in during inspiration (See Figure 5.5). Reduced O_2 saturation (<95%) – due to impaired gaseous exchange. Pulse oximeters measure % oxygen saturation of haemoglobin. *Note: anaemic children may have 100% O_2 saturation but still be in respiratory distress.* Finger clubbing – due to proliferation of tissue in finger tips, lifting the nail base. Associated with prolonged hypoxaemia and/or suggestive of chronic lung disease. Peak Expiratory Flow Rates (PEFR) L/min – The simplest of the lung function tests which can be measured with a peak flow meter in children who are able to reliably coordinate the necessary forced expiration. Usually from 4–5 years of age. Readings are compared to height and individual norms to detect changes in resistance to air flow.

Modified from: Whaley & Wong (1999) and Betz *et al.* (1994).

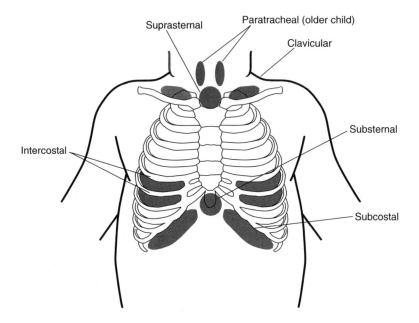

Figure 5.5 Location of Soft Thoracic Tissue Retractions

Source: Reprinted from *Nursing Care of Infants and Children*, Whaley and Wong, copyright 1999, with permission from Elsevier.

change with age and should be assessed with the knowledge of the normal variations (See Table 5.1). Respiratory pauses become less frequent with maturation of the respiratory centre in the brain stem. Tachypnoea (rapid rate) is the most common alteration in breathing and most important clue to respiratory dysfunction (Wohl, 1994). The presence of disease and hypoxia often require the patient to take frequent small breaths to lessen the work of breathing and facilitate gas exchange. Conversely, obstructive upper airway conditions (eg, choanal atresia – a congenital narrowing or blockage of the nasal airway by membranous or bony tissue) require prolonged inspiration and higher pressures which result in indrawing, or retractions, of soft thoracic tissues. Lower airway obstruction (eg, bronchiolitis) is associated with prolonged expiration, and often accompanied by an audible wheeze. Shallow irregular breathing or periodic breathing indicates cerebral dysfunction or drug intoxication.

Increased work of breathing manifests with nasal flaring, grunting, and retractions (intercostal, suprasternal and substernal). This may be accompanied by dyspnoea (laboured respiration) (see Table 5.2). Thoracic retractions, particularly in *infants* and *younger children*, can be extreme because of the compliant nature of the cartilaginous chest wall, which can lead to impaired gas exchange because of ventilation/perfusion mismatch (see Figure 5.5). This condition is also associated with the posture of the child, airway and alveolar structure and the complexity of the control of breathing. Paradoxical, or asynchronous, movement of the chest and abdomen is a sign of chest wall muscular weakness or immaturity, and/or diaphragmatic fatigue. This phenomenon is commonly observed in the *newborn* or *premature infants*. Hyperinflation of the chest indicates lower airway obstructive disease with air trapping or pneumothorax under tension, and may be evident as an increase in the anteroposterior (AP) diameter of the chest. Consequent to a unilateral pneumothorax is the unilateral increase in chest size pertaining to the affected side, which may almost be diagnostic of the condition. A decrease in AP diameter suggests lung hypoplasia, restrictive lung disease or thoracic cage malformation. Thoracic asymmetry is present in children who have asymmetric air entry or exit secondary to a pneumothorax, paralysed diaphragm, bronchial obstruction (in condition such as asthma or cystic fibrosis), lobar collapse or foreign body with air trapping.

Auscultatory Assessment of Respiratory Status

Auscultation is a useful way to assess distribution of ventilation. Breath sounds can be evaluated with and without a stethoscope. The presence or absence of grunting, stridor, wheezing (sound on expiration) or rhonchi (presence of secretion in the peripheral airways) should be noted. The thinner chest wall of a *young child* facilitates easier access to airway sounds but the small dimensions of the chest wall result in referred 'noise' and can hinder localization of abnormalities. In older subjects, cough is present in conditions associated with production of sputum such as bronchitis, whereas in *young children*, cough is consistent with infection and conditions such as aspiration, gastric oesophageal reflux and cystic fibrosis.

Evaluation of Gas Exchange

Gas exchange is routinely monitored with blood gases. Although either arterial or capillary blood gases are the routine method of monitoring, both have the disadvantages of causing distress and discomfort to children. Furthermore, blood gas results provide static rather than continuous monitoring.

The introduction of pulse oximetry has enabled continuous online monitoring of peripheral oxygen saturation (SpO_2) in clinical practice. It is both non-invasive and relatively simple to use. The pulse oximetry sensor, comprising a light emitting diode (LED) and a photodetector, is programmed to detect variations in light transmission and absorption with diastolic and systolic changes in the pulse wave. Once the photometric sensor is placed on the finger, hand, toe or foot, there is no warm-up time and readings can be immediately obtained. Hence oximetry can be used for spot readings as well as continuous monitoring. Accuracy is extremely good at oxygen saturations greater than 60 per cent, below this the readings can be falsely high (O'Rourke, 1992). In general, although a SpO$_2$ level between 95 and 99 per cent denotes haemoglobin being adequately saturated with oxygen, caution is required when monitoring *premature infants* receiving oxygen therapy. This is because oximetry is insensitive to hyperoxia, which potentially is a dangerous situation for the *premature infant* at risk for developing retinopathy of prematurity (retrolental fibroplasia). The main clinical limitations of pulse oximetry are encountered in conditions such as extreme peripheral vasoconstriction, temperature <30C, extreme anaemia (reduced haemoglobin concentration), which reduces the oxygen carrying capacity of the blood, or polycythemia (increase in haemoglobin concentration). Interference from external light or movement of the extremity can be a technical problem. Figure 5.6 shows the relationship between haemoglobin oxygen saturation and partial pressure of oxygen in the blood.

Capnography, or measurement of end tidal CO$_2$ (ETCO$_2$), is a less commonly used method of monitoring the partial tension of CO$_2$ within the blood (P$_{CO2}$) in conscious children. A sampling sensor is placed in the nose, or in the endotracheal tube, to detect CO$_2$ elimination in the form of a graph or curve. An initial upward slope is followed by a plateau, which represents the end tidal P$_{CO2}$ value. The slope of the initial curve can be used to evaluate the pattern of exhalation, providing important information about air movement in the small airways (O'Rourke, 1992).

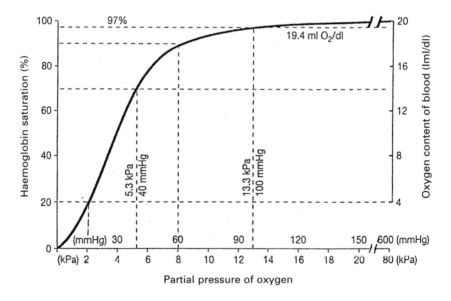

Figure 5.6   Relationship of Haemoglobin Oxygen Saturation to Partial Pressure of Oxygen

Note: The oxygen–haemoglobin dissociation curve (shown by the solid line) is applicable when pH is 7.4, P$_{CO2}$ is 5.3 kPa (40 mmHg) and blood is at 37°C.

Infections of the Lung

Infections occur more frequently in the respiratory tract, in particular the upper airways, than in any other organ. This might not be surprising due to the constant environmental exposure to which the lung is subjected by breathing.

The lung is normally a sterile environment. However, infection occurs when there is alteration in normal host defence mechanisms, diminution in the individual's immune status or when an immunocompetent individual is exposed to a virulent organism that overwhelms the host defences. *Infants* and *children* are more vulnerable to infections since they have a relatively less mature immune system, fewer specific antibodies than adults and a narrower bronchial tree allowing for easier obstruction in the presence of extra secretion, inflammation or oedema of the airways.

Respiratory Tract Disorders During Infancy and Childhood

Although respiratory infections occur more frequently during the autumn and winter months, there is no evidence that low temperatures or 'cold airs' *per se* either promote the spread of viruses or decrease our resistance to them (Herendeen and Szilagy, 2000). Any condition that increases airway resistance, or decreases compliance, results in increased work of breathing (increased respiratory rate, retractions, nasal flaring). If respiratory muscle fatigue develops, respiratory failure may follow. Table 5.3 summarizes some of the common respiratory tract conditions that occur during infancy and childhood.

Conclusion

This chapter has explored the development and assessment of the respiratory system from the antenatal period through to infancy and early childhood. The normal structure and function of the respiratory system has been reviewed, including, where relevant, particular characteristics present during early development, followed by an exploration of pre- and postnatal development. It is clear that there are particular periods of vulnerability to respiratory disease, from the premature baby whose lungs have not fully developed and who may experience long-lasting effects, to the bottle fed baby with an increased incidence of respiratory infections as they do not receive the protection of antibodies in breast milk and the young child who may be exposed to viruses and bacteria to a greater degree during attendance at nursery. In the young child the ability to cope with such infections is also compromised by the developmental stage of the respiratory system. The smaller size of the airways creates a higher peripheral resistance to air flow

Table 5.3 Summary of Common Respiratory Disorders in Infancy and Early Childhood

Respiratory disorders	Characteristics	Causative agents
Rhinitis, pharyngitis/ nasopharyngitis	Common in infants and children; significant cause of nasal inflammation. Rhinorrhoea, pyrexia; older children may also complain of sore throat, earache, cough with phlegm, diarrhoea/ vomiting.	Rhinovirus; parainfluenza viruses, respiratory syncytial virus (RSV), adenovirus, coronaviruses.
Laryngitis	Common in infants and children Pyrexia, hoarseness, loss of voice, acute stridor.	Parainfluenza viruses.
Laryngo-tracheobronchitis ('croup')	Affects children <5 years of age, most commonly aged 6 months to 2 years; more common in boys than girls. Starts as a viral infection, increasingly prominent barking cough, progressive stridor, pyrexia, tachycardia, increasing recession and restlessness, hypoxia.	Viral parainfluenza B.
Epiglottitis	Occurs mostly in children 6 months to 6 years of age, with a peak incidence at 2–3 years. Sore throat, restlessness, hyper-pyrexia, toxicity, rapidly worsening stridor, drooling without a cough, increase difficulty in breathing, hypoxia.	Haemophilus influenzae type b, although becoming rare due to availability of vaccine. In rare cases involving older children and adults: Staphylococcus aureus and pneumococci.
Bronchiolitis	Annual epidemics during late autumn, winter and early spring. Most common during first year of life. Restless and distressed, hyperpyrexia, tachypnoea, hyper-expanded chest, hypoxia, cyanosis may be present. Apnoea may occur in younger infants and the premature.	Mainly caused by RSV, other cases due to parainfluenza viruses, rhinovirus, adenovirus.
Viral pneumonia	Common in infants <6 months old, peak incidence between 2–3 years. Usually occurs in late winter and early spring. Early signs may be non-specific. Pyrexia, tachypnoea, intercostal, subcostal and supra-sternal retractions, nasal flaring and use of accessory muscles.	RSV (in infancy), adenoviruses, parainfluenza virus (older infants and toddlers), influenza B, adenovirus.

Continued on next page

Table 5.3 (*Cont.*)

Respiratory disorders	Characteristics	Causative agents
Bacterial pneumonia	More common in children with underlying chronic illness such as cystic fibrosis or immunological deficiency. In *younger children* – acute illness; pyrexial, looks toxic, wheezing *Older children* often have a cough which may produce purulent sputum, tachypnoea, grunting, nasal flaring and cyanosis, often have referred shoulder tip or abdominal pain.	In the *newborn* – group B streptococci (associated with septic shock), gram negative bacilli (e.g. Klebsiella and Pseudomonas) from the birth canal. In *younger children* – Haemophilus influenza, Streptococcus pneumoniae, Staphylococcus aureus. In *older children and adolescents* – Streptococcus pneumoniae, mycoplasma pneumoniae.
Asthma	Occurs throughout the childhood years. During an asthmatic exacerbation: worsening shortness of breath, cough, wheezing, chest tightness. Airways narrow due to broncho-spasm, mucosal oedema, mucus plugging with air being trapped behind obstructed or narrowed airways. The child hyperinflates his lungs in an attempt to keep airways open and allow gas exchange to take place. Hypoxia may occur during acute episodes because of mismatching of ventilation and perfusion.	Triggers likely to precipitate or aggravate asthmatic exacerbations: allergens such as grasses, spores, pollens or dust mites; irritants include tobacco smoke, sprays and chemicals. Other triggers: cold air, food additives, exercise, colds and infections, pets, strong emotions such as fear; environmental changes eg moving home, starting new school.
Cystic fibrosis	Characterized by the exocrine gland dysfunction; increased viscosity of bronchial mucus causes obstruction in airways, stagnation of mucus favours bacterial colonization resulting in frequent infections, lung tissue destruction, bronchial wall weakness, peribronchial fibrosis and diffused bronchiectasis; atelectasis and emphysema may occur. Impaired gas exchange leads to variable degree of hypoxia and hypercapnia.	Frequently infected by bacteria such as Haemophilus influenza, Staphylococcus aureus, Pseudomonas aeruginosa and Streptococcus pneumoniae.

and is more easily blocked by inflammation and mucous secretions, explaining the increased incidence of lower airway disease in children. All of which highlights the need for accurate assessment of respiratory function in the infant and young child. Much can be learned through a thorough visual assessment, which can be augmented by auscultation, pulse oximetry and, where necessary in the more critically ill child, more invasive assessments such as blood gas analysis. Where chronic respiratory problems are encountered, children may also be referred for lung function tests – a description of which is beyond the scope of this book.

Review Questions

1. What is the sequence of prenatal respiratory development?
2. What factors contribute to the infant's vulnerability to retractions of the rib cage?
3. What advice would you give to new parents to help reduce the risk of respiratory infection in early childhood?
4. How can respiratory function in children be assessed visually?
5. What tools are currently used to assist with the assessment of respiratory function and how do these work?

Further Reading

Hinchliff, S, Montague, SE and Watson, R (eds) (1996) *Physiology for Nursing Practice*, 2nd edn. London: Baillière Tindall. A good basic anatomy and physiology book which provides many links to clinical practice, although not specifically for children.

Prasad, SA and Hussey, J (eds) (1995) *Paediatric Respiratory Care – A Guide for Physiotherapists and Health Professionals*. London: Chapman and Hall. Written by physiotherapists, clinicians and radiologists, this book provides useful information on development and physiology of children's respiratory system, assessment of respiratory function, paediatric chest imaging, and the care and management of children with respiratory disease.

Silverman, M (ed.) (1995) *Childhood Asthma and Other Wheezing Disorders*. London: Chapman and Hall Medical. For readers who would like to read more about respiratory disorders in childhood.

Hughes, JMB and Pride, NB (eds) (1999) *Lung Function Tests: Physiological Principles and Clinical Applications*. London: WB Saunders. For further information on the assessment of respiratory function.

West, JB (1995) *Respiratory Physiology – The Essentials*, 5th edn. Baltimore: William and Wilkins.

West, JB (1998) *Pulmonary Pathophysiology*, 6th edn. Baltimore, Williams and Wilkins. The above two books provide more detailed accounts of the physiology and patho-physiology of the respiratory system.

References

Aubard, Y and Magne, I (2000) Carbon monoxide poisoning in pregnancy. *BJOG*, 107(7), 833–8.

Baraldi, E, Filippone, M, Trevisanuto, D, Zanardo, V and Zacchello, F (1997) Pulmonary function until two years of life in infants with bronchopulmonary dysplasia. *Am J Respir Crit Care Med*, 155, 149–55.

Barker, DJP, Godfrey, KM, Fall, C, Osmond, C, Winter, PD and Shaheen, SO (1991) Relation of birth weight and childhood respiratory infection to adult lung function and death from chronic obstructive airways disease. *BMJ*, 303, 671–5.

Barker, DJP (1994) The undernourished baby. In *Mothers, Babies and Disease in Later Life*, pp. 121–39. London: BMJ Publishing Group.

Betz, CL, Hunsberger, M and Wright, S (1994) *Family-Centered Nursing Care of Children*, 2nd edn. Philadelphia: WB Saunders.

Brooke, OG, Anderson, HR, Bland, JM, Peacock JL, Stewart, CM (1989) Effects on birth weight of smoking, alcohol, caffeine, socioeconomic factors, and psychosocial stress. *BMJ*, 298, 795–801.

Burri, PH (1994) Structural development of the lung in the fetus and neonate. In MA Hanson, JAD Spencer, CH Rodeck and D Walters (eds), *Fetus and Neonate: Physiology and Clinical Applications; vol 2: Breathing*, pp. 3–19. Cambridge: Cambridge University Press.

Chan, KN, Noble-Jamieson, CM, Elliman, A, Bryan, EM, Silverman, M (1989) Lung function in children of low birthweight. *Arch Dis Child*, 64, 1284–93.

Chaudhry, B and Harvey, D (2001) *Mosby's Colour Atlas and Text of Paediatrics and Child Health*. London: Mosby Inc.

Cherukupalli, K, Larson, JE, Rotschild, A and Thurlbeck, WM (1996) Biochemical, clinical and morphologic studies on lungs of infants with bronchopulmonary dysplasia. *Pediatr Pulmonol*, 22, 215–29.

Coates, AL, Bergsteinsson, H, Desmond, K, Outerbridge, EW, Beaudry, PH (1977) Long-term pulmonary sequelae of premature birth with and without idiopathic respiratory distress syndrome. *J Pediatr*, 90, 611–16.

Collins, MH, Moessinger, AC and Kleinerman, J (1985) Fetal lung hypoplasia associated with maternal smoking: a morphometric analysis. *Pediatr Res*, 19, 408–412.

Couriel, JM (1994) Passive smoking and the health of children. *Paed Resp Med*, 1, 12–16.

Cushing, AH, Samet, JM, Lambert, WE, Skipper, BJ, Hunt, WC, Young, SA *et al.* (1998) Breastfeeding reduces risk of respiratory illness in infants. *Am J Epidemiol*, 147(9), 863–70.

Dezateux, C, Stocks, J, Wade, AM, Dundas, I, Fletcher, ME (2001) Airway function at one year: Association with premorbid airway function, wheezing and maternal smoking. *Thorax*, 56, 680–6.

Dunnill, MS (1962) Postnatal growth of the lung. *Thorax*, 17, 329–33.

Ellis, H, Logan, BM, Dixon, AK (eds) (1994) *Human Sectional Anatomy*, p. 106. London: Arnold.

Enhorning, G, Duffy, LC and Welliver, RC (1995) Pulmonary surfactant maintains patency of conducting airways in the rat. *Am J Respir Crit Care Med*, 151, 554–6.

Galdes-Sebaldt, M, Sheller, JR, Grogaard, J and Stahlman, M (1989) Prematurity is associated with abnormal airway function in childhood. *Pediatr Pulmonol*, 7, 259–64.

Gross, SJ, Iannuzzi, DM, Kveselis, DA and Anbar, RD (1998) Effect of preterm birth on pulmonary function at school age: a prospective controlled study. *J Pediatr*, 133(2), 188–92.

Haglund, B, Cnattingius, S (1990) Cigarette smoking as a risk factor for Sudden Infant Death Syndrome: A population based study. *Am J Public Health*, 80, 29–32.

Harding, R (1994) Fetal breathing: Relation to postnatal breathing and lung development. In MA Hanson, JAD Spencer, CH Rodeck and D Walters (eds), *Fetus and Neonate: Physiology and Clinical Applications; vol 2: Breathing*, pp. 63–84. Cambridge: Cambridge University Press.

Harsten, G, Prellner, K, Heldrup, J, Kalm, O and Kornfalt, R (1990) Acute respiratory tract infections in children. A three-year follow-up from birth. *Acta Paediatr Scand*, 79, 402–9.

Herendeen, NE and Szilagy, PG (2000) Infections of the upper respiratory tract. In RE Behrman, RM Kliegman and HB Jenson (eds), *Nelson Text Book of Pediatrics*, pp. 1261–6. Philadelphia: W.B. Saunders Company.

Hislop, AA (1995) Developmental anatomy and cell biology. In M Silverman (ed.), *Childhood Asthma and Other Wheezing Disorders*, pp. 35–54. London: Chapman and Hall Medical.

Hislop, AA and Haworth, SG (1989) Airway size and structure in the normal fetal and infant lung and the effect of premature delivery and artificial ventilation. *Am Rev Resp Dis*, 140, 1717–26.

Hislop, A, Wigglesworth, JS and Desai, R (1986) Alveolar development in the human fetus and infant. *Early Hum Dev*, 13(19), 1–11.

Hjalmarson, O and Sandberg, K (2002) Abnormal lung function in healthy preterm infants. *Am J Respir Crit Care Med*, 165, 83–7.

Hogg, JC, Williams, J, Richardson, JB, MacKlem, PT, Thurlbeck, WM (1970) Age as a factor in the distribution of lower airway conductance and in the pathological anatomy of obstructive lung disease. *N Engl J Med*, 282, 1283–7.

Hoo, A-F, Henschen, M, Dezateux, C, Costeloe, K and Stocks, J (1998) Respiratory function among preterm infants whose mothers smoked during pregnancy. *Am J Respir Crit Care Med*, 158(3), 700–5.

Howie, PW, Forsyth, JS, Ogston, SA, Clark, A and du V Florey, C (1990) Protective effect of breast feeding against infection. *BMJ*, 300, 11–16.

Jeffery, PK and Hislop, AA (1995) Embryology and growth. In RAL Brewis, B Corrin, DM Geddes and GJ Gibson (eds), *Respiratory Medicine: vol 1*, pp. 3–21. London: W.B. Saunders.

Kirkpatrick, BV and Mueller, DG (1998) Respiratory disorder in the newborn. In V Chernick, TF Boat and EL Kendig (eds), *Kendig's Disorders of the Respiratory Tract in Children*, 6th edn, pp. 328–64. Philadelphia: W.B. Saunders.

Kosch, PC and Stark, AR (1984) Dynamic maintenance of end-expiratory lung volume in full-term infants. *J Appl Physiol*, 57, 1126–33.

Lum, S, Hoo, A-F, Dezateux, CA, Goetz, I, Wad, AM, DeRooy, L *et al.* (2001) The association between birthweight, sex and airway function in infants of non-smoking mothers. *Am J Respir Crit Care Med*, 164: 2078–84.

Merkus, PJFM, ten Have-Opbroek, AAW and Quanjer, PH (1996) Human lung growth: A review. *Pediatr Pulmonol*, 21: 383–97.

Mok, Q (1999) Special needs of the critically ill child. In AJ MacNab, DJ MaCrae and R Henning (eds), *Care of the Critically Ill Child*, pp. 6–11. London: Churchill Livingstone.

Openshaw, P, Edwards, S and Helms, P (1984) Changes in rib cage geometry during childhood. *Thorax*, 39, 624–7.

O'Rourke, PP (1992) Assessment and monitoring of respiratory function. In BP Fuhrman and JJ Zimmerman (eds), *Pediatric Critical Care*, pp. 411–23. St Louis: Mosby Inc.

Papastamelos, C, Panitch, HB, England, SE, Allen, JL (1995) Developmental changes in chest wall compliance in infancy and early childhood. *J Appl Physiol*, 78, 179–84.

Robertson B (1993) Corticosteroids and surfactant for prevention of neonatal RDS. *Ann Med*, 25(3), 285–8.

Saetta, M and Turato, G (1999) Lung structure and function. *Eur Respir Mon*, pp. 1–19. ERS Journals Ltd.

Segedin, E (1999) Epidemiology of severe illness in childhood. In AJ MacNab, DJ MaCrae, R Henning (eds) *Care of the Critically Ill Child*, pp. 12–23. London: Churchill Livingstone.

Stark, AR, Cohlan, BA, Waggener, TB, Frantz, IID and Kosch, PC (1987) Regulation of end expiratory lung volume during sleep in premature infants. *J Appl Physiol*, 62 1117–23.

Wadsworth, ME and Kuh, DJ (1997) Childhood influences on adult health: A review of recent work from the British 1946 national birth cohort study, the MRC National Survey of Health and Development. *Paediatr Perinat Epidemiol*, 11(1), 2–20.

Walters, DV (1994) Fetal lung liquid: secretion and absorption. In MA Hanson, JAD Spencer, CH Rodeck and D Walters (eds), *Fetus and Neonate: Physiology and Clinical Applications; vol 2: Breathing*, pp. 42–62. Cambridge: Cambridge University Press.

Watkins, CJ, Leeder, SR and Corkhill, RT (1979) The relationship between breast and bottle feeding and respiratory illness in the first year of life. *J Epidemiol Community Health*, 33: 180–2.

Whaley, LF and Wong, DL (eds) (1999) *Whaley & Wong's Nursing Care of Infants and Children*, 6th edn. St. Louis: Mosby Inc.

Wohl, ME (1994) Manifestations of pulmonary disease. In ME Avery and LR First (eds), *Pediatric Medicine*, pp. 259–72. Baltimore: Williams and Wilkins.

Wohl, ME (1998) Developmental physiology of the respiratory system. In V Chernick, TF Boat and EL Kendig (eds), *Kendig's Disorders of the Respiratory Tract in Children*, 6th edition, p 19–27. Philadelphia: W.B. Saunders.

Wong, DL (1999) The child with problems related to transfer of oxygen and nutrients. In LF Whaley and DL Wong (eds), *Whaley & Wong's Nursing Care of Infants and Children*, 6th edn, pp. 1415–55. St Louis: Mosby Inc.

CHAPTER 6

Internal Transport: Blood and Haemostasis

Alexandra Lewandowska and Dr Craig Smith

Contents

- Reviewing the Basics.
- Development of the Blood
- Prevention and Control of Bleeding
- Assessment of the Function of the Blood in Childhood
- Transfusion
- Chapter Conclusion
- Review Questions
- Further Reading
- References

Learning Outcomes

At the end of the chapter you will be able to:

- Understand of the basic physiology of blood and related tissues.
- Discuss the development of the blood from embryonic life through into childhood.
- Outline the normal function and values of blood at different ages.
- Discuss some of the physiological origins of disease affecting blood.
- Identify some of the more common blood diseases through assessment of the child.

Introduction

Humans are large, successful multi-cellular organisms. Our large genome contains highly evolved or preserved genes coding for a programme of cellular differentiation that allows some groups of cells to develop very specific functions at the expense of losing other functions. Highly differentiated cells are grouped together into organs, and are sited where they may perform their special functions most efficiently. Herein lies the importance of blood. The bloodstream supports this 'multi-organ system of life' and carries individual highly specialized cells and signals to all the other cells in the body.

The aim of this chapter is to provide the reader a basic understanding of the normal physiology of blood, the development of blood from embryological life through to childhood and an insight into some of the processes that lead to disease.

Reviewing the Basics

Before the development of the blood can be explored the functions of blood, the circulation and the constituents of the blood will be reviewed.

The Functions of Blood

The blood provides the body with the means to accomplish a wide range of activities. These include the transport of substances around the body, communication with body cells and organs, the circulation of chemicals and cells which help to protect the body against infection and those which help to maintain haemostasis (see Table 6.1 for further examples).

Table 6.1 The Functions of Blood

Transportation
  Oxygen and nutrients
  Carbon dioxide and waste materials
Communication
  Hormones, cytokines
Infection control
  Leucocytes, immunoglobulins, complement
Haemostasis
  Platelets, clotting factors

The Circulation of Blood

The right heart pumps blood a short distance into the very extensive set of vessels known as the pulmonary circulation, which are intimately adjacent to pulmonary cells, and the air spaces of the outside world. The size and intimacy of the pulmonary vascular bed allows for the rapid unloading of carried carbon dioxide, water and heat and then the acquisition of oxygen. This rapid process is facilitated by the unique properties of red blood cells. Oxygenated blood then returns the same short distance to the left heart, which pumps it via larger vessels to all the organs of the body. Cellular congestion is eased by the elastic properties of the vessels. As blood passes through organs, the liquid component of blood may leave the vessels and enter the space between vessels and cells. The individual cells of organs exchange ions and molecules with the blood along concentration gradients or with the help of specialized transport mechanisms.

The Constituents of Blood

Plasma, the liquid component of the blood, is made up of water, electrolytes and other molecules including proteins of widely differing function. Proteins include albumin, immunoglobulins, hormones, complement, coagulation factors and inflammatory signals. In addition, food components and other chemicals are in solution in plasma or carried bound to transporting proteins. The other component of blood is cellular and includes red cells (erythrocytes), white cells (leucocytes) and platelets (see Table 6.2).

Supporting Tissues

These should be included or considered as part of blood, in the way that stations are part of the railway system (see Figure 6.1). Cellular components develop, enter and leave at these points. These organs continuously support the quality and quantity of circulating blood (see Table 6.3).

Table 6.2   Cellular Components of Blood

Cellular component	Function
Red blood cells	Responsible for oxygen transportation.
Platelets	Membrane-enclosed fragments of cells important for haemostasis.
White blood cells (leucocytes)	A group of cells with different roles in our immune response to real or perceived invasion or damage.

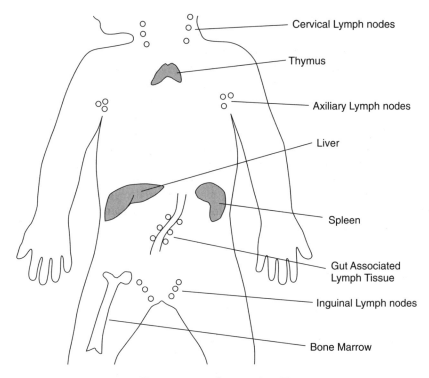

Figure 6.1 Supporting Tissues

Table 6.3 The Functions of Supporting Tissues

Bone marrow
  Red cell, white cell and platelet production
Thymus
  Maturation of lymphocytes
Lymph nodes and lymph vessels
  Infection control
Spleen
  Infection control and red cell turnover
Liver
  Phagocytosis

Development of the Blood

Embryology and Cell Specialization

Shortly after conception and implantation in the uterine wall, groups of cells known as blood islands within the yolk sac begin the path of division and differentiation towards being either blood cells or vascular system cells (Hann *et al.*, 1991). Blood cells are initially pluripotent ie, they retain the potential for varying specialization. However, their descendents become committed to an increasingly specialized form and function. These blood cells are part of the early development of the liver, spleen and bone marrow and make up a significant percentage of these organs at this time. The liver, in particular, is host to the majority of blood cell division and differentiation during the *first two trimesters* of pregnancy. The spleen plays a small part and the bone marrow an increasing one, taking over as the main site in the *last trimester*. The bone marrow in *infancy* and *early childhood* consists mainly of haemopoietic cells (cells from which blood cells are formed), however their relative proportion falls as they are slowly replaced by marrow fat with increasing age. By *late adulthood* only a small part of the available marrow space is required for haemopoiesis. At any time in life, if extra haemopoiesis is required, the marrow spaces again fill with haemopoietic cells. If this isn't sufficient then the liver and spleen can contribute to haemopoiesis again (extramedullary haemopoiesis).

Box 6.1   Sites of Haemopoiesis During Development

- The liver is the site of the majority of blood cell division and differentiation during the *first two trimesters* of pregnancy.
- The bone marrow takes over as the main site in the *last trimester*.
- The amount of bone marrow involved in haemopoiesis falls during childhood as by late adulthood only a small part of the available marrow space is needed for haemopoiesis.
- If extra haemopoiesis is required at any time, more of the marrow can resume its haemopoetic function and may be joined by the liver and the spleen if needed.

The actual content of circulating blood changes *during fetal life* (Hann *et al.*, 1991; Roberts and Murray 2001). Smaller non-nucleated red cells replace primitive, larger nucleated red cells. A rapid rise in their numbers occurs at the end of the *first trimester* and again *at term*. The percentage of blood composed of cells compared to surrounding fluid (packed cell volume) rises from 20 to 60 per cent, with this increase in cell numbers. The amount of haemoglobin in red cells also rises. Granulocytes, eosinophils and basophils (all types of white cell) increase in number. Histiocytes and macrophages (phagocytes) are not seen circulating before the *second trimester*. Megakaryocytes (platelet producing cells) and platelets are seen early on and platelet numbers begin to rise in the *second trimester*. See Table 6.4 for an overview of blood count values from *birth* to the beginning of *adolescence*.

The Production and Maturation of Blood Cells

Haemopoiesis refers to the production and maturation of the cellular components of blood (see Figure 6.2). The main site of haemopoiesis from infancy onwards is the bone marrow. It is a continuous process and proceeds through numerous intermediate stages (Hoffbrand *et al.*, 2001; Pallister, 1999). All of the components of blood are formed from a progenitor cell – a cell that has the ability to mature into any blood cell. These cells lead to pluripotent stem cells. The pluripotent stem cells are the precursors of the main cell lines and

Table 6.4 Normal Full Blood Count Values Through Childhood

Age	Haemoglobin (g/dl)	Haematocrit (packed cell volume)	WBC ($\times 10^9$/L)	Platelets ($\times 10^9$/L)
Birth	15–24	0.47–0.75	10–26	150–400
6 months	10–13	0.30–0.38	6–17	210–560
12 months	10–13	0.30–0.38	6–16	200–550
2–6 years	11–14	0.32–0.40	6–17	210–490
6–12 years	11–15	0.32–0.43	5–15	170–450

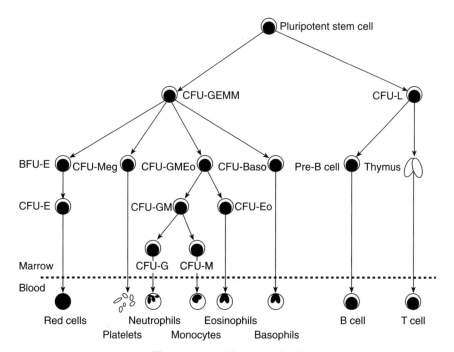

Figure 6.2 Haemopoiesis

are referred to as colony-forming units *(CFU)*. These can either parent the lymphoid line (CFU-L, colony forming unit-lymphoid) or the non-lymphoid line (CFU-GEMM, CFU-granulocyte, erythroid, macrophage, megakaryocyte). Further differentiation leads to unipotential cell lines, capable of producing single cell types.

The Regulation of Haemopoiesis

Each cellular element is continually replaced and the equilibrium of this mechanism is dependent on a complicated system, which is influenced by the life cycle of the cell and ongoing changes in demand for the cell type. Colony-stimulating factors and the interleukins are the two main categories of haematopoietic growth factors responsible for this equilibrium. These glycoproteins act at different sites along the differentiation process. Interleukin 3 (IL-3) and granulocyte-macrophage colony stimulating factor (GM-CSF) for example, together act on the colony forming unit GEMM thus stimulating the production of erythrocytes, basophils, eosinophils, monocytes, neutrophils and platelets. The combination of other interleukins and colony stimulating factors specific to each stage continues throughout differentiation.

Erythropoiesis, the production of red blood cells (Dame and Juul, 2000; Hanspal, 1997; Palis and Segal, 1998; Dame 2000) is mainly controlled by erythropoietin *(EPO)*, a hormone secreted by the kidney. A feedback system monitors the body's demand for oxygen. EPO is synthesized by the kidneys when there is a reduced number of circulating red blood cells, resulting in reduced oxygenation. EPO binds to the committed progenitor cell that will differentiate into forming the mature red cell, thereby stimulating production. The production of platelets is regulated by thrombopoeitin *(TPO)*. TPO is synthesized in the liver or kidneys and can increase the number of megakaryocytes, the maturation process and the subsequent release of platelets. Interestingly platelet production includes the unique process of endomitotic replication, where the parent cell becomes increasingly large and polyploid before platelets are released.

The process of B and T lymphocyte differentiation (major cell groups of the immune system) is regulated by the presence of antigens and inflammatory signals.

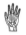

Decreased production of one or more of the haemopoietic lineages can occur. If red cells, white cells and platelets are all involved, the blood film appearance is termed pancytopenia. There are two main types of bone marrow failure (Vlachos and Lipton, 1996); arising from either hereditary (eg, Fanconi's anaemia) or acquired causes such as viral infections, drugs, toxins or immune disorders (eg, acquired aplastic anaemia). The term congenital is used to refer to those presenting early in life from either group. Single cell lines may be affected. If only the red cell line is involved, Diamond–Blackfan anaemia results, appearing in *the first few months of life*. In addition, the marrow may be disturbed by myelodysplastic disorders and leukaemia, which replace normal marrow cells and their production of normal blood cells.

Nutritional Factors and Red Cell Development (Erythropoiesis)

There is a constant requirement for the production of new blood cells. This process requires a constant supply of essential nutrients. Iron, vitamin B_{12} and folate are essential nutritional factors for blood cell production. Deficiency of these factors will produce symptoms and signs in the blood system as well as other body systems. Anaemia is the main consequence in the blood system.

Iron

Iron is essential to all cells. It is so important that we have evolved specific mechanisms for absorption, transportation and recycling. It is used in haem containing compounds such as haemoglobin and myoglobin as well as in important enzymes that are essential to metabolism (eg, the cytochromes). Iron is found in red meat, liver, fish and some green vegetables as either inorganic iron or iron within haem containing compounds ie, myoglobin. Inorganic iron is absorbed more readily as the active ferrous Fe^{2+} ion in the upper small bowel whereas iron within haem compounds is absorbed within the compound. Iron absorption is regulated at the mucosal surface. The mucosal cells contain stored iron (ferritin) in proportion to total body stores, when these are low more iron is absorbed and released into the blood stream. The opposite is true when stores are high. Iron released into the blood stream is picked up by a specific carrier protein, transferin, which transports it to the bone marrow where it is incorporated into haem as part of the production of haemoglobin. Excess iron is stored in the liver, bone marrow and tissue macrophages as ferritin. There is no mechanism for iron excretion.

Therefore, iron overload may occur from over supplementation or from repeated blood blood transfusions. Iron is lost from the body by regular bleeding (eg, menstruation, gastrointestinal bleeding) leading to iron deficiency and then anaemia.

The *fetus* obtains a good iron store from its mother. This occurs predominantly during the *last trimester*. The store at this time is usually 1.5–2.0 times the requirement. However, growth is so rapid in the *first months of life* that the stores are quickly utilized by new cells. Iron is very efficiently absorbed from breastmilk, facilitated by lactoferrin, which binds with two molecules of iron enhancing intestinal absorption. By the age of *6 months* iron from fetal stores and breastmilk is no longer sufficient to meet the infants demands (Department of Health, 1994). It is during this period of rapid growth and a simple weaning diet that dietary intake of iron may be insufficient to maintain a normal haemoglobin. A similar problem can occur during the *pubertal growth spurt*. Absorption can be enhanced by Vitamin C and intake of protein in the same meal or inhibited by phytates in cereals and legumes and tannins in tea and coffee (Department of Health, 1994).

Box 6.2   Factors Influencing Iron Absorption

- Absorption is enhanced by Vitamin C intake in the same meal as iron containing foods.
- Absorption is inhibited by:
  - a) phytates in cereals and legumes; and
  - b) tannins in tea and coffee.

Therefore consumption of fresh fruit and vegetables high in vitamin C should be encouraged from an early stage in weaning, while the drinking of tea and coffee should be discouraged in young children. The latter two drinks have no specific nutritional value to children and may contribute to the development of iron deficiency anaemia. Diets high in fibre from cereals and pulses are not advised in children *under 2 years.*

Source: Department of Health (1994).

The introduction of solids to the breast feeding infant's diet or the use of iron fortified formula milk is usually sufficient to meet the demands of rapid growth.

 Iron deficiency anaemia (Lilleyman *et al.*, 1999, Wharton, 1999) is the commonest nutritional disorder of *early childhood* in the UK (Department of Health, 1994). If non-fortified or low iron food and milk (cow's milk) are used iron deficiency may occur during *the first 2 years of life. Premature babies* have smaller iron stores as they are born before the majority of iron is transferred. They require active iron supplementation for at least the first year. During *the early school years*, growth is less rapid. The finding of iron deficiency is more worrying at this time, as it may represent poor nutrition or chronic blood loss. Causes of blood loss include gastrointestinal bleeding from gastritis (Helicobacter pylori infection), inflammatory bowel disease or a Meckel's diverticulum. In tropical countries, hookworm infestation and schistosomiasis lead to blood loss and iron deficiency anaemia in children.

Vitamin B_{12}

Hydroxocobalamin is the main dietary form of vitamin B_{12}. It is an essential co-enzyme in metabolism. It is found in red meat, liver, kidney and dairy products. It is absorbed across the distal small bowel after binding to intrinsic factor produced by the gastric parietal cells. The number of intrinsic factor receptors in the ileum indirectly determines the amount of vitamin B_{12} that is absorbed. Vitamin B_{12} is transported to the bone marrow attached to transport proteins known as transcobalamines. Developing cells have receptors to bind transcobalamines. The majority of B_{12} is stored in the liver.

Folic acid

The role of the dietary factor folate is similar to vitamin B_{12}. In different molecular forms it also acts as an important co-enzyme to processes essential to cell production and survival. Folates are found in leafy vegetables, eggs and liver. Unlike vitamin B_{12} they are very sensitive to the process of cooking. Folates are absorbed from the upper small bowel and then transferred to the bone marrow. Folate is also stored in the liver, however the reserves are more quickly exhausted than those for vitamin B_{12}. Folate is essential to DNA and RNA synthesis and therefore cell division and survival. The role of folate in this process is dependent upon the presence of vitamin B_{12} as a co-enzyme.

Megaloblastic Anaemia's are less common in *children* and may arise from deficiencies or inborn errors in metabolism of vitamin B_{12} or folate (Lilleyman *et al.*, 1999).

Haem Synthesis

Haem is a porphyrin that is made within the mitochondria of cells and is essential to life. It combines with globin chains to make haemoglobin. The formation of haem begins in the cytoplasm, with the combination of succinyl-CoA and glycine to produce aminolaevulinic acid (ALA). This important first step is catalysed by the enzyme ALA synthetase which is rate limiting to the subsequent steps. Two ALA molecules form a pyrrole. Four pyrrole molecules form a tetra pyrrole molecule. This is stabilized and becomes a porphyrin ring. The final step involves the insertion of a ferrous ion into the protoporphyrin IX molecule. Each of these steps is enzyme controlled.

Deficiencies of the enzymes of haem biosynthesis lead to a group of disorders known as the porphyrias. These arise from an overproduction of haem precursors as the body strives to maintain haem synthesis. Presenting symptoms (skin lesions, acute neurovisceral crises) can help distinguish the type of porphyria. These conditions are rare in *children*.

Red Blood Cells (Erythrocytes)

In health, the bone marrow produces red cells, white cells and platelets. The absolute number of each group varies with age. Red cells are the most numerous of the three cell lines. Their development and specialization within the bone marrow, involves a number of sequential cell divisions, which lead to a reduction in cell size and the loss of all their nuclear material. The number of cell divisions is affected by the adequate presence of vitamin B_{12}, folic acid and iron. While nuclear material is still present, protein synthesis continues, producing haemoglobin and the red cell enzymes. The reticulocyte is the name given to the near mature red cell as it is released from the bone marrow. The highly differentiated cell, which emerges into the circulation, is small and flexible. It contains the proteins and enzymes essential for its unique function. Without nuclear material it has a limited life span of up to 120 days before it is removed from the circulation. The cell membrane defines the shape and flexibility of the red cell. The majority appear as biconcave discs. A greater normal variability of shape is seen in the *neonatal period*. The normal size and shape of red cells allows their safe passage through capillary beds less than half their normal diameter of 8μm. Red cells are often removed from the circulation as they pass through the spleen.

The red cell membrane

Haemoglobin and the red cell enzymes are packaged in a lipid bilayer studded with numerous protein molecules. The membrane allows some small molecule movement across it. The actual constituents of the inner and outer lipid layer can vary during the life of the red cell and can affect their shape. Phospholipids and unesterified cholesterol molecules are the main constituents. Glycolipids are located at the outer layer where they form part of the surface glycoproteins (including the blood group proteins or antigens). The phospholipid content of the inner and outer membrane is similar but varies and includes sphingomyelin, phosphatidyl choline, phosphatidyl serine, phosphatidyl ethanoamine and the phosphinositides.

In some disease states eg,. sickle cell disease, the normal distribution of phospholipids can change and make the outer membrane more likely to stimulate clotting or complement-mediated lysis.

Red cell membrane proteins may function as identifiers, receptors or simply as important structural components. Exposed proteins contribute to the many blood group antigens. Proteins, which cross the outer and inner membrane, may also act as transport channels or contribute to the cytoskeleton and final shape of the cell by binding to internal structural proteins. Spectrin is the main protein of the cytoskeleton and consists of alpha and beta subunits, arranged in different forms. Ankyrin, another structural protein, binds to spectrin and membrane proteins.

Proteins, which act as transport channels are important as they maintain intracellular cation concentrations, which determine water content and cell volume, and therefore cell shape and deformity. Normal red cell deformability is important and enables rapid passage through small vessels. Any process that alters deformability of the red cell can lead to a shortening of red cell survival.

Changes in the red cell membrane which lead to an alteration in size, shape and flexibility of the red cell can lead to a shortened red cell life and a haemolytic anaemia. In hereditary spherocytosis, an autosomal dominant disorder, the proteins of the cytoskeleton or membrane (spectrin, ankyrin and band 3) are deficient or abnormal. This leads to a resorption of membrane but no change in cell volume. The circulating red cells are spherical instead of biconcave. Eventually they become trapped and die in the spleen. Clinical features include jaundice and splenomegaly, in addition to the haemolytic anaemia. Hereditary elliptocytosis is a similar disorder. These membrane changes however do confer a survival advantage against malaria and are common in malarial parts of the world.

Red blood cell antigens are surface proteins. They have the ability to be recognized as foreign and are grouped together in the blood group systems (ABO, Rhesus, Kell etc) based on their variations between people. Some blood groups are more important than others and become relevant clinically when blood from different people is mixed (during a transfusion or a feto-maternal bleed in pregnancy) or if your own immune system recognizes them as foreign (autoimmune disease).

Fifteen percent of the Caucasian population is Rhesus antigen negative. If a Rhesus negative mother carries a Rhesus positive baby she will develop anti-bodies to the Rhesus antigen if it enters her circulation during pregnancy or delivery (Urbaniak and Greiss, 2000). Once exposed, an immune memory for the antigen is available in the event of a second exposure, often during a subsequent pregnancy. IgG antibodies cross the placenta and bind to fetal red cells, triggering their early destruction. Severe anaemia *in utero* may develop leading to cardiac failure, oedema and death (hydrops fetalis). Alternatively, ongoing red cell destruction can lead to haemolytic anaemia and jaundice *after birth*. High levels of unconjugated bilirubin enter the brain and can permanently damage it (kernicterus). Other blood group incompatibilities can also occur. ABO group incompatibility is common. Here the mother raises anti-A or anti-B antibodies to surface antigens. The presence of maternal antibody in the neonatal circulation is detected by the Coomb's test.

Red cell contents

Red cells do not contain nuclear material but they do contain Haemoglobin, enzymes and other chemicals, which are central to red cell function. Haemoglobin is a large protein complex. It consists of two pairs of globin chains. Each globin chain is bound to a haem molecule. The resulting larger molecule has a unique final shape and chemical properties, which allow it to carry out the vital functions of binding and releasing oxygen under different conditions. Haemoglobin has a hydrophobic core and a hydrophilic surface.

The structure of haemoglobin

The primary structure of globin chains: The alpha globin 'gene cluster' on chromosome 16 and the beta globin 'gene cluster' on chromosome 11 code for globin polypeptide chains. A pair from each region is required. Each region codes for *embryonic* and *adult* forms of globin. In addition each region may code for different variations in the final globin chain. As a result nearly 700 haemoglobin variants have been described. The actual amino acid sequence that is coded for is very important. The amino acid residues, which bind haem or form bonds with adjacent globin chains in the final structure, determine the functional success of the molecule. If these essential residue positions are wrong or different, then the final structure and function of the molecule will be different and its relationship with oxygen will change. Variations in non-essential residues can occur without significantly altering function. The 'alpha gene' produces a 141 residue chain and the 'beta gene' produces a 146 residue chain.

The secondary and tertiary structure of a globin chain: Both polypeptide chains contain non-helical and helical segments. The beta chain has eight helical segments designated A to H. The alpha chain is similar but has no D helix. Haem binds to the F helices. The non-helical segments allow bending in the final structure. When the chain bends at the non-helical segments, distant residues become adjacent to each other producing a 3-D spherical structure.

The quaternary structure of globin chains: The relationship between two pairs of globin chains and their bound haem is determined by many different chemical bonds between the four adjacent globin-haem molecules. Each alpha globin has an interface with both beta globin chains. The relationship of the alpha1 and beta2 interface changes when oxygen is bound. The deoxy form (T-form) is tighter and more stable than the oxy-form (R-form) which has fewer bonds. In addition the oxy-form is more able to bind more oxygen. This relationship with oxygen is modified further by chemical changes in the local environment. Together these forces determine the ability of haemoglobin to pick up, hold on to or to give up oxygen. In the lungs it will preferentially bind oxygen whereas this is reversed in the tissues where oxygen is needed. When oxygen is unloaded, the globin interface changes enough to allow 2,3-diphosphoglycerate (2,3-DPG) to bind to haemoglobin. This new temporary state of haemoglobin has a reduced affinity for oxygen making it more likely to give up rather than take up oxygen. This state is preferable while it passes through organs that need oxygen. Acidosis (high hydrogen ion concentration) and high carbon dioxide tension also reduce the affinity of haemoglobin for oxygen. These two chemical states are also more likely in tissues that require more oxygen. The relationship between haemoglobin and oxygen can be represented in the haemoglobin oxygen dissociation curve (see Figure 6.3).

The sigmoid shape of this curve defines the relationship between the arterial oxygen tension and the percentage haemoglobin saturation. In the presence of increased amounts of 2,3-DPG, carbon dioxide or hydrogen ions, haemoglobin is less likely to bind oxygen. Therefore the arterial oxygen tension of the blood has to be higher for the haemoglobin to bind the same

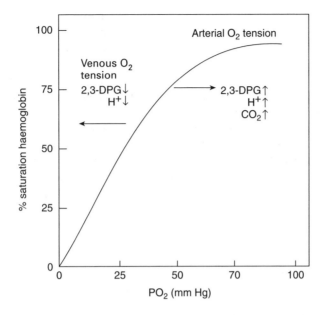

Figure 6.3 The Haemoglobin–Oxygen (O$_2$) Dissociation Curve

amount of oxygen compared to when these three chemicals are at their normal concentrations. The reverse is also true when their levels are lower than normal. Finally oxygen affinity is higher or lower depending upon the presence of a haemoglobin variant. Sickle cell haemoglobin has a lower affinity for oxygen whereas fetal haemoglobin has a high affinity. Fetal haemoglobin does not bind 2,3-DPG.

Variation in the amino acid sequence in globin chains alters the structure and function of haemoglobin (Olivieri, 1997). Some changes in the red cell, including haemoglobin, confer a survival advantage against malaria. This may explain why some of the haemoglobin variants have been preserved in relatively high frequency. For example in sickle cell disease the B-globin chain amino acid sequence is altered by the insertion of a valine residue for a glutamic acid residue. This small change alters the characteristics of the haemoglobin molecule particularly when deoxygenated. The gene for this mutation is found in areas where malaria is common. The heterozygote state produces a mixture of normal and sickle cell type haemoglobin which confers both the normal function of haemoglobin and the survival advantage against malaria. This is known as sickle cell trait. Sickle cell disease occurs when the individual is homozygous for the sickle cell gene or heterozygous for the gene but with the other gene also coding for another different abnormal haemoglobin. The homozygous state (SS disease) is severe. The haemoglobin S molecules change shape on deoxygenation forcing the biconcave red cell to become an elongated sickle shape. This shape is much less flexible and will get stuck in capillary beds leading to its much shorter life span (haemolysis) and vessel occlusion. Hypoxia, infection and dehydration may all precipitate sickling episodes.

Red cell chemistry

The 120-day life span of the red cell depends upon its ability to maintain a stable chemical intracellular environment. Red cell metabolism is directed at maintaining the normal structure and function of haemoglobin and the red cell membrane. Iron is kept in the active ferrous form, oxidative damage is prevented and the membrane is maintained. Glucose enters the red cell and is converted to lactate through a number of steps known as the Embden–Meyerhof pathway (glycolysis) (see Figure 6.4). For each molecule of glucose used, two molecules of adenosine triphosphate (ATP) are generated. These molecules are the currency of energy within the cell and can be used to fuel the processes that maintain red cell volume and shape and therefore function. The movement of

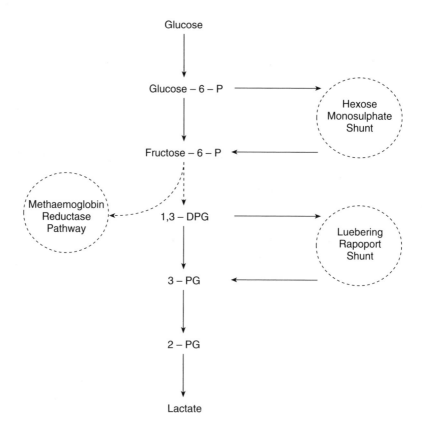

Figure 6.4   Red Cell Chemistry – the Embden–Meyerhof Glycolytic Pathway

sodium and potassium ions across the membrane is energy dependent. In addition this pathway generates reduced nicotinamide-adenine dinucleotide (NADH) which supports normal haemoglobin function. At the beginning of this pathway some molecules may be diverted along a brief diversion known as the hexose monophosphate shunt which allows generation of reduced nicotinamide-adenine dinucleotide phosphate (NADPH) which also supports haemoglobin function. This support is the enzyme-mediated maintenance of iron in the functionally active state. NADPH may also combine with glutathione to maintain the sulphydril groups in haemoglobin and the red cell membrane, which are important for their respective functions. A second diversion towards the end of the pathway between glucose and lactate known as the Luebering–Rapoport shunt generates 2,3-DPG, which regulates haemoglobin's oxygen affinity along with hydrogen ion and carbon dioxide concentrations.

Abnormalities of enzymes within these pathways may be functionally significant and lead to disease (glucose-6-phosphate dehydrogenase deficiency and pyruvate kinase deficiency).

White Blood Cells

The five members of the white blood cell group can be divided into two main categories; phagocytes and immunocytes. Neutrophils, eosinophils and basophils are known as the granulocytes due to their cytoplasmic granules. Granulocytes and monocytes are the phagocytes. B and T lymphocytes are known as the immunocytes. See Figure 6.5 for diagrams of blood cells.

Phagocytes

Neutrophil: The neutrophil cell contains small granules, which on staining show as pink-blue or grey-blue colour (Hann, 1996). The nucleus is multi-lobed. The identified precursors of neutrophils are myeloblasts, the promyelocyte, myelocyte, and then the metamyelocyte which finally differentiates into a juvenile neutrophil. By *adulthood* the neutrophils account for approximately 60 per cent of the white cells. The lifespan of the neutrophil in the blood stream is only 10hrs. The neutrophil count *at birth* is higher than the *adult* value. It then decreases and plateau's *after 7 days*. The *adult* average number is $1.5–6.0 \times 10^9/l$.

Eosinophil: The eosinophil cell contains slightly larger cytoplasmic granules than the neutrophil. The stain used to identify the cell is called acidic dye eosin, a deep red colour, from which the name eosinophil arises. The nucleus of the cell is generally bilobed. In the adult the eosinophils account for approximately 1 per cent of the white blood cells. *Adult* levels are usually $0.05–8.0 \times 10^9/l$, and are seen *early in the first year*.

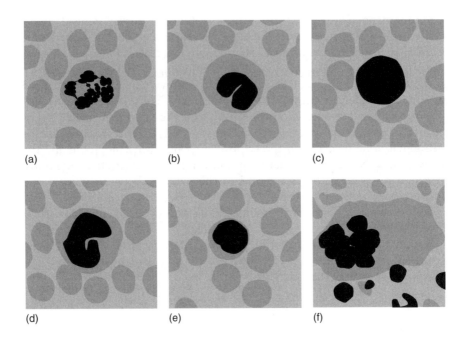

Figure 6.5   Diagrams of Blood cells
(a) neutrophil
(b) eosinophil
(c) basophil
(d) monocyte
(e) lymphocyte
(f) megakaryocyte

Basophil: The basophil cell contains large dark cytoplasmic granules that cover the nucleus. On staining the basophil is a pale grey blue. Generally they are not seen in the blood stream. In the tissue, they develop into mast cells. Basophils account for about 1 per cent of the white blood cells. The normal number of basophils remains constant from *birth* to *adulthood* (0–0.2 × 10⁹/l).

Monocyte: The monocyte cell is usually bigger than all the other white blood cells. The nucleus can be kidney shaped or indented and the cytoplasmic granules very fine. Mature monocytes are found in the blood stream where they can be maintained for approximately 10 hours. However when they enter the tissue they mature into macrophages. The lifespan of the macrophage can be several months or years and can take on specific functions. Monocytes account for about 5 per cent of the white blood cells. Adult range (0.15–1.3 × 10⁹/l) is seen from *2 years*.

Function of phagocytes

Granulocytes and monocytes are the primary defence against bacterial infections. When the neutrophil and eosinophil enter the tissue both play a general role in fighting bacterial and fungal infections. Basophils mediate inflammatory responses (Falcone *et al.* 2000). Monocytes remove bacteria and debris through the process of phagocytosis and are involved in the process of activating antigens and directing them to T lymphocytes. The function of neutrophils and monocytes can be described through a three-phase reaction. The phagocyte is initially mobilized to the site of infection or damage (chemotaxis), the bacteria is then engulfed (phagocytosis) and finally the bacteria is killed and digested. Eosinophils play an important role in controlling parasite infection, but are also associated with allergic disease where their activity may do more harm than good. Further detail on the process of phagocytosis can be found in the chapter on protecting children from infection.

Immunocytes

Lymphocytes are essential for providing specific immunity. Generally the lymphocyte is a small cell with a round nucleus that fills most of the cell. Lymphocytes account for about 33 per cent of the white blood cells. The number of lymphocytes present *at birth* is slightly higher than the *adult* value. There are two main types of lymphocytes that have different specific actions within the immune process, B-lymphocytes and T-lymphocytes. There are two stages of cell development (lymphopoiesis). Primary lymphopoiesis is the division of the stem cell in the bone marrow and thymus (T cell only) and secondary lymphopoiesis is the process, which follows exposure to an antigen. This takes place in the lymph nodes and spleen in conjunction with other lymphoid tissue or in the blood stream and tissue spaces with other lymphocytes.

B-lymphocytes: are responsible for immunity against bacteria. This is referred to as humoral immunity. Twenty per cent of lymphocytes are B-lymphocytes. The mature B-lymphocyte binds to antigens by receptors present on the surface of the cell, which recognize the antigen and trigger production of specific antibodies directed at the antigen. Mature cells producing antibodies are known as plasma cells. Memory cells are also developed in this process that will in the future react rapidly to the same antigen. T cells assist this humoral immunity.

T-Lymphocytes: Primary lymphopoiesis of T-lymphocytes commences from the stem cell in the bone marrow but the immature cells are processed through the thymus. Secondary lymphopoeisis is antigen specific but activation depends upon a macrophage processing and presenting the antigen to the immature cell. T-lymphocytes are responsible for immunity against intracellular infections (bacteria, viruses, protozoa and fungi) and foreign bodies (transplant organs). This is historically referred to as cell-mediated immunity. Eighty per cent of lymphocytes are T-lymphocytes. Mature T-lymphocytes can be divided into four groups. Helper cells (T_H), lymphocytes that are involved in delayed type hypersensitivity reactions (T_{DTH}), suppressor cells (T_S) and cytotoxic cells (T_C). Lymphocytes can be identified by their surface molecules in a scheme called cluster designation (CD). After designation, they may be referred to by their CD number eg, CD_4 and CD_8 cells.

Complement proteins

These serum proteins are involved in both non-specific and specific immune responses. They can be activated by direct bacterial contact or by antibody–antigen immune complexes. Their activation can lead to increasing inflammation, direct damage to cell membranes or to assisting phagocytosis by opsonization. Opsonization is the coating of antigen, to make it more 'attractive' to phagocytes.

The human immune system is both complex and variable. It strives to distinguish self from non-self as quickly as possible. In doing so, it must be able to respond to a very wide range of possible infecting organisms. Inherited and acquired faults do exist, but are usually uncommon. Age plays an important role. The *newborn* is protected by maternal IgG antibodies, which have crossed the placenta. In *infancy*, humoral responses are poor, predisposing this age group to certain organisms eg, Neisseria meningitidis, Haemophilus influenzae, streptococcus pneumoniae et., and variable responses to vaccinations. Due to the complexity of the immune system a wide range of congenital and acquired abnormalities can occur, a few examples of which are given below.

- Failure of T and B cell function leads to death in infancy – known as severe combined immunodeficiency (SCID).
- Absence of the thymus in Digeorge syndrome predisposes the child to infection.
- Reduction in the adhesion molecules of leucocytes, which normally enable these cells to leave the blood and enter damaged tissue to facilitate repair, as in leucocyte adhesion deficiency (LAD), results in delayed separation of the umbilical cord *after birth* and a predisposition to bacterial infections.
- Mutations in the gene for Bruton tyrosine kinase in X-linked agammaglobulinaemia, results in a failure of B cell development, exposing these boys to significant bacterial infections from *infancy.*
- Acute Lymphoblastic Leukaemia, the commonest childhood malignancy with an incidence of 4/100,000 children, peaking between *2 and 5 years of age*, is a biologically heterogeneous disease with no single aetiology (Kersey, 1997). Suggested causative agents include genetic factors, immune deficiency, environmental factors, radiation, electromagnetic fields, chemicals, drugs and infection (viral). B-cell leukaemia's account for 85 per cent of cases.
- Neutropenia – a low neutrophil count, can occur at any age and predispose the child to significant infection. *Premature babies* may be neutropenic following severe growth retardation or maternal illness.

Platelets

Platelets originate from the progenitor cell in the bone marrow. The precursor cell, megakaryoblast, differentiates to produce the megakaryocyte and then the platelet. This process does not occur through cellular differentiation but DNA replication with each stage of the process. Therefore rather than splitting, the cell gets larger with the increase of nuclear lobes in multiples of two. This replication is called endomitotic synchronous nuclear replication. A mature megakaryocyte contains eight nuclear lobes. At this stage the lobes release themselves within the cell and form into the structure that will become the platelet. The platelets are then finally released into the blood stream. About 4000 platelets are produced by each megakaryocyte. The spleen holds about a third of all new platelets.

The platelet is disc shaped and contains granular cytoplasm but no nucleus. The surface of the platelet contains glycoproteins (Ia, Ib, IIb, IIIa,) that are essential for adhesion and aggregation during the process of clot formation. The life span of the platelet is about 12 days. The platelet count at birth is comparable to adult values ($150-440 \times 10^9/l$). Platelets are essential for haemostasis.

Disorders leading to changes in the quantity or quality of platelets lead to problems such as petechiae, bruising and bleeding. Neonatal thrombocytopenia is defined as a platelet count of $<150 \times 10^9/L$. It includes specific genetic abnormalities and diseases of the *perinatal period*, which lead to a low platelet count. Some examples are given below:

- Intrauterine infections can lead to thrombocytopenia *at birth* presenting as petechiae in association with other abnormalities including hepatosplenomegaly, chorioretinitis and intracranial calcification (eg,. TORCH syndromes).
- When passive transfer of maternal antiplatelet antibodies to maternal and fetal platelets occurs, a low platelet count results which usually recovers within a month of birth and is often insignificant. This is known as maternal autoimmune thrombocytopenia.
- In neonatal alloimmune thrombocytopenia, a mechanism similar to Rhesus or ABO incompatibility occurs. Maternal antibodies are directed against fetal platelets producing a severe thrombocytopenia and a high risk of significant bleeding, including intracranial haemorrhage.
- More commonly, thrombocytopenia is a feature of certain *neonatal* diseases, particularly infection and necrotising enterocolitis (NEC).

Later in childhood, the commonest cause of thrombocytopenia is Immune thrombocytopenic purpura (ITP). These children are otherwise well apart from extensive petechiae and bruising in the absence of significant trauma. The platelet count is very low. Platelet survival time is reduced as they are prematurely removed from the circulation because of some inappropriate immune mechanism. Recovery is usually spontaneous, but severe bleeding can occur.

Prevention and Control of Bleeding

As large multicellular organisms, we rely on the circulation of blood between organs. This is partly dependent on the physical properties of blood and the vessels. If a vessel tears or is disrupted by trauma, blood in its normal fluid state, will quickly leak into surrounding tissues or out of the body. However blood contains clotting factors which when alerted to such an event contribute to local clotting ie a conversion of blood into a solid phase which plugs the bleeding point and prevents blood loss. This process involves many clotting factors and signals from adjacent tissues as well as the vessel wall itself. There exists a fine balance between switching on and switching off the formation of appropriate clots. Both sides of this balance are cascades. Abnormalities in these cascades can lead to uncontrolled bleeding or coagulation, which can be life threatening.

The vessel

If the vessel wall is torn or damaged blood loss can be minimized by local vessel constriction. The vessel constricts in response to local chemicals/vasoactive substances. Exposure of chemicals within the wall of the torn vessel to the clotting factors in the blood or wall lead to the local production of a clot where it is most needed. This process also involves the activation and aggregation of platelets.

Platelets

Exposure of a damaged vessel wall leads to the rapid adherence of platelets. The process of adherence leads to a change in shape and function of the platelets. Chemicals usually residing within platelet granules are released locally promoting further adhesion and aggregation of more platelets leading to a haemostatic plug in the vessel wall preventing blood loss. Coagulation factors within the blood and the platelets themselves lead to the formation of a supporting scaffold of fibrin fibres around the platelet plug to stabilize it and prevent re-bleeding.

Coagulation factors

The vessel wall, platelets and blood contain the coagulation factors that are involved in the cascade system that prevents bleeding and maintains vessel patency (see Figure 6.6). These factors are active enzymes and proenzymes waiting to be activated or catalysts waiting to activate the proenzymes. Once

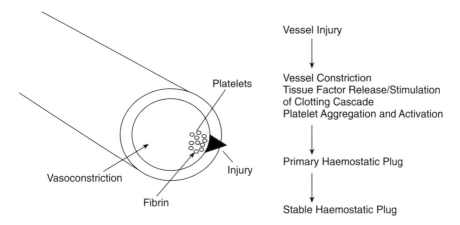

Figure 6.6 Diagram of Early Haemostasis

stimulated the cascade's function is to convert the soluble protein fibrinogen into the insoluble scaffold of fibrin, which supports the platelet haemostatic plug. The cascade has traditionally been viewed as two separate pathways (intrinsic and extrinsic) leading to a common final pathway. Our three dimensional understanding of this process comes from our knowledge of the relevant importance of individual factors or steps within this cascade. More recently, this two-sided view has been replaced by the view that the formation of the tissue factor -factor VII complex, is central to the involvement of other coagulation components.

Traditional view of the extrinsic pathway

Tissue damage releases tissue factor (TF). In the presence of calcium, TF binds with factor VII to form activated TF: VII complexes. This is the most important step in activating clotting. This complex activates factor X and IX.

Traditional view of the intrinsic pathway

If circulating factor XII comes in contact with exposed components of a damaged vessel wall it becomes activated and in turn activates factor XI which in turn activates factor IX. Factor IX once activated forms a complex with factors VIII and X, calcium and platelet membrane phospholipid (The Tenase complex) which leads to the activation of factor X.

Common pathway

The above responses both lead to the activation of factor X. It then forms a complex with factor V, calcium ions, phospholipid and prothrombin (the prothrombinase complex) which leads to the release of active thrombin, which can convert insoluble fibrinogen into fibrin. Thrombin then activates factor XIII that helps stabilize the fibrin scaffold with the formation of cross-links. In addition thrombin can further activate factor IX.

Modern view of the coagulation system (see Figure 6.7)

At the site of vessel injury, factor VII binds to tissue factor and is immediately activated. This results in a 'two-unit enzyme'. The activated factor VII being the catalytic component and the tissue factor being the regulatory component. This tissue factor/factor VIIa complex binds and activates factor X. The activated factor X, in the presence of factor V, Ca++ and the platelet membrane, converts prothrombin to thrombin, which in turn converts fibrinogen to fibrin. As well, the factor VII/tissue factor complex also activates factor IX. The activated factor IX, in the presence of factor VIII, Ca++, and the platelet membrane, activates more factor X which generates more thrombin. Some of this thrombin activates factor XI which then accelerates the activation of factor IX. The net result is an amplification process with the ultimate, localized generation of large amounts of thrombin and the conversion of fibrinogen to a fibrin clot.

The relative importance of some clotting factors

Some clotting factors are more important than others. Their relative concentrations have an effect on the activity of each other. Some of the factors determine

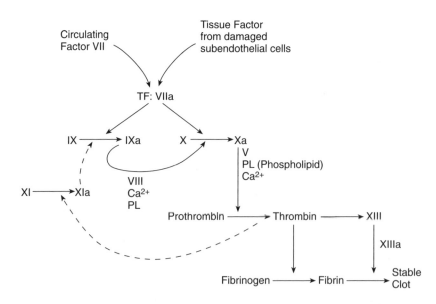

Figure 6.7   Coagulation

the success of the ongoing cascade. Their absence (VIII and IX) can lead to clinically significant bleeding disorders.

Defects in the Factor VIII and IX genes are responsible for the hereditary bleeding disorders haemophilia A and haemophilia B. Decreased or absence of factor VIII or IX will result in prolonged bleeding. These factors affect the same part of the coagulation cascade, making these deficiencies clinically indistinguishable, although haemophilia A is more common. Both are X-linked recessive genes and nearly always affect males only.

Some disease processes involve more than one part of the clotting mechanism. For example, Von Willebrand Disease, which is the most common hereditary bleeding disorder. The gene for von Willebrand factor (VWF) is on chromosome 12 and the majority of cases are inherited in an autosomal dominant pattern with variable penetrance. VWF serves as a carrier protein for factor VIII, but it is also essential for initiating the involvement of platelets in haemostatic plugs. Deficiency of VWF leads to mucosal bleeding, easy bruising and heavy menstruation.

The role of vitamin K

Vitamin K is required for the essential modification (carboxylation) of the clotting proteins II, VII, IX, X, protein C and protein S. This modification allows the clotting factors to bind calcium and phospholipid. Vitamin K is a fat-soluble vitamin. The *newborn* is born with only a small store of this vitamin and unfortunately breast milk only provides very small quantities.

Bleeding can occur at the *end of the first week*, but may occur anytime in *the* *first few* months for breast fed babies. This is known as Vitamin K deficiency bleeding of the newborn which can be prevented by oral or intramuscular vitamin K *at birth*. Vitamin K may also not be absorbed *during childhood* if fat absorption is poor eg. cystic fibrosis.

Blood coagulation inhibitors

Once fully activated the coagulation pathway needs controlling. Excess activation would lead to over formation of clots and tissue damage. Continued activation can also lead to the exhaustion or consumption of clotting factors, which would predispose to uncontrolled bleeding in the event of further vessel damage. Inhibitors of blood coagulation attempt to tailor the coagulation response. Anti thrombin III binds and inactivates thrombin and other serine proteases. Heparin cofactor II specifically inactivates thrombin. Tissue factor pathway inhibitor (TFPI) binds to activated factor X and activated TF: VII to interrupt the cascade at those points. Protein C is activated by thrombin in the presence of the co-factor thrombomodulin. It inactivates factor VIII and V and thereby reduces further thrombin formation. Protein C is also involved in fibrinolysis. The activity of protein C is enhanced by forming a complex with protein S.

The fibrinolytic system

This smaller cascade controls the break-up of the fibrin clot. Plasminogen is activated to plasmin by components within the fibrin clot (tissue plasminogen activator). Plasminogen and plasmin bind both fibrin and fibrinogen affecting their function. If fibrinolysis occurs too rapidly a successful fibrin clot will never form. Therefore fibrinolysis is controlled by inhibitors of plasmin (α2-antiplasmin, α2 macroglobulin) and plasminogen (plasminogen activator inhibitors). The degradation of fibrinogen and fibrin lead to fibrinogen degradation products.

Activated partial thromboplastin time (APTT)

This test on plasma measures the time required to generate thrombin and fibrin polymers via the intrinsic pathway. It assesses the function of factors I, II, V, VIII, IX, X, XI and XII. It is commonly used to monitor the effects of heparin, an anticoagulant, on coagulation.

Prothrombin time (PT)

This test measures the time to generate a fibrin clot from plasma, as a measure of extrinsic pathway function. It assesses the function of factors I, II, V, VII and X. It is commonly used to monitor oral anticoagulant therapy (warfarin) and liver dysfunction. The INR (International Normalized Ratio) is the ratio of the patients PT to the control PT.

Assessment of the Function of the Blood in Childhood

The three cell lines produced by the bone marrow have specific functions and produce specific symptoms during disease. When red cell production is impaired or red cell survival time is reduced, then children become pale. The measured haemoglobin concentration is low and confirms anaemia. Anaemia may present in association with jaundice as a result of increased red cell destruction. Impaired white cell function manifests as severe or recurrent infections. Low platelet counts and low clotting factors lead to bruising and bleeding. The pattern of symptoms, their severity and the age of the child help point the way to particular diagnoses. In addition, the involvement of the lymph nodes, liver or spleen is a feature of some diseases which may be detected at initial assessment through physical examination of the child. In addition to the above signs and symptoms of blood function in the child, it is obvious from the preceding chapter content that much of the more detailed assessment of the blood in childhood has to be conducted through the results of blood testing (Geaghan,

1999; Lilleyman *et al.*, 1999). Some of the more common investigations are listed below:

- Full blood count (haemoglobin, white cell count, differential count and platelets);
- Reticulocyte count (number of young red cells);
- Film (shape, size and colour of cells);
- Clotting studies (ability to clot compared to control);
- Blood group (common red cell antigens);
- Direct Coombs' test.

Transfusion of Blood Products

The transfusion of donor blood/blood products is a central component of the management of haematological problems in childhood. Special care must be taken in choosing the right product and preparation that is safe for the individual (Perotta and Snyder, 2001). This is particularly true for *neonates* and the immunocompromised.

Summary

The successful multicellular organism is dependent on the circulation of blood. Nutrients, waste materials and signals are transported from one organ to another. In addition blood is essential for immunity and haemostasis. The properties of the liquid and cellular components of blood are highly evolved and designed to support these diverse functions. Congenital and acquired diseases affect the blood via a number of different mechanisms including genetic disorders. The function of the blood can be assessed initially through observation and examination of the child. However this will only provide indications of likely problems, more detailed assessment by blood testing is always needed.

Review Questions

1 Discuss the changing sites of haemopoiesis during development from conception to adulthood.
2 Discuss the vulnerability of children to iron deficiency anaemia across the age range.
3 Explain the events which occur in rhesus incompatibility between a pregnant woman and her unborn child.
4 Outline the changes in the coagulation cascade.
5 Discuss the contribution of blood investigations to the assessment of blood disorders in children.

Further Reading

Hoffbrand, A, Pettit, J and Moss, P (2001) *Essential Haematology*. Oxford. Blackwell Science. This book is one of a series of books designed for medical students. However its comprehensive coverage of haematology, presented in an easy to read format, makes it valuable for all students of the topic who are looking for a basic text to provide the foundations on the subject. It includes genetics, classification, clinical presentations and treatment.

Lilleyman, JS, Hann, IM and Blanchette, VS (1999) *Pediatric Hematology. 2nd edn.* Edinburgh: Churchill Livingston. This book provides a comprehensive and referenced overview of the diagnosis and treatment of blood disorders in childhood, including a useful section listing normal values for paediatric haematological variables.

References

Dame, C and Juul, SE (2000) The switch from fetal to adult erythropoiesis. *Clinics in Perinatology*, 27(3), 507–26.

Department of Health (1994) *Report on Health and Social Subjects 45. Weaning and the Weaning Diet. Report of the Working Group on the Weaning Diet of the Committee on Medical Aspects of Food Policy.* London: HMSO.

Falcone, FH, Haas, H and Gibbs, BF (2000) The human basophil: A new appreciation of its role in immune responses. *Blood*, 96(13), 4028–38.

Geaghan, SM (1999) Hematologic values and appearances in the healthy fetus, neonate, and child. *Clinics in Laboratory Medicine*, 19(1), 1–37.

Hann, IM (1996) *Colour Atlas of Paediatric Haematology*. Oxford. Oxford Medical Publications.

Hann, IM, Gibson, B and Letsky, E (1991) *Fetal and Neonatal Haematology*. London: Bailliere Tindall.

Hanspal, M (1997) Importance of cell-cell interactions in regulation of erythropoiesis. *Current Opinion in Hematology*, 4(2), 142–7.

Hoffbrand, A, Pettit, J and Moss, P (2001) *Essential Haematology*. Oxford. Blackwell Science.

Kersey, JH (1997). Fifty years of studies of the biology and therapy of childhood leukemia. *Blood*, 90(11), 4243–51.

Lilleyman, JS, Hann, IM and Blanchette, VS (1999) *Pediatric Hematology. 2nd edn.* Edinburgh: Churchill Livingston.

Olivieri, NF (1997) Fetal erythropoiesis and the diagnosis and treatment of hemoglobin disorders in the fetus and child. *Seminars in Perinatology*, 21(1), 63–9.

Palis, J and Segel, GB (1998) Developmental biology of erythropoiesis. *Blood Reviews*, 12(2), 106–14.

Pallister, C (1999) *Biomedical Sciences Explained. Haematology.* Oxford: Butterworth Heinemann.

Perrotta, PL and Snyder, EL (2001) Non-infectious complications of transfusion therapy. *Blood Reviews*, 15(2), 69–83.

Roberts, IAG and Murray, NA (2001) *Haematology in the Newborn*. Singapore: World Scientific Publications Co.

Urbaniak, SJ and Greiss, MA (2000) RhD haemolytic disease of the fetus and the newborn. *Blood Reviews*, 14(1), 44–61.

Vlachos, A and Lipton, JM (1996) Bone marrow failure in children. *Current Opinion in Pediatrics*, 8(1), 33–41.

Wharton, BA (1999) Iron deficiency in children: Detection and prevention. *British Journal of Haematology*, 106(2), 270–80.

CHAPTER 7

Internal Transport: Heart and Circulation

Barbara Novak

Contents

- Development of the Cardiovascular System
- Assessment of Cardiovascular System in Children
- Summary
- Review Questions
- Further Reading
- References

Learning Outcomes

At the end of this chapter you will be able to:

- Outline the key stages in the embryonic and fetal development of the cardiovascular system.
- Describe the changes in circulation that occur at the time of birth.
- Compare the circulation of blood in the fetus with that in a child.
- Describe the methods of assessment of cardiovascular function in the infant and child in health.

Introduction

The cardiovascular system can be considered as an efficient transport network supported by a rhythmically pulsatile four-chambered heart. Its role is to transport blood within the closed circuit of semi-compliant vessels, delivering nutrients and metabolic substrate to the tissue and removing metabolic waste products from the tissue. Thus the cardiovascular system has a key role in ensuring that all cells are supported in their normal function.

Development of the Cardiovascular System

The Systemic and Pulmonary Circulation

The circulatory system can be divided into two functional compartments, the systemic circulation supported by the left ventricle, and the pulmonary circulation, which is supported by the right ventricle. Both, the right and the left ventricle work in harmony. The systemic circulation transports oxygenated blood and nutrients from the left ventricle of the heart through the aorta to the systemic arteries and capillaries. By contrast, the pulmonary circulation receives its deoxygenated blood from the right ventricle. This blood is then pumped through the pulmonary artery (Figure 7.1) to lungs. Here a complex capillary bed surrounds the alveoli and these facilitate gaseous diffusion across the capillary–alveolar membranes. As a consequence of this gaseous diffusion, oxygenated blood is carried back to the left atrium by way of venules, which ultimately fuse giving rise to four pulmonary veins that attach to the posterior wall of the left atrium. The fundamental difference between the pulmonary and systemic circulation is the purpose of the circulating blood. The systemic circulation supplies blood to all organs supporting the metabolic requirements of the tissue, while the pulmonary circulation serves as an important component of the gas exchange unit ensuring that the blood returning to the left ventricle is fully oxygenated.

Embryonic and Fetal Development

The heart and its corresponding blood vessels develop from the splanchnopleuric mesoderm (embryonic tissue adjacent to the endoderm) in the cardiogenic region. The underlying endoderm contributes to this development by signalling to the primitive angioblastic cords to converge and form a pair of lateral endocardial tubes. The subsequent folding of the embryo brings the pair of endocardial tubes closer together and into the future thoracic region. A gradual fusion of these tubes results in the formation of a single primitive heart tube (Figure 7.2), which undergoes a sequenced process of folding, reshaping and septation which transforms the single

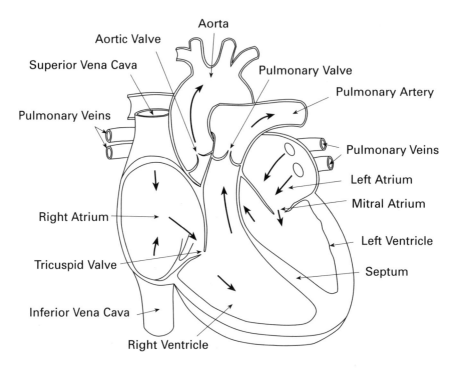

Figure 7.1   A Cross-section of the Heart Depicting the Flow of Blood

lumen into the four chambers of the definitive heart. The initial chambers are primitive, as outlined in Figure 7.3.

The primitive heart tube consists of endothelium, which forms a series of expansions and shallow ridges and crevices, known as sulci, which shape the framework of the primitive heart. By *day 22* a thick mass of splanchnopleuric mesoderm surrounds this heart tube and then differentiates into two distinctive layers, the myocardium and the cardiac jelly. Larsen (2001) defines this cardiac jelly as a layer of thick acellular matrix synthesized by the developing myocardium. Populations of mesothelial cells derived independently from the splanchnopleuric mesoderm form the visceral pericardium. These cells are believed to migrate onto the surface of the developing heart from the regions of the septum transversum or the sinus venosus.

As of *day 23*, the single heart tube begins to elongate and simultaneously loop, and fold (Figure 7.2c and d). The bulbus cordis is displaced to the *right*. This displacement simultaneously adjusts the position of the primitive ventricle to the *left* and allows the primitive atrium to move in an upward direction. The complex embryonic cardiac folding is believed to be completed by *day 28* of gestation. Larsen (2001) claims that this highly organized looping of the primitive heart tube may be 'intrinsically motivated'. That is, signals for the looping may come from the state of hydration of the cardiac jelly, the active

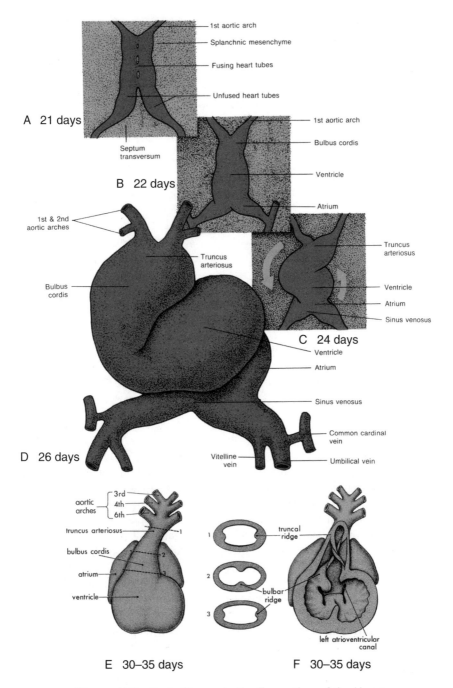

Figure 7.2 Early Stages in the Formation of the Heart

Source: Reprinted from *Before We Are Born: Essentials of Embryology and Birth Defects*, 4th ed. Moore and Persaud, copyright 1993 Mosby, with permission from Elsevier.

migration, and development, of the primitive myocytes (cardiac muscle cells) or alternatively be induced by the haemodynamic forces of the circulating blood.

The primitive heart begins to contract on approximately *day 22* (Larsen, 2001), and within the next two days blood begins to circulate through the primitive embryonic vessels. Although the first blood cells found in the embryo's circulation are formed in the yolk sac, normal embryonic and later fetal haematopoiesis occurs in the liver, spleen, thymus and, of course, eventually the bone marrow.

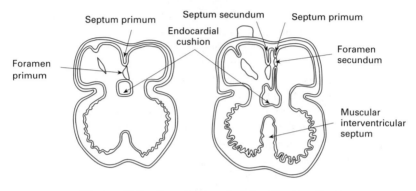

Figure 7.3   Development of the Cardiac Septa

Source: Reprinted from *Mosby's Clinical Nursing*, 3rd ed, Thompson, McFarland, copyright 1993, with permission from Elsevier.

The Developing atria

Remodelling of the right atrium occurs during the *fourth and fifth weeks* of gestation. This process begins with the incorporation of the enlarged right sinus horn and the developing venae cavae (Figure 7.2). Similarly in the left atrium, a single pulmonary vein sprouts and then divides forming the right and left pulmonary veins. These pulmonary veins grow in the direction of the lung tissue and eventually join up with smaller pulmonary veins that develop around the primitive bronchial tissue. The right and left pulmonary veins are eventually reconstructed to form, in most instances, four pulmonary veins, which are incorporated into the posterior wall of the primitive left atrium.

As the atria and the common atrioventricular canal divide, a definitive separation of the systemic and pulmonary blood flow is established. But this process depends on a gradual and systematic fusion of the septum premum and the septum secundum (Figure 7.3). The septum premum establishes a firm interatrial muscle and the septum secundum contributes to the development of the foramen ovale, or oval widow. Throughout the embryonic and early fetal life all septal structures form large openings that allow blood to flow in a specific direction. The most significant of those is the foramen ovale, which permits shunting of blood from the right atrium to the left atrium. This allows the blood to bypass the right ventricle, the pulmonary artery and its tributaries. The foramen ovale normally closes soon after birth largely due to the abrupt cessation of fetal circulation *at birth*, the first breath and the eventual dilatation of the pulmonary vessels. These mechanisms reverse the pressure difference between the atria and push the flexible membraneous septum against the less conforming muscular septum thus closing the foramen ovale and blocking any shunting of blood from the right to the left atrium.

Division and shaping of the common atrioventricular canal by the septum intermedium (the middle segment of the intraventricular septum) into the right and left atrioventricular canals ensures that the right atrioventricular canal aligns the right atrium with the right ventricle and the left atrioventricular canal aligns the left atrium with the left ventricle. Division and reshaping of the common atrioventricular canal begins the developmental process of the primitive left ventricle which establishes a firm contact with the proximal portion of the truncus arteriosus, a major vessel, which is ultimately divided to form the future aorta and the main pulmonary artery. The four main cardiac valves begin to form in the *fifth week* of gestation, almost immediately following the division of the atrioventricular canal, and the septation of the truncus arteriosus. Proliferating cells that surround these orifices form the mitral and tricuspid valves. This process is initially supported by growth and shaping of ventricular muscle from below.

The development of the ventricles

Both the right and the left ventricle are composite structures. According to Larsen (2001) the right ventricle is derived predominantly from the inferior aspects of the bulbus cordis and the right aspect of the conus cordis (Figure 7.2). The left ventricle develops mainly from the primitive ventricle and the left wall of the conus cordis. The division of the two ventricles and the establishment of their corresponding outflow tracts, the aorta and the main pulmonary artery, completes the morphogenesis of the heart and its major vessels.

The intraventricular septum is thought to form as a result of the developing right and left ventricular walls opposing one another (Collins, 1995; Larsen, 2001). However, growth of this muscular septum is halted just before the superior edge meets the inferior membraneous surface of the septum intermedium, the middle segment of the intraventricular septum (Figure 7.3). This arrest in growth allows for blood flow between the ventricles and prevents the left ventricle being occluded from its outflow tract. The flow of blood between these two chambers appears to contribute to the development of the ventricles. As the ventricular septum develops, the myocardium itself begins to enlarge forming characteristic ventricular trabeculae (ridges in the myocardium). The ventricular chambers and their outflow tracts are carefully coordinated as the heart evolves into a competent mechanical pump.

The main cardiac outflow pathway is the truncus arteriosus, (Figure 7.4) that is divided by a septum establishing thereby the right and left outflow tract for the respective ventricles. The separation of the aorta from the main

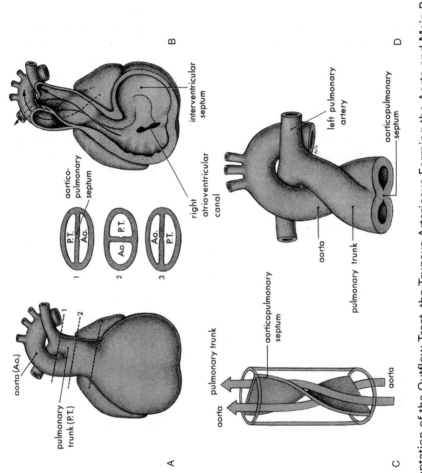

Figure 7.4 Septation of the Outflow Tract, the Truncus Arteriosus Forming the Aorta and Main Pulmonary Artery

pulmonary artery is followed by the appearance, at their base, of three distinctive swellings. These swellings (tubercules) are believed to evolve, during the *sixth week* of gestation, into the characteristic semilunar valves, otherwise known as the aortic and the pulmonary artery valves. Development of these valves is not complete until the *ninth week* of gestation (Larsen, 2001). The function of these valves is to prevent backflow of blood from the aorta and the pulmonary artery trunk into the respective left and right ventricle.

The final stage in the intracardiac development involves the growth of the membraneous interventricular septum, which is originally derived from the inferior endocardial cushion (Figure 7.3). This membraneous septum fuses with the muscular interventricular septum to eliminate any flow between the right and the left ventricles at about *8 weeks* of gestation. The earlier establishment of the aorta and the pulmonary artery ensures that both ventricles can now function autonomously with respect to their own outflow tracts.

Where complete fusion of these two important structures fails a membraneous ventricular septal defect (VSD) will persist. This is the most common type of congenital cardiac anomalies that can occur in children.

The development of the valves

The atrioventricular valves begin their development in the *fifth week* of gestation with the formation of the cusps within the atrioventricular canals. The free edge of these cusps attaches to the sinew-like cordae tendinae which in turn insert into the papillary muscles. The design of these valves is such that on folding back during diastole they allow blood to flow from the atria to the ventricles, but on closing tightly during systole they prevent a backflow of blood into the atria. Generally, the left atrioventricular valve has only two cusps, which form the bicuspid valve, which is also known as the mitral valve. The right atrioventricular valve, usually, but not always, develops three cusps and these give rise to the tricuspid valve.

Box 7.1   The Development of the Heart at 8 Weeks

The heart and circulation develop early in embryonic life because of its critical function in supporting the growth and development of the fetus. By 8 weeks gestation the heart has developed as follows:

- The atrioventricular valves have formed on the left and right sides of the heart.
- The ventricular septum is complete.
- The basic shape of the heart has appeared with its four chambers.

- The aorta and pulmonary trunk have divided separating the flow of blood leaving the heart from the two ventricles.
- The heart beats rhythmically.

The remaining period of gestation facilitates growth and maturation of the cardiovascular structures.

Such early development makes the heart vulnerable to teratogens as much of its fundamental development has taken place before pregnancy is confirmed.

The vascular connection

On *day 17* of gestation primitive blood vessels begin to appear in the splanchnopleuric mesoderm of the yolk sac. On *day 18* a similar aggregation of cells, commonly referred to as blood islands, initiates the formation of blood vessels in the embryonic disc. The early development and subsequent shaping of the endocardial tubes allows a pair of dorsal aortas to attach to their cranial axis and so form the first pair of aortic arches (Figure 7.2). During the *fourth and fifth weeks*, four additional aortic arches develop connecting the rudimentary aortic sac, or truncus arteriosus to the dorsal aortas, these fuse later to form the median dorsal aorta. This complex network of the aortic arches is eventually remodelled to establish arteries within the upper thorax, neck and head. The dorsal aorta gives rise to three distinctive sets of arterial vessels (Collins, 1995; Larsen 2001):

- The ventral arteries which supply the gut and the lateral arteries which supply the retroperitoneal organs such as the kidneys and the gonads.
- The intersegmental arteries, which supply, in part, the head, the neck and body walls.
- The arteries supplying the gastrointestinal tract are derived from remnants of vitelline arteries and the vitelline duct, which anastomose with the paired dorsal aortae. The dorsal aortae in turn connect to the umbilical arteries, which carry blood from the embryo and later the fetus to the placenta.

The primitive venous system consists of three major components:

- the cardinal veins, which drain the head, neck, body walls and limbs;
- the vitelline veins, which initially drain the yolk sac; and
- the umbilical veins, which carry oxygenated blood from the placenta to the embryo/fetus.

All three set of veins initially drain into the right and left sinus horns, (Figure 7.2) but their extensive modification gives shape to a more defined systemic venous connection with the right atrium. The left sinus horn is eventually transformed into the coronary sinus and the oblique vein of the left atrium. The coronary sinus receives most of the venous blood returning from the coronary vascular bed. The vitelline venous system gives rise to the liver sinusoids and the portal system that transports venous blood from the intestinal tract to the liver. The vitelline system further subdivides within the liver establishing the ductus venosus, a small vessel that directs the embryonic and later fetal blood from the umbilical vein directly into the inferior vena cava.

By approximately *day 55* of human gestation (just under 8 weeks) the basic shape of the heart has been attained (Larsen, 2001). The remaining period of gestation facilitates growth and maturation of the cardiovascular structures. Myocardial cells proliferate in conjunction with the rapid accumulation and availability of contractile proteins and metabolic substrates.

The Fetal Circulation

During pregnancy the placenta meets the metabolic demands of the fetus in terms of gas exchange, delivery of nutrients and the elimination of metabolic waste products. This process requires, however, a high blood flow from the fetal heart to the placenta. Maternal blood flows freely through the intervillous spaces of the placenta, and the fetal blood flows through chorionic villi capillaries which protrude into the intervillous spaces. Although the maternal and fetal blood do *not* mix, water and other metabolic substrates diffuse easily. As the fetal haemoglobin has a higher oxygen affinity than adult haemoglobin it facilitates efficient diffusion and uptake of oxygen. Water, electrolytes and other nutrients such as proteins of low molecular weight cross the placental barrier selectively in both directions.

A diagrammatic outline of fetal circulation can be seen in Figure 7.5. The fetal blood is normally 'incompletely' (70–75 per cent) saturated with oxygen in the placenta and this blood then flows through the umbilical vein contained within the umbilical cord. Most of this blood passes through the ductus venosus into the inferior vena cava, where it mixes with the deoxygenated blood returning from the lower part of the fetus. A smaller quantity of blood enters the left branch of the portal vein to perfuse the liver. This volume of blood then enters the inferior vena cava. The mixed blood, (oxygen content of 60–65 per cent) is then transported to the right atrium via the vena cava. Almost all of this blood passes directly through the foramen ovale to the left atrium bypassing the right ventricle and lungs. From the left atrium the blood is transported to the left ventricle and then pumped into the aorta.

The deoxygenated blood returning to the heart via the superior vena cava is directed primarily through the right atrium to the right ventricle and then the main pulmonary artery. However, as the fetal lungs are fluid filled and offer high resistances to this blood flow the pressure in the main pulmonary

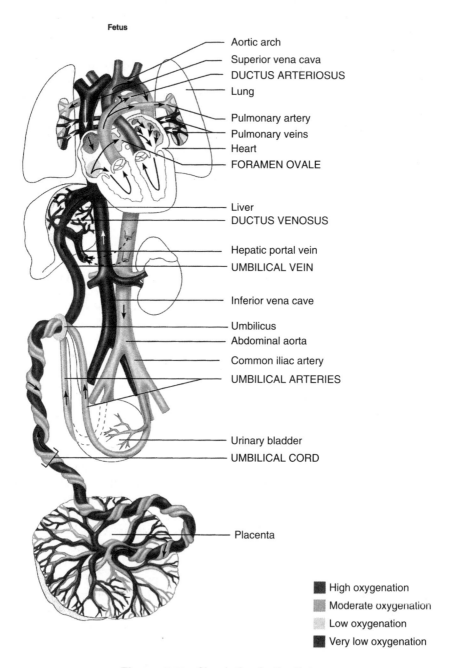

Fetus

- Aortic arch
- Superior vena cava
- DUCTUS ARTERIOSUS
- Lung
- Pulmonary artery
- Pulmonary veins
- Heart
- FORAMEN OVALE

- Liver
- DUCTUS VENOSUS

- Hepatic portal vein
- UMBILICAL VEIN

- Inferior vena cave

- Umbilicus
- Abdominal aorta
- Common iliac artery
- UMBILICAL ARTERIES

- Urinary bladder
- UMBILICAL CORD

- Placenta

■ High oxygenation
▨ Moderate oxygenation
░ Low oxygenation
■ Very low oxygenation

Figure 7.5   Circulation in the Fetus

Source: Pearson Education from *Human Anatomy and Physiology*, 6th ed, Fig. 28.13, p.1127, by Elaine N Marieb. Copyright 2004 by Pearson Education, Inc.

artery during systole is transiently higher than the pressure in the aorta. As a result most of the right ventricular blood is directed through the ductus arteriosus to the aorta. As the ductus arteriosus opens into the aorta distal to the point where the arteries to the neck, head and upper limbs branch off, these parts of the body are supplied with more highly oxygenated blood than the rest of the body.

Only a small quantity of blood flows through the pulmonary capillaries returning to the left atrium by way of the pulmonary veins. It is important to remember that this pulmonary venous blood is deoxygenated during fetal life.

The pair of umbilical arteries branch off the iliac arteries, and the blood is divided between the umbilical cord, the placenta, and the lower parts of the body.

Changes in Circulation Following Birth

At birth the blood flow through the single umbilical vein and the pair of umbilical arteries ceases (Figure 7.6), and this has a number of mechanical consequences. (see Table 7.1) The cessation of blood flow through the umbilical arteries increases peripheral resistance a physiological mechanism that could be attributed to local, reflex vasoconstriction; which in turn raises the aortic pressure. The loss of contact with the placenta increases the partial pressure of carbon dioxide in the newborn infant's blood and this stimulates the infant's respiratory centre, which initiates active respiration. The initial respiratory efforts begin the process of lung expansion and inhalation of atmospheric air. As the infant's pulmonary fluid is eliminated and displaced, resistance to blood flow through the lungs decreases ensuring a more efficient blood flow through the air-filled lungs. This facilitates more efficient gas diffusion, which contributes to the significant increase in the oxygen content of the blood. The improved oxygen saturation in turn gradually reduces pulmonary vascular resistance and so pulmonary arterial pressure falls.

Closure of the ductus arteriosus and foramen ovale

During fetal life the lungs are essentially bypassed by the ductus arteriosus. However, as the lungs inflate, and oxygen content in the blood increases the pressure in the pulmonary artery reduces. The concomitant increase in the aortic pressure reverses the blood flow through the ductus arteriosus. The high oxygen content of blood appears to induce gradual contraction of the oxygen sensitive muscle that makes up the ductus arteriosus. The narrowing of the lumen of this small vessel eventually obliterates the blood blow and contributes to its atrophy and occlusion (Case, 1985, Gluckman and Heymann, 1996). This closure is a slow process, taking place over the next 7 to 10 days. The advantage in this slow closure is that it permits some blood

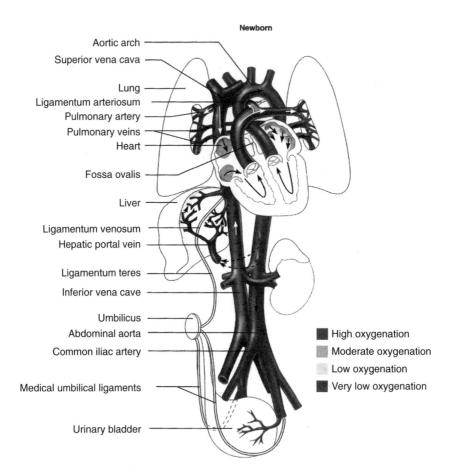

Figure 7.6   Circulation in the Newborn

Source: Adapted from Marieb (2004).

to flow through the ductus arteriosus, ensuring adequate lung perfusion at the time when the normal pulmonary circulation is being established and adjusted in keeping with the ongoing pulmonary changes, which occur at this stage. The ductus arteriosus closes permanently at approximately *4 months* postnatally.

The changes in the direction of the blood flow that occur after birth lead to a fall in the right atrial pressure, while the pressures in the left atrium rises due to the increased pulmonary venous return. This new pressure gradient, with higher pressure in the left atrium to that found in the right atrium, causes the valve guarding the foramen ovale to move tightly against the left atrial wall, effecting a closure of the interatrial communication. Local tissue reconstruction eventually reforms this valve and contributes to its successful, permanent fusion with the surrounding septal tissue.

Table 7.1 Changes in the Function of Fetal Circulation at Birth

Anatomical Structure	Function before Birth	Functional changes at Birth
A single umbilical vein	Transports oxygenated blood from the placenta to the fetal liver and heart.	Is obliterated by the cutting of the umbilical cord. Eventually becomes a ligament of the liver.
A pair of umbilical arteries	Transport arterio-venous blood from the fetus to the placenta.	Become obliterated by the cutting of the umbilical cord. Eventually form the bladder ligaments on the anterior abdominal wall.
Ductus venosus	Shunts oxygenated blood into the inferior vena cava.	Is obliterated by the cutting of the umbilical cord. Eventually forms the ligamentum venosum.
Ductus Arteriosus	Shunts oxygenated and some deoxygenated blood from the pulmonary artery to the aorta.	Become gradually smaller and is eventually obliterated forming the ligamentum arteriosum.
Foramen Ovale	Shunts oxygenated blood from the right atrium to the left atrium.	The normal increase in left atrial pressure compresses the membraneous flap against the septum closing the small aperture. Fibrous tissue eventually ensures the closure of this septal window.

Box 7.2   Major Differences Between the Fetal and Postnatal Circulation

The purpose of the cardiovascular system is the transport of oxygen, nutrients and waste products around the body. The fetal circulation is substantially different from that of the postnatal baby because this exchange takes place in the placenta. Major differences in fetal circulation are:

- Blood flows between the fetus and the placenta via umbilical veins and arteries.
- Blood flow between the right and left atria occurs which effectively bypasses the pulmonary circulation which supplies the lungs.
- Due to the high resistance to flow in the lungs, most of the blood from the right ventricle and the main pulmonary artery flows through the ductus arteriosus into the aorta, also bypassing the lungs.
- Fetal haemoglobin has a high oxygen affinity as it takes up oxygen at a lower level of concentration.

Postnatal Development

The normal position and shape of the heart

In *infants and young children*, the heart is a small rounded three-dimensional pyramid, which lies in the mediastinal cavity more horizontally than in the adult (Figure 7.7). The apex of the heart is higher, in the fourth left intercostal space, extending only to the fifth intercostal space by *7 or 8 years* of age. The base of the heart lies in an oblique position behind the sternum. It consists of the atria and their respective auricles (small pouches in the wall of each atrium). The two ventricles form the inferior aspect of the cardiac silhouette coming together to form the apex (Figure 7.7).

A mature heart weighs between 230 and 340 grams but this is only achieved between *17 and 20 years of age* (Gabella, 1995). In childhood the heart is considerably smaller, and varies with age and body surface area. The heart is suspended in a pericardial sac by its attachments to the aorta and the pulmonary artery. This leaves the apex of the heart relatively free which allows the ventricles, during contraction, to move the apex forward, allowing it to strike against the left side of the chest wall. This characteristic thrust is felt as the apex beat.

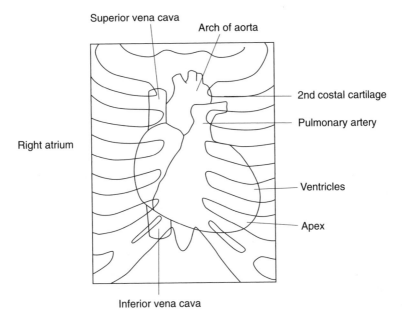

Figure 7.7   Normal Position of the Heart in the Thorax

The framework of the heart

The walls of the heart consist of three anatomically distinctive layers:

- The outer layer known as the pericardium;
- The middle layer known as the myocardium; and
- The inner layer known as the endocardium.

The pericardium   The fibrous pericardium, encloses, and to some extent, offers protection for the heart. It merges with the adventitia of the veins and arteries that communicate with the heart. The serous pericardium is a double-layered membrane that consists of flat secretary epithelium, connective tissue and some adipose tissue. In *young infants and children* the quantities of this adipose tissue is insignificant. The two layers of the serous pericardium form a small pericardial cavity holding a small volume of serous fluid, which lubricates this cavity.

The myocardium   or the contractile muscle of the heart is composed of highly specialized contractile proteins, sarcoplasmic reticulum, numerous nerve fibres and sensory nerve endings. Myocardial mass increases fairly rapidly during fetal life as a result of increase in cell number, hyperplasia. The composition of the myofibrils within the myocytes increases rather more slowly throughout *fetal life* and *early infancy*, giving rise to what is known as myocyte hypertrophy – increase in cell size. *After birth*, in children of all ages, there is only a limited capacity for myocyte hyperplasia, but myocyte hypertrophy continues up to *20 years of age*.

Sources of chemical energy for the myocardium   The chemical energy for the contraction of heart muscle is derived from the metabolism of carbohydrates and fatty acids. Metabolism of fatty acids requires approximately 11 per cent more oxygen than carbohydrates in order to produce an equivalent quantity of adenosine triphosphate, so fatty acids are not as efficient as glucose in terms of providing metabolic fuel or energy. However, the adult myocardium has a strong preference for fatty acids and this contrasts with *fetal* and *neonatal* myocardium, which appears to be an obligatory user of carbohydrates or glucose. This may have clinical significance in circumstances of severe hypo-glycaemia, when myocardial contractility and cardiac function in *neonates* (and possibly *young children*) may be affected adversely (Gluckman and Heymann, 1996). There is no evidence concerning the timing of this transition from the use of glucose to fatty acids as the dominant metabolic fuel, but it is possible that this transition is a gradual process influenced by dietary factors.

The endocardium   is composed of endothelium and a layer of fibroelastic connective tissue that lines the inner surfaces of the heart including the four cardiac valves. Characteristically, the endocardium is thicker in the atria than the ventricles and this may have a functional significance.

The functional features of the heart

The coordinated contraction of heart muscle provides the mechanical energy for the transportation of blood throughout the entire vasculature. The strength of myocardial contractility and electrodynamic controls are brought about by sophisticated cellular mechanisms, which are crucial in the mecha-nisms commonly known as excitation–contraction coupling.

In the *fetus*, the right ventricle ejects approximately 60 per cent of blood while the left ventricle ejects only 40 per cent of the total cardiac output. As both ventricles pump blood against a similar vascular resistance there is little differ-ence in the thickness of the myocardium as the two ventricles develop. In some instances, the right ventricular wall is slightly thicker in comparison to the thick-ness of the left ventricular wall and this persists for some time after birth. Electrocardiographic (ECG) recordings reflect this phenomenon as a relative right ventricular dominance. This physiological right ventricular hypertrophy is generally attributed to the workload of the right ventricle during *fetal life*, which is stimulated by the physical development of the right ventricular myocardium. A clear distinction must, however, be made between the physiological right ventricular hypertrophy and a hypertrophy initiated by some form of patho-physiological changes that may affect the heart of the *neonates and infants*.

Heart rate

Table 7.2 shows how the resting heart rate varies with age. The faster heart rate in *babies and children* is largely attributed to the smaller size of the ventricular chambers, which are only capable of ejecting a small amount of blood, commonly referred to as stroke volume, on each contraction. However, as the child's metabolic demands are high and these have to be met by an effective cardiac output (the quantity of blood pumped by the left ventricle per minute), the potential deficits created by the small stroke volume are corrected by the higher heart rate. As children grow older, their hearts become larger, the stroke volume increases, and this contributes to the significant reduction of the heart rate. It is important to appreciate that the heart rate and stroke volume fluctuate with activity.

Table 7.2 Normal Range of Heart Rates in Children at Rest

Age of the child	Normal range Beats per minute	Average range Beats per minute
Newborn–6 months of age	90–160	120
6–12 months of age	80–140	110
1–3 years	80–120	100
3–6 years	75–115	90
6–9 years	70–110	90
9–11 years	70–105	85
11–14 years	65–100	80

The cardiac cycle

Cardiac cycle is defined as the time spanning from the beginning of one heart beat to the beginning of the next. Each cycle is initiated and governed by an action potential generated within the sinoatrial node. This action potential is rapidly conveyed to both atria but there is a fractional delay in the passage of the impulse from the atria to the ventricles. This mechanism allows the atria to contract before the ventricles, and ensures that the blood is pumped into the ventricles increasing the ventricular volume, which in turn increases the stroke volume. The four actions or phases of the cardiac cycle (see Figure 7.8) are commonly known as:

- contraction (phase I) Figure 7.8a, b
- ejection or systole (phase II) Figure 7.8c
- relaxation (phase III) Figure 7.8d
- filling or diastole (phase IV) Figure 7.8e

Although the rhythmic pulsation of the heart is intrinsically generated (a mechanism frequently referred to as myogenic), the ultimate harmonizing

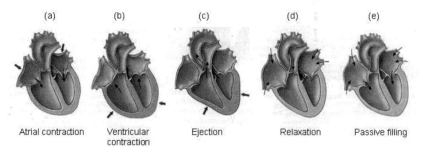

(a)	(b)	(c)	(d)	(e)
Atrial contraction	Ventricular contraction	Ejection	Relaxation	Passive filling

Figure 7.8   Blood Flows During the Phases of the Cardiac Cycle

Source: Reprinted from *Fundamentals of Anatomy and Physiology*, 6th ed, by Frederic H. Martini. Copyright 2004 by Frederic H. Martini, Inc. Reprinted by permission of Pearson Education, Inc.

of the cardiac cycle, in terms of rate, force of contractility and volume output is achieved by the autonomic nervous system. The autonomic nerves have a direct effect on the nodal tissue, the coronary vessels, atrial and ventricular myocardium and thus to some extent, augment and support the cardiac function. Physical activities or crying will also increase the child's heart rates significantly by, among other factors, increasing oxygen demand.

At the onset of ventricular contraction the atrial and ventricular pressure are fairly equal. However, as the ventricular blood volume increase and the ventricular pressure rises, the atrioventricular valves close completely, giving rise to the first heart sound (lub). Since the pulmonary artery and aortic valves remain closed the ventricles are said to be in isovolumetric contraction. This raises the ventricular pressure further and causes a bulging of both the semilunar and the atrioventricular valves. The semilunar valves open when the left ventricular pressure exceeds the aortic pressure and the right ventricular pressure exceeds the pulmonary artery pressure. The rapid expulsion of blood during the early phase of systole raises the ventricular pressures further establishing a maximum ejection point. This is followed by the last systole phase, which influences the gradual decline in the ventricular and aortic pressures, and the onset of ventricular diastole or early isovolumetric relaxation which culminates in the closure of the semilunar valves and the initiation of second heart sound (dub).

The volume of blood that is ejected at each ventricular contraction is defined as the stroke volume. Cardiac output is defined as the amount of blood ejected by the heart during each minute, that is cardiac output = stroke volume × heart rate/min. By contrast, the cardiac index takes into consideration the body surface area and is a measure of the cardiac output per square meter of body surface area. The cardiac index values continue to rise to above $4.0L/min/m^2$ up to *10 years of age*, and then decline, falling to a new lower normal value of about $2.4 \ L/min/m^2$ (Guyton and Hall, 1996). This phenomenon may be attributed to the normally high metabolic rate in younger children. Exercise and crying will also influence the child's stroke volume and cardiac output or index but this is usually transitory. Factors that have a more significant impact on cardiac output are the child's age, size, metabolism and body surface area.

While the function of the heart shows some degree of adaptability, only five factors are perceived as critical to the ultimate control of the cardiac output. These are the heart rate, myocardial contractility, the preload (the volume of blood that returns to and stretches the ventricles prior to contraction), after-load (the resistance to the ejection of blood from the ventricle into the great vessels), and total peripheral resistance. The heart rate and myocardial contractility are of cardiac origin. Both are sensitive to, and augmented by, neural and humoral mechanisms. By contrast, the preload and afterload are dependent on blood volume, and factors such as the size of the heart and the dimension of the blood vessels. There is however, a cyclical nature to this, in that both preload and afterload are important determinants of cardiac output; on the other hand, both factors are determined by myocardial contractility and cardiac output.

Assessment of the Cardiovascular System in Children

The status of the cardiovascular system is often reflected in a child's general health and appearance. But this cannot be assumed without careful physical assessment and evaluation. A typical assessment should consist of inspection, palpation, auscultation, accurate documentation and critical evaluation of the evidence.

Inspection provides opportunities for noting the child's general appearance, body size, proportions, skin colour, visible pulsations and exaggerated shapes to the thorax. The child's response to stimuli or the surrounding environment will indicate that normal developmental milestones have been reached. Observation of the respiratory rate and pattern will also contribute to the assessment of cardiovascular function.

In health, the body temperature is relatively constant at 36.0°C to 37.5°C at the core and the peripheral temperature is no lower than 34°C to 35°C. Lower values at the periphery may suggest low environmental temperatures or that the child's peripheral perfusion is being compromised.

Palpation uses tactile skills to evaluate the child's haemodynamic status. The pulse can be palpated in superficial arteries such as the brachial or radial artery. Pulse qualities that can be identified are:

- frequency;
- rhythm;
- amplitude;
- sharpness; and
- tension.

The child's apex beat is often visible, but always palpable. In health, the apex beat is synchronous with the carotid and radial pulse, and the first heart sound. See Table 7.2 for the normal range of heart rates in children at rest.

In children, an arterial pulse is usually palpable as a gentle but definitive wave over a bony orifice such as the radius. Pulse waves may be felt at the carotid or femoral arteries or dorsalis pedis. Pulses may be difficult to feel in neonates and young children because of the relatively low arterial resistance to blood flow generated by the relative thinness of the tunica media within the walls of the arteries and arterioles.

 In children under 1 year of age heart rate should be assessed over the apex of the heart using a stethoscope rather than by palpation of the radial pulse as it may not be possible to reliably feel the radial pulse.

However, as the child grows older, the muscle fibres of the tunica media (the middle layer of blood vessel walls) increase, augmenting the internal diameter of the arteries and raising the resistance to arterial blood flow, which in turn influences the magnitude of the pulse wave.

Intensity of a pulse may be rated on a scale of 0 to 4 as follows:

- an absent pulse is graded as 0;
- a palpable but weak and easily obliterated pulse is graded 1;
- a normal easily palpable pulse is graded as 2;
- a full pulse is graded as 3; and
- a bounding pulse that is easily visible is graded as 4.

Blood pressure – this term generally applies to the arterial pressure in the systemic circulation. It fluctuates with each heart beat between a maximum value (systolic pressure) achieved during cardiac systole, and a minimum value (diastolic pressure) which reflects the diastole phase of the heart. It can be measured directly using arterial invasive methods by inserting a needle, attached to a monitoring device into a peripheral artery. More commonly however, blood pressure is measured externally, or is estimated indirectly by using an inflatable cuff on the upper arm or sometimes below the knee, on the leg. In order to ensure accuracy of the measurement taken, the size of the cuff must be proportional (2/3 of the limb must be covered, e.g. on the upper arm this is 2/3 of the distance between the shoulder and the elbow) to the size and dimensions of the child's limb. The Doppler percutaneous flow probe is helpful in measuring the systolic and a diastolic pressure, as it detects cessation of blood flow very accurately. The difference between the systolic pressure value and the diastolic value is known as the pulse pressure. The major physiological factors that affect the pulse pressure are the stroke volume, the force of ventricular ejection, and the compliance of the arterial vascular network. The greater the stroke volume, the greater is the amount of blood that must be accommodated in the arterial network. This produces a rise in the systolic pressure and a fall in the diastolic pressure, which will culminate in a wider pulse pressure.

Blood Pressure – Control and Influences

The factors that influence blood pressure values are complex. They include functional development and maturation of the sympathetic and parasympathetic nervous system, as well as the maturation of the cardiovascular reflex mechanisms, and the degree of smooth muscle development in the resistance vessels. There is some evidence to support the assumption that intrauterine environment which influences low birth weight may contribute to the development of hypertension in adulthood (Barker *et al.*, 1993).

In health, blood pressure parameters are variable during infancy and childhood. Under normal physiological conditions however, the growing and developing child should show a gradual increase in the systolic and diastolic pressures according to age (Table 7.3).

Adaptation and maintenance of normal blood pressure is attributed principally to baroreceptors present in the carotid and aortic bodies, which are believed to augment and sustain the systemic blood pressure by reflex.

Table 7.3   Blood Pressure in Childhood

Age of the child	Systolic Blood Pressure mm Hg	Diastolic Blood Pressure Mm Hg
Newborn	73	55
6 months	90	53
1 years	90	56
3 years	92	55
6 years	96	57
9 years	100	61
12 years	107	64
15 years	114	65

Note: Readings are the 50th centile for boys (taken from Second Task Force on Blood Pressure Control in Children, 1987)

Auscultation involves listening to the heart sounds that are generated by the systematic opening and closing of valves and the vibration of blood against the walls of the heart and major blood vessels. In health, it is common to distinguish two heart sounds, which are heard as S_I and S_{II}. Under normal circumstances S_1 is louder at the apex of the heart in the mitral and tricuspid valve area. Conversely, S_{II} is best heard near the base of the heart in the pulmonary artery and the aortic valve area. Two further heart sounds may be audible and these are known as S_{III} and S_{IV}. S_{III} is produced by vibrations caused during ventricular filling and may be heard in some children and young adults. S_{IV} is generally attributed to the reduction in vibration initially caused by atrial contraction at the end of diastole. This sound is seldom heard but when audible further cardiac evaluation should be considered. Cardiac murmurs are another important group of heart sounds in neonates and young children. Many of these are of no significance but profound and persistent cardiac murmurs may suggest underlying cardiac or major blood vessel anomaly that will require further evaluation and systematic screening of the entire cardiovascular system.

Chest Radiography can determine the position of the heart, its size, shape and chamber enlargement; the condition of the lungs particularly in terms of pulmonary blood flow, venous return and air entry.

Electrocardiography records the changes in the electrical potentials during cardiac activity (Figure 7.9 and Table 4.4). Such data also provide information about the anatomical orientation of the heart, the relative size of the chambers of the heart, heart rate, rhythm and origin of excitation; the spread of the impulse, and any disturbances in the above events suggestive of cardiac problems.

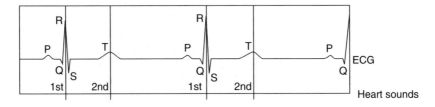

Figure 7.9 Electrocardiograph of the Heart

Table 7.4 Electrocardiograph Recording of the Function of the Heart as a Pump

Electrocardiographic event	Corresponding physiological event in the heart
P wave	Depolarization (excitation) of the atria prior to their contraction. The depolarizing action potential or impulse is initiated in the sinoatrial node. It spreads through the muscle of the atria to the atrioventricular node.
P–R segment	Atrial depolarization and conduction of impulses through the atrioventricular node.
QRS complex	Depolarization (excitation) of the ventricles, the repolarization (relaxation) of the atria is masked by the ventricular depolarization.
S-T segment	End of ventricular depolarization and the beginning of the ventricular repolarization
T wave	Repolarization (relaxation) of the ventricles

Electrocardiography also reflects age-related changes. A summary of the age-related significant points may be detailed as follows:

- At birth the thickness in the right ventricular muscle exceeds the thickness of the left ventricular muscle. But the significant increase in the left ventricular workload after birth gradually augments this. Thus, the right ventricular dominance seen in *newborn infants* is gradually replaced by left ventricular dominance in *later childhood*. The ratio of left to right ventricular muscle mass in young adults is believed to average at 2.5:1 (Berne and Levy, 2001; Park and Guntheroth, 1987) and the electrocardiography recording reflects this ratio.
- The overall increase in the size of the heart allows the heart to 'manage' a greater quantity of blood volume, and the stroke volume and cardiac output are increased and heart rate decreases.
- Consequently in conjunction with the decreasing heart rate all lengths and intervals (PR interval, QRS duration, QT interval) of the cardiac cycle increase (Berne and Levy, 2001).

Echocardiography – This technique uses high frequency sound waves to document detailed images, from which the heart valves, the atria, ventricles, the septal tissue and the great vessels can be identified and their dimensions measured. Most congenital cardiovascular defects may be identified using this technique and their size and complexity critically assessed.

Box 7.3 Methods of Assessment of Cardiac Function in Children

Cardiac function in children can be assessed in the following ways:

- History taking – information gathering from the child (when able to communicate) and parents/carers;
- Inspection – observation of the child's appearance including body size indicating growth, body shape, central and peripheral colour and respiratory rate and pattern;
- Palpation – pulses at the apex and peripherally;
- Auscultation – to listen to heart sounds and record blood pressure;
- Chest radiography – to determine the position, size and shape of the heart, and the condition of the lungs;
- Electrocardiography – to record the electrical potentials during cardiac activity; and
- Echocardiography – to provide detailed images of the structure of the heart.

Summary

The cardiovascular system begins its embryonic development on the *day 17 of gestation*. Though not fully developed the heart establishes its independent function early in order to support the metabolic needs of the rapidly developing and growing embryo. By the end of the *eighth week of gestation* the heart and its vascular connections are fully formed and in a position to support the fetal circulation.

Appropriate anatomical construction of the heart is critical to its function as a pulsatile pump, capable of supporting the independent demands of the pulmonary and systemic circulations. The right atrium and right ventricle are aligned to receive deoxygenated systemic blood, which is transported to the lungs by way of the pulmonary artery. Here oxygenation takes place and the oxygenated blood returns to the left atrium by way of the four pulmonary veins. The blood from the left atrium is emptied into the left ventricle and from here the blood flow is directed to the aorta and the systemic circulation. The pulsatile contraction of the heart can be described as the cardiac cycle consisting of a systole and a diastole.

Review Questions

1. Outline the sequence of embryonic development of the heart and the great vessels.
2. Describe the essential constituents of the fetal circulation.
3. Outline the physiological mechanisms involved in the establishment of normal circulation after birth and explain why this adaptation is important to extrauterine life.
4. Describe the normal anatomical position and shape of the heart in children.
5. Identify the common methods used in the assessment and evaluation of a child's cardiovascular function.

Further Reading

Berne, R and Levy, M (2001) *Cardiovascular Physiology*. Baltimore: Mosby. This text offers an invaluable account of cardiovascular physiology as seen in healthy adults.

Campbell, A. and McIntosh, N. (1998) *Forfar and Arneil's Texbook of Paediatrics*. NewYork: Churchill Livingstone. This textbook offers an invaluable account of knowledge and skills required in assessing newborn infants and children. It also provides a helpful account of common congenital cardiovascular pathophysiology.

Nolan, G (1998) Transcription and the broken heart. *Nature*, 392, p. 129–30. This article offers an invaluable insight into some of the factors that may influence the development of the embryo's heart.

Smith, J, Ley, S, Curley, M, Elixson, E, and Dodds, K (1996) Tissue Perfusion. In M Curley, J Bloedel Smith and P Moloney-Harmon (eds), *Critical Care Nursing of*

Infants and Children. Ch. 9, pp. 155–245, W.B. Saunders Company. This chapter provides an informative account of the many factors, that are known to influence tissue perfusion.

Srivastava, D and Olson, EN (2000) A genetic blueprint for cardiac development. *Nature,* 407, 221–6. This article offers an invaluable insight into some of the genetic factors that may influence the development of the embryo's heart.

References

Barker, DJP, Osmond, C, Golding, J, Kuh, D and Wandworth, MSJ (1993) Growth in utero, blood pressure in childhood and adult life, and mortality from cardiovascular disease. In DJP Baker (ed.), *Fetal and Infant Origins of Adult Disease.* London: British Medical Journal.

Berne, R and Levy, M (2001) *Cardiovascular Physiology.* The Mosby Physiology Monograph Series. Missouri: Mosby Inc St. Louis.

Case, RM (1985) *Variations in Human Physiology.* Manchester: Manchester University Press.

Collins, P (1995) Neonatal anatomy and growth. Ch 4, pp. 343–75. In L Bannister, *et al.* (eds), *Grays Anatomy.* New York: Churchill Livingstone.

Gabella, G (1995) Cardiovascular system. In L Bannister *et al.* (eds), *Grays Anatomy.* New York: Churchill Livingstone.

Gluckman, . and Heymann, M (1996) *Paediatrics and Perinatology: The Scientific Basis.* London: Arnold.

Guyton, A and Hall, J (1996) *Textbook of Medical Physiology.* Philadelphia, London: W.B. Saunders Company.

Larsen, W (2001) *Human Embryology.* London: Churchill Livingstone.

Park, M and Guntheroth, W (1987) *How to Read Paediatric ECGs.* Baltimore: Mosby Year Book.

Second Task Force on Blood Pressure Control in Children (1987) Normal blood pressure readings for boys. Bethesda, MD: National Heart, Lung and Blood Institute.

CHAPTER 8

Feeding the Body in Childhood

Julie Wilcox

Contents

- Prenatal Development
- Development During Infancy and Childhood
- Assessment of Gastrointestinal Function
- Conclusion
- Review Questions
- Further Reading
- References

Learning Outcomes

At the end of the chapter you will be able to:

- Describe key features in the embryological development of the gastrointestinal system.
- Describe the physiological development of the gastrointestinal system from infancy to adolescence.
- Identify the benefits of breast feeding and describe the physiological rationale behind current recommendations for weaning.
- Discuss the assessment of the gastrointestinal function.

Introduction

The main body system involved in the transformation of food into the cells, tissues and structures of the body is the gastrointestinal system. This system is involved in the intake, breakdown and absorption of food and the elimination of waste. It also plays an important role in protecting the body against micro-organisms and other potentially harmful substances that could be ingested. Digestive processes may be described as mechanical (eg, breakdown by chewing or churning) or chemical (eg,breakdown by enzyme activity – see Table 8.1).

Although the structures of the gastrointestinal system are well developed at birth, many functions are immature. The ability to eat and digest the same foods as an adult is acquired gradually over many months. Infants and children are vulnerable to particular disturbances of the gastrointestinal tract, due to their immaturity. This chapter aims to review the development of the gastrointestinal system from conception through to adolescence.

Prenatal Development

In utero, nutrition and the elimination of waste products are carried out by the placenta. Nevertheless, the digestive system does not lie dormant, activity does take place. The development of the digestive system is a fascinating and complex process, consequently only a summary can be given here. More detail can be found in human embryology texts such as Moore and Persaud (1998) and Larsen (1997), which are major sources for this section.

Research into prenatal development is, generally, limited to non-invasive methods of investigation on the healthy developing fetus. Consequently some of current understanding is taken from animal studies, 'in vitro' (laboratory) tissue tests, or postmortem studies, from which conclusions about normal human development are drawn.

Early Embryonic Development

As early as the *fourth week* of embryonic life a primitive gut tube develops as the embryonic disc folds into a more cylindrical shape. As the tube develops it differentiates into a variety of more complex structures and is described as having three regions (see Figure 8.1):

1 *The foregut*, which develops into the oral cavity, tongue, salivary glands, pharynx, oesophagus, stomach, part of the duodenum, liver and biliary system and pancreas (and also part of the respiratory system, see Chapter 5);

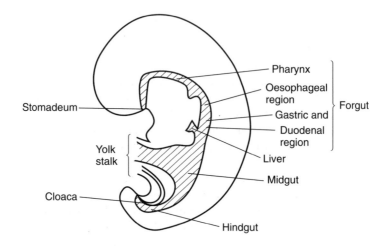

Figure 8.1   The Embryo at 4 Weeks

2 *The midgut*, which forms most of the duodenum, the rest of the small intestine and part of the colon; and

3 *The hindgut*, which forms the remainder of the colon, the rectum and the anus (and also part of the genitourinary system (see Chapter 9).

Box 8.1   Early Embryonic Development

The development of the gastrointestinal tract begins very early in embryological development, with the following events taking place often before the woman is aware she is pregnant:

3rd week of gestation:
The pharynx begins to emerge from pharyngeal arch tissue.

4th week of gestation:
• A primitive gut tube forms with three regions, foregut, midgut and hindgut.
• The oesophagus, stomach, pancreas and liver begin to develop from the foregut.
• Blood cells may begin to develop in the embryonic liver.
• The caecum is distinguishable as a bulge in the midgut.
• The tongue begins to develop from pharyngeal arch tissue.
• The face begins to form.

Growth of the gut tube occurs throughout fetal life. However, the *third trimester* is the period of greatest growth-rate when the gut doubles in length (Touloukian and Smith, 1983).

The Oral Cavity and Pharynx

The tongue arises from pharyngeal arch tissue and begins to develop during the *fourth week*. Three swellings, the tongue buds, merge to form a single structure. The fusion of the two median buds results in the groove (median sulcus) which can be seen in the centre of the tongue.

The salivary glands develop from ectoderm and endoderm in the primitive oral cavity. The parotid glands develop first, early in the *sixth week*, secreting fluid from about *18 weeks*. The submandibular glands develop later in the *sixth week*, beginning to secret from about *16 weeks*. The sublingual glands develop during the *eighth week*. Salivary amylase is secreted early in fetal life, gradually increasing with gestational age (Murray *et al.*, 1986), although this is still at a relatively low level at birth.

The lips, gums and jaws are formed as part of the development of the face. The face forms from several distinct prominences, beginning early in the *fourth week*:

- the maxillary prominences grow towards each other and fuse anteriorly;
- the medial nasal prominences, develop and fuse similarly, together these form the upper lip, gum and maxilla;
- the mandibular prominences form lower lip and jaw.

Cleft lip results from abnormal development of the maxillary prominences.

The palate develops in two main stages. First, early in the *sixth week*, a primary palate develops as a projection from the floor of the nasal cavity. A secondary palate then develops from two projections, called palantine shelves. These grow towards each other from the maxillary processes, at the sides of the primitive oral cavity. They fuse with each other and the primary palate, beginning in the *ninth week* anteriorly, continuing posteriorly, where the uvula is formed in the *twelfth week*. The nasal septum also develops during this period. The anterior part of the palate becomes ossified, forming the hard palate, while the posterior part, the soft palate, develops a muscle layer.

Cleft palate results from the failure of the palantine shelves to develop and/or fuse. It occurs frequently in association with cleft lip.

The teeth develop from tissues of the oral cavity. The enamel arises from the ectoderm and the other dental structures from the surrounding mesenchyme. The anterior teeth begin to develop first, in the *sixth week*, but the process continues for many years. *At birth*, the teeth are still in an immature form and have not erupted through the gum.

The pharynx arises mainly from pharyngeal arch tissue, beginning to develop from the *third week*. The tonsils develop here from pharyngeal pouch tissue from the *third month*. Lymph follicles, however, do not form until the *final trimester*. From *11–12 weeks*, the fetus is capable of sucking and swallowing amniotic fluid. This is thought to help regulate amniotic fluid volume.

Disorders preventing the fetus from swallowing (for example, oesophageal atresia) are often accompanied by polyhydramnios (excessive amniotic fluid volume) (Schmitz, 1991).

Amniotic fluid contains protein, carbohydrates, triglycerides, growth factors and other molecules that may be important for the healthy development of the gut (Kelly and Newell, 1994). From *18–24 weeks* sucking movements are seen, and the 'thumb-sucking fetus' is a much loved image used in television documentaries about prenatal life.

If born before *34–35 weeks* gestation, sucking is not usually sufficiently mature for effective feeding, and is known as 'non-nutritive sucking'.

The Oesophagus

The oesophagus develops from the foregut. During the *fourth week*, a pouch grows from this region, developing into the lung bud. The trachea and other respiratory structures develop from this outgrowth (see Chapter 5). The oesophagus then elongates rapidly. The smooth muscle layer arises from the surrounding splanchnic mesenchyme. The circular muscle layer is present by *five weeks* and the longitudinal muscle layer at *8 weeks*. The epithelial lining and glands develop gradually from surrounding endoderm. The mature lining, of stratified squamous epithelium appears around *25 weeks* (Grand *et al.*, 1976).

Oesophageal atresia (blind-ended oesophagus) and tracheo-oesophageal fistula (connection between the oesophagus and trachea) are congenital abnormalities that occur when the oesophagus and trachea fail to develop normally.

The Stomach

The stomach can first be identified in the *fourth week* as a swelling of part of the foregut. During the following 2 weeks, the dorsal (posterior) wall grows more rapidly than the ventral (anterior) wall, starting to develop the characteristic shape of the mature stomach (see Figure 8.2). During the *seventh and eighth weeks*, the stomach rotates so that the greater curvature (previously the dorsal wall) is situated towards the right, and the lesser curvature (previously the ventral wall) is situated towards the left. The rotation of the stomach helps to move the dorsal mesentery (part of the peritoneum which carries blood and lymph vessels and nerves to the abdominal organs) into place, forming the various folds such as the greater and lesser omentum (part of the peritoneum rich in fatty tissue which protects abdominal organs). The rotation also helps to place the nerve supply, with the right vagus nerve supplying the posterior wall of the stomach, and the left vagus nerve supplying the anterior wall.

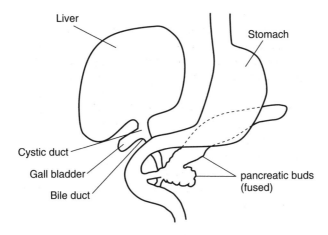

Figure 8.2   The Development of the Upper Gastrointestinal System at
6 Weeks

Secretory cells become evident in the stomach between *weeks 10 and 12*. By
the *end of the first trimester*, gastric pits and glands can be identified in the
gastric epithelium, which soon produce pepsin, lipase, hydrochloric acid,
gastrin, intrinsic factor and renin (Kelly *et al.*, 1993; Ménard *et al.*, 1995,
Weaver, 1991).

The Pancreas

The pancreas also develops from the foregut, beginning on approximately
day 26. Initially, two pancreatic buds form which fuse into a single structure late in the *sixth week* (see Figure 8.2). During this period, ducts
develop within each bud, fusing to form the pancreatic ducts, joining with
the bile duct at the proximal end. Insulin can be secreted from as early as
10 weeks. Pancreatic acini, the exocrine cells of the pancreas, begin to differentiate from blunt ended tubules from about the *twelfth week* (Grand *et al.*,
1976).

The Liver and Biliary system

The liver, gall bladder and bile duct system develop mainly from the foregut.
During the *fourth week*, an outgrowth, the hepatic diverticulum, appears.
During the *fifth week*, an outgrowth at the base of the hepatic diverticulum
appears which develops into the gallbladder and cystic duct. At the same time,
the stalk uniting the cystic and hepatic ducts elongates to form the common

bile duct (see Figure 8.2). The liver grows rapidly from the *fifth to the tenth weeks*, filling most of the abdominal cavity. It has an important role in the formation of blood cells during fetal life and this may begin as early as the *fourth week*. Bile formation begins during the *twelfth week*, although in limited quantities as bile is not needed to emulsify fats until solid feeding begins, as breastmilk is already emulsified. See Box 8.5 for a discussion of the differences between breastmilk and infant formula.

Biliary atresia results from failure of bile duct development. Without surgery and/or transplantation this condition is fatal. Assessment of the neonate must include observation for the initial symptoms of persistent jaundice.

The Small Intestine

During the *fifth week* a region of the midgut begins to elongate, growing more rapidly than the abdominal cavity, pushing it into a loop. The upper limb of this loop forms the small intestine, the lower limb forms the first portion of the large intestine. By *week 6*, the gut loop protrudes out of the abdomen, into the umbilicus. During the following two weeks, the loop continues to grow, rotating by 90° in a clockwise direction, as viewed anteriorly. During the *tenth to twelfth weeks*, the loop returns to the abdominal cavity, which has grown sufficiently to accommodate it. As it returns, it rotates by a further 180° in a clockwise direction, placing the small intestine and colon ready to develop towards their final anatomical position. The factors responsible for the movements and rotations of the gut are not yet well understood.

Exomphalos results when the intestine protrudes (herniates) through the abdominal wall into the base of the umbilicus into an umbilical sac and the intestine fails to return to the abdominal cavity.

Gastroschisis is different, as here, the intestine develops outside the abdomen. The intestine is not enclosed in a sac as it does not protrude through the umbilicus but beside it. It appears to be an abnormality of closure of the muscles of the abdominal wall.

Villi and crypts (projections and indentations in the intestinal mucosa), in the small intestinal wall, begin to develop during the *ninth week*. Immature enteroendocrine and goblet cells appearing during the *ninth and tenth weeks* (Lacroix *et al.*, 1984a). Sucrase, maltase, isomaltase and trehalase are present by *10 weeks* and are almost at mature levels by *14 weeks*. Lactase is present by *10 weeks* but its activity remains low in utero. Glucoamylase is present from *13 weeks*. Peptidases are also thought to be secreted from around the *tenth week*, with the exception of enterokinase, which activates pancreatic enzymes being secreted from about the *twenty-sixth week* (Antonowicz and Lebenthal, 1977; Lebenthal and Lee, 1980; Mènard, 1994). See Table 8.1 for a summary of key aspects of chemical digestion.

Lymphoid cells start appearing at around the *twelfth week*, developing into Peyer's patches (oval masses of lymphoid tissue in the mucous membrane of

Table 8.1 Summary of the Timetable of Development of Key Aspects of Chemical Digestion

Source	Factor	Main nutrient digested	Approximate age first detected (weeks gestation)*	Approximate activity in term neonate (% of adult)*
Mouth	Lingual lipase	Fat	30 weeks	100
	Salivary amylase	Carbohydrate	16 weeks	10
Stomach	Gastric acid	Activates Pepsinogen converting it to pepsin – see below.	13 weeks	not known?
	Gastric lipase	Fat	10 weeks	not known?
	Pepsinogen/Pepsin	Protein	16 Weeks	<10
Pancreas	Proteases (eg, trypsinogen, chymotrypsinogen)	Protein	26 weeks	10–60
	Lipase	Fat	30 weeks	5–10
	Glucoamylase	Carbohydrate	(4 months postnatal)	0
Liver	Bile	Fat	12 weeks	50
Small intestine –	Peptidases (eg, aminopeptidase, dipeptidase)	Protein	10 weeks (except enterokinase – 26 weeks)	100
Brush border	Dissacharidases (eg, sucrose-isomaltase, lactase, maltase)	Carbohydrate	100–14	100

* see text for details and references.
Source: Adapted from Lebenthal *et al.* (1983).

the small intestine) at around *16 weeks* (Orlic and Lev, 1977). The musculature begins to develop with the formation of the circular muscle layer,
followed by the longitudinal muscle layer, between *weeks six and eight*
(Weaver, 1991). The autonomic nerve supply appears from *week nine* and
peristalsis may occur from *week thirteen*.

The Large Intestine and Anus

The caecum, vermiform appendix, ascending colon and the first part of the
transverse colon develop from the midgut. The caecum is distinguished as a
bulge in the midgut during the *fourth week*. The vermiform appendix develops as a blind ended tube from the primitive caecum during the *sixth week*.
The herniation of these developing structures into the umbilicus and their
rotations, are described above. As they return to the abdominal cavity, the
shortening and folding of the mesenteries helps to fix the structures in place.

The remainder of the transverse colon, the descending and sigmoid colon,
the rectum and upper part of the anal canal, form from the hindgut. The lower
portion of the hindgut is an expanded region known as the cloaca. During the
fourth week, a wedge of tissue, the urorectal septum, begins to grow into
the cloaca. This forms a partition dividing the cloaca into two distinct tubes
by the *eighth week*; a lower tube which forms the rectum and upper anal canal,
and an upper tube which forms part of the urinary system (see Chapter 9).
The lower part of the anal canal develops from the upward growth of the anal
pit, an indentation in the outer surface of the embryo which grows upwards
towards the lower part of the hindgut. The anal canal is established when the
anal membrane, between the anal pit and the hindgut, ruptures at the end of
the *eighth week*.

Cloacal exstrophy occurs when the cloaca fails to divide and develop
normally. A variety of serious problems can arise, such as the exposure of the
bladder and anorectal canal through the abdominal wall.

Imperforate anus, a blind-ended rectum, may result from failure of the anal
pit to form, leading to complete anal agenesis. Alternatively, the main canal
and musculature of the anus may develop, but the anal membrane fails to
rupture.

The musculature develops from the *eighth week*, with the circular muscle
layer appearing first, about two weeks before the longitudinal layer. The gut
wall becomes innervated by neuroblasts, primitive neurons, from the *fifth
week*, although mature distribution of the ganglion cells is not achieved until
the *sixth month* (Weaver, 1991).

Hirschsprung's disease arises when innervation of a segment of the bowel,
most commonly in the sigmoid colon, fails to develop. Normal peristalsis
cannot occur in the affected segment, leading to chronic constipation (if the
segment is small) or bowel obstruction (if the segment is large when it may be
detected at birth as a meconium ileus).

The lining shows longitudinal folds from the *eighth week*. Initially villi are present in the lining of the large intestine, but these disappear during the *second trimester*. Enteroendocrine cells develop from *10 weeks* and goblet (mucous secreting) cells from *12 weeks*. Brush-border enzymes are secreted in the large intestine from the *tenth week*, increasing up to *20 weeks*, after which they decline, though they may still be detected by the *twenty-eighth week* (Lacroix *et al.*, 1984b).

Development During Infancy and Childhood

The gastrointestinal system has to adapt abruptly *at birth* to help the infant change from receiving nourishment passively through the fetal blood supply to an active process of feeding, digestion and absorption. This section provides an overview of what is known about the development of gastrointestinal activities in the different parts of the system during infancy and childhood.

Reflexes Associated with Feeding

Various reflexes are present at birth related to feeding, including, rooting, gag, sucking, swallowing and biting. These are summarized in Table 8.2.

Various factors can inhibit these reflexes. For example, they may be absent or inefficient in *preterm infants*. Sedation of the mother during labour, for example with pethidine, can delay the initiation of sucking and swallowing (Nissen *et al.*, 1995). Birth trauma, neurological damage and other perinatal problems can also inhibit the reflexes.

The Development of the Mouth, Pharynx and Larynx

At birth, the mouth is suited to sucking and swallowing a liquid diet. The tongue is stubby and rounded, developing a more pointed shape later with chewing and speech. *Infants* have a small oropharynx, as *at birth* the tongue is relatively large and wholly in the mouth. During the first *5 years of life* the posterior part descends into the larynx (Moore and Persaud, 1998). The cheeks contain fatty pads which assist with feeding but also contribute to the smallness of the oral cavity. The soft palate and the arytenoid mass (in the region of the vocal cords) are also relatively large in infancy. The larynx is relatively high in the neck during *infancy*, opposite the fourth cervical vertebra, descending to the level of the fifth cervical vertebra as the neck elongates during *childhood* and the sixth cervical vertebra in *adulthood* (see Figure 8.3). The epiglottis, which closes the airway during swallowing, is long during *infancy*, protecting against aspiration of the liquid diet, allowing the baby to feed safely in a recumbent position (Fink et al., 1979; Stevenson and Allaire, 1991).

Table 8.2 Reflexes Associated with Feeding

Reflex	Area of Stimulation	Effect	Purpose	Duration
Rooting	Touching cheek or upper lip	Baby turns head to side and opens mouth	Assists baby to locate food	From 28 wks gestation, strongest in first 2–3 wks of life. May persist for months (Milla, 1991). Transition to voluntary act occurs from 2 months of age (Iwaynama and Eishima, 1997).
Gag	Food or fluid on mid third of tongue in young infants and posterior third from 7 months (Stevenson and Allaire, 1991)	Contraction of muscles of the pharynx.	Protects respiratory tract from inhalation of food or other materials.	Persists throughout life.
Sucking	Hard palate.	Sucking may occur spontaneously during sleep.	Milk feeding	From 18–24 wks gestation persisting throughout life.
Swallowing	Food on posterior portion of the tongue.	Swallowing	Ingestion of food and fluid.	Throughout life. Voluntary control develops between 6–12 wks.
Biting	Pressure on upper or lower gums.	Rhythmic bite and release movement.	Starts liquid flowing into the mouth during breast feeding (Stevenson and Allaire, 1991)	Incorporated into chewing from 5 months of age (Milla, 1991).

(a)   (b)

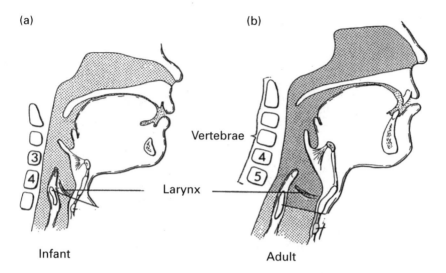

Vertebrae

Larynx

Infant   Adult

Figure 8.3 Comparison of the Infant (a) and Adult (b) Larynx

Source: Reprinted from *Nursing Care of the Critically Ill Child*, 2nd edition, Hazinski MF, copyright 1992, with permission from Elsevier.

Chemical digestion in the mouth

Salivary amylase has been detected in *preterm infants*, the concentration increasing with gestational age (Murray *et al.*, 1986). Although enzyme activity is relatively low in *early infancy*, it does not appear to be inactivated by gastric acid when swallowed, consequently it may be able to contribute to the digestion of starches in the stomach and small intestine.

Between *4 and 6 months of age* saliva production increases, helping to moisten food, promoting digestion, when weaning is introduced (see Box 8.6). Those involved with feeding infants will observe that babies appear to be able to distinguish between different tastes. However, little is known about the sense of taste and its development during infancy (Milla, 1991)

Mechanical digestion in the mouth

The teeth: The eruption of teeth, combined with development of the neuro-muscular control involved in chewing, allows for increasing variability in the texture of food. Primary teeth (deciduous, 'milk teeth' or 'baby teeth') begin to erupt from the *sixth month of life*, coinciding with increased saliva production. The timing and pattern are variable, but the typical order is shown in Figure 8.4. The tooth erupts through the gum as the growth of the root, dentin and pulp of the tooth exerts pressure. This process, known as 'teething', may be painful and is often accompanied by drooling and biting on hard objects. There is some controversy over whether other symptoms such as

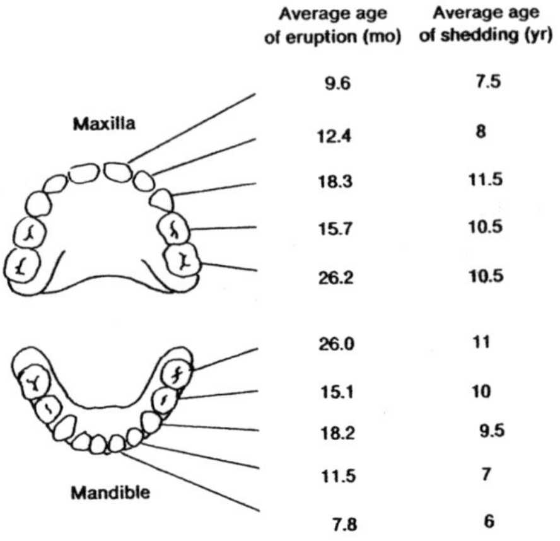

	Average age of eruption (mo)	Average age of shedding (yr)
	9.6	7.5
Maxilla	12.4	8
	18.3	11.5
	15.7	10.5
	26.2	10.5
	26.0	11
	15.1	10
	18.2	9.5
	11.5	7
Mandible	7.8	6

Figure 8.4   Eruption of Primary 'Milk' Teeth

Source: Reprinted from *Dentistry for the Child and Adolescent*, 5th ed, McDonald and Avery, copyright 1987, with permission from Elsevier.

fever, diarrhoea, respiratory symptoms and earache can be attributed to teething. One study did demonstrate a mild fever before the eruption of the first tooth (Jaber *et al.*, 1992) but there is a danger of attributing fever, or other symptoms, to teething without ruling out other causes.

Box 8.2   Teething

The emergence of the first teeth begins from around the *sixth month of life*. Known as 'teething', it may cause pain as the tooth emerges through the gum. Other symptoms are also often attributed to teething such as fever, diarrhoea, respiratory symptoms and earache. Jaber *et al.* (1992) did find an association between a mild fever and the eruption of the first tooth. But there is a danger of attributing fever, or other symptoms, to teething without ruling out other causes as more serious illness may be missed in its early stages as a result.

The deciduous teeth are shed between *ages 6–13 years* and are followed by the eruption of permanent teeth (Figure 8.5). Losing teeth is an important social milestone for some children and may be accompanied by cultural practices (for example, in Britain, receiving money from a 'tooth fairy').

The Mechanisms of Feeding and Eating

Feeding is a complex activity, requiring the integration of sucking, swallowing, breathing and the appropriate muscular activity of the oesophagus and

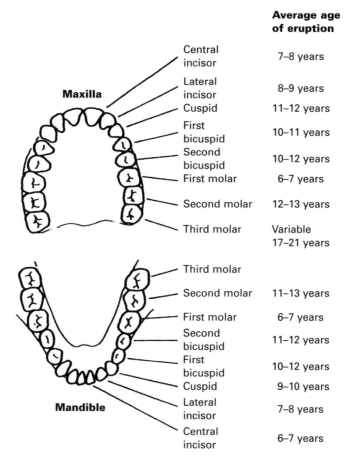

Average age of eruption

Maxilla		
Central incisor	7–8 years
Lateral incisor	8–9 years
Cuspid	11–12 years
First bicuspid	10–11 years
Second bicuspid	10–12 years
First molar	6–7 years
Second molar	12–13 years
Third molar	Variable 17–21 years

Mandible		
Third molar	
Second molar	11–13 years
First molar	6–7 years
Second bicuspid	11–12 years
First bicuspid	10–12 years
Cuspid	9–10 years
Lateral incisor	7–8 years
Central incisor	6–7 years

Figure 8.5   Eruption of Secondary or Permanent Teeth

Source: Reprinted from *Dentistry for the Child and Adolescent*, 5th ed, McDonald and Avery, copyright 1987, with permission from Elsevier.

stomach. An effective sucking pattern, known as 'nutritive sucking', develops in the *term infant* within a few days of birth. Sucking is rhythmic, in burst of 10–30 sucks, with 1–4 swallows per burst. After swallowing, the oesophagus propels feed into the stomach by peristalsis, which is coordinated with relaxation of the lower oesophageal sphincter. There is a difference in tongue and jaw action between bottle- and breast-fed babies due to the differences in the shape and structure of the breast and artificial teat. Some infants do not adapt readily between the two different modes, either sucking inappropriately at the human nipple after bottle feeding, or refusing the bottle after breast feeding (Lang *et al.*, 1994).

Box 8.3   'Nipple Confusion'

In some families a breastfeeding mother may express milk so that another member of the family, often the father, can also share in the pleasurable activity of feeding the baby. However some infants do not adapt readily between the two different modes, either sucking inappropriately at the human nipple after bottle feeding, or refusing the bottle after breast feeding (Lang *et al.*, 1994), often referred to as 'nipple confusion'. This may be related to the difference in tongue and jaw action required due to the differences in the shape and structure of the breast and the artificial teat.

Sucking and swallowing action matures in early infancy. In the *first 4 months*, the lips tend to be held loosely during sucking and feed may dribble from the corner of the mouth during feeding. From about four months onwards, the lips and jaw close firmly during sucking. Swallowing matures between about *6–12 weeks* when the tongue moves upward and backward to help form a bolus (Milla, 1991).

Although sucking and swallowing are reflexes *at birth*, development of feeding is a learned activity. Spoon feeding of pureed solids is generally introduced when lip control begins to develop, replacing primitive reflex movements (Milla, 1991). Initially, the infant sucks from the spoon with the same action as drinking the liquid feed (Stevenson and Allaire, 1991). From *6 months*, cup feeding can be successfully introduced. The biting reflex has gone and the jaw may be stabilized on the cup by muscular control. Elevation of the tongue tip during swallowing at this stage also aids successful cup drinking. However, full control of cup drinking is not achieved until *2–3 years of age* (Milla, 1991) and young children, up to the age of about *2 years* frequently bite on the cup to compensate for lack of jaw stability (Stevenson and Allaire, 1991). Cup feeding of *neonates and preterm babies* is practised in some centres to avoid using an artificial teat. Here the baby 'laps' the milk delivered carefully to its lips in a small cup (Lang *et al.*, 1994).

Chewing develops from the biting reflex at about *5 months of age*. From *6–7 months of age* increasing coordination of tongue, lip and jaw movements enable the tongue to move food from side to side. By *7 months*, the infant can brush one lip over the other to clear food from the lips. Around the age of *1 year*, rotary movements of the jaw develop, control is gained over lip closure and the cheek muscles are able to direct food towards the molar teeth. By *2 years of age*, a mature chewing action is usually achieved, with coordination of the tongue, lips, jaws and cheeks. However, development of feeding skills may continue throughout childhood. Schwartz *et al.* (1984) identified maturational changes in tongue movements and swallowing between *4 and 5 years of age* with *adult* swallowing patterns being acquired still later.

Progression through the various stages is variable and may be influenced by many factors. Alexander (1991) suggested that the tendency of *infants* to put items in their mouth helps to modify the gag reflex and prepare the baby for foods of different textures.

Infants who are not able to put their fingers, or objects, in their mouths, such as those with motor disabilities may develop oral hypersensitivity and feeding difficulties (Stevenson and Allaire, 1991).

Development of feeding will be partly paced by physical development, but social, cultural and interpersonal factors play an important role in the development of feeding skills (Stevenson and Allaire, 1991).

The Oesophagus

Development of structure

At birth the oesophagus is approximately 10cm in length and 0.5cm in diameter (Weaver, 1991). The portion of the oesophagus within the abdominal cavity is only a few millimetres long *at birth*, lengthening to about 15mm by about *2 years of age*. The angle between the stomach and the oesophagus, the 'angle of His', is less marked in *young infants* and does not achieve the acute angle seen in adults until the *second or third year of life* (Milla, 1996). This is directly related to the changing shape of the stomach from transverse in *infancy* to the vertical *adult* stomach.

Mechanical digestion in the oesophagus

The upper oesophageal sphincter (UOS) is a ring of muscle located about 6–8cm from the nostrils in *infants*. The UOS is normally closed between swallowing, preventing air entry into the oesophagus during breathing and protecting the lung from aspiration of refluxed gastric contents. The sphincter relaxes during swallowing, vomiting, retching, belching and gagging. It would appear that the sphincter is present even in *preterm infants*, exhibiting mature function in the *newborn period* (Grybowski, 1965).

The lower oesophageal sphincter (LOS) is located at the junction between the oesophagus and stomach. The LOS helps to prevent reflux of gastric contents into the oesophagus. It is a region of high pressure, approximately 1cm in length in *young infants*, 1.6cm in *infants over 1 year of age* and 2–4cm in *adults*. Although it is described as a sphincter, a 'muscle ring' is not anatomically present.

The tendency to gastrointestinal reflux in *young infants* was thought to be related to the immaturity of the LOS, but it is now generally agreed that LOS pressure, which partly determines its function, is relatively mature *at birth*, although the length of the sphincter does increase during childhood (Moroz *et al.*, 1976; Nurko, 1991).

In *preterm infants*, however, LOS pressure is relatively low, correlating with gestational age (Newell *et al.*, 1988).

Peristalsis is initiated by swallowing. The presence of striated (voluntary) muscle in the upper two thirds of the oesophagus enables peristalsis to be initiated voluntarily when swallowing becomes a voluntary act during *early infancy*. Relatively little is known about the development and function of the body of the oesophagus (Milla, 1996), but we do know that motor activity is poorly coordinated in *preterm infants*, peristalsis maturing with postnatal age and experience of feeding (Grybowski, 1965).

No chemical digestion takes place in the oesophagus.

The Stomach

Development of structure

In the *newborn* the stomach has a capacity of approximately 30mls, increasing rapidly during infancy. The shape also changes as noted above.

Mechanical digestion in the stomach

Four different modes of motor activity have been described related to the stomach:

1 receptive relaxation to receive a feed;
2 contraction of the antrum following feeding;
3 gastric emptying following feeding; and
4 gastric emptying during fasting.

The best studied of these activities in *infants* is gastric emptying following feeding (Milla, 1996) which is affected by the composition of feeds. Increasing the fat content (long-chain triglycerides) delays emptying and therefore feeds supplemented with fat may remain in the stomach longer. An increase in the overall caloric density of the feed also delays gastric emptying, although one study demonstrated that despite this *infants* receiving the higher caloric feeds did absorb more calories over time than those on an unsupplemented feed (Siegal *et al.*, 1984). Gastric emptying is slower in *preterm infants* than in *term infants*. Breast milk has been demonstrated to empty significantly faster than formula feed (Ewer *et al.*, 1994; Splinter and Schreiner, 1999; Tomomasa *et al.*, 1987). This is likely to be a result of the lower fat content, finer emulsion and lower casein:whey ratio in breastmilk, which results in a softer curd (Thomas, 1994) (see Box 8.5). This may be very beneficial to *preterm infants* who have feeding intolerance related to delayed gastric emptying.

 Due to the faster stomach emptying time of breastmilk, when infants are fasted prior to surgery, those on formula are fasted for longer than breast fed infants (Splinter and Schreiner, 1999).

Chemical digestion in the stomach

Gastric acid helps protect the gut from microorganisms and aids digestion. Secretion by the parietal cells in the gastric mucosa occurs from early in fetal life. Concentrations in *preterm infants* may be lower than *at term* (Marino *et al.*, 1984). Studies on the amount of gastric acid production over the *early months of infancy* have produced conflicting results. Several studies suggest that acid production is relatively high in the *first 10 days of life*, then declines until about *day 30*. Adult levels appear to be achieved by about *3 months of age* (Wershil, 1991).

Gastrin is a hormone produced in the gastric mucosa. In *adults*, it stimulates gastric acid production. *Infants* have significantly higher concentrations of gastrin than adults, persisting until at least *4 months of age*, although gastrin concentrations do not rise after feeding, as they do in adults (Moazam *et al.*, 1984). The role of gastrin as a trophic hormone, promoting the maturation of gut function, is probably of most importance *in infancy* (Wershil, 1991).

Pepsinogen, produced by chief cells in the stomach, is converted to pepsin by hydrochloric acid and promotes the digestion of proteins in the stomach. Secretion is below adult values in *early infancy*, increasing with postnatal age. *Premature infants* have lower secretion, relative to their maturity (Adamson *et al.*, 1988). Demand for pepsin is likely to be lower prior to weaning as breastmilk does not contain complex proteins.

Gastric lipase prepares fat for further lipolysis by pancreatic lipase (Manson and Weaver, 1997). Secretion has been demonstrated in *preterm infants* and it is thought to reach mature concentration by *3 months of age* (Ménard, 1994). Gastric lipase is active in the relatively low pH of the infant's stomach and inactivated either by the lower gastric pH from *3 months of age* or in the duodenum by pancreatic trypsin.

Intrinsic factor, a small glycoprotein secreted by the parietal cells of the stomach, is necessary for the absorption of vitamin B_{12} in the intestine. Secretion appears to increase during the *first 2 weeks of life* to half adult concentrations, reaching adult concentrations by *3 months of age*. *Preterm infants* also appear to secrete intrinsic factor. Secretion appears to be unaffected by feeding or fasting (Marino *et al.*, 1984).

The Liver

The liver contributes to fat digestion by the secretion of bile into the duodenum. Bile acid formation occurs at a low rate in *newborns*. Bile acids are conjugated with the amino acids taurine or glycine to form bile salts. *In infancy*, conjugation with taurine occurs more readily, as breast milk provides a good source of taurine. *After birth*, the bile acid-conjugating enzymes gradually increase. Normal bile metabolism requires the cycling of bile products from the liver into the small intestine, absorption into the hepatic portal vessels and reuptake by liver cells. In *early infancy*, bile salt secretion into the intestine is reduced, limiting fat digestion, especially long-chain fatty acids. However, as breastmilk is already emulsified the need for bile for fat digestion is limited. Intestinal reabsorption is immature, partly due to immature active transport mechanisms in the ileum. This may be further impaired in *preterm infants* where gut motility is uncoordinated. Bile acid uptake and clearance by the liver is reduced and the *newborn* has relatively high serum bile acid concentrations (Shaffer, 1991).

The liver is also a major organ of nutrient metabolism. *At birth*, the liver is functionally immature in a number of areas. For example, amino acid metabolism is limited and more of the amino acids are 'essential' from the diet. In addition to the eight amino acids considered essential in adults, *infants* are also thought to require a dietary supply of histidine, taurine, tyrosine and cystine (Macleod, 1994).

The Pancreas

The exocrine function of the pancreas does not mature until *late infancy*. Pancreatic amylase is produced in the pancreatic acini from *birth* where it accumulates until it is released into the duodenum from *4–6 months of age* (Lebenthal and Lee, 1980). Significant levels of activity are not achieved until *9–12 months of age* (Milla, 1986). Pancreatic lipase is produced from *30 weeks gestation* in low concentrations until well into the *first year of life*. It requires the presence of colipase and bile salts to function effectively. Pancreatic lipase does not hydrolyse milk fats well, although this is significantly improved if the milk has been predigested by gastric lipase (Manson and Weaver, 1997). Pancreatic proteases are secreted from *26 weeks gestation* but activity is low in the *first few weeks of life*, increasing 10 fold by *9 months of age* (Milla, 1986).

The immaturity of the pancreas during the first few months of life, is an important factor in the recommendation by the Department of Health (1994) to delay the introduction of weaning until 4 months.

The Small Intestine

Development of structure

The normal length of small intestine in *term neonates* is approximately 200–250cm (Warner and Ziegler, 1993). The mature length is known to be very variable in adults, from 300–850cm, similar differences are likely to exist in children (Nightingale, 1994; Vanderhoof, 1995).

In the *newborn period*, in both term and preterm babies, the epithelium is relatively permeable, allowing the absorption of whole sugars and proteins. This matures rapidly, generally within the *first 4 days*, with the tightening of junctional complexes and loss of pinocytosis. It is not clear whether this is an adaptive process, facilitating the uptake of antibodies and other useful macromolecules in the vulnerable postnatal period, or if it is simply a matter of structural immaturity (Weaver *et al.*, 1984). It may also provide a possible route for allergens (Cusson,1994).

Chemical digestion in the small intestine

The brush border enzymes, sucrase and maltase are present in mature concentrations *at birth*. There is also a high level of glucoamylase activity, with one study demonstrating that infants at *1 month of age* have levels comparable with *5 year olds* (Lebenthal and Lee, 1980). Lactase activity is also high during *early infancy*, stimulated by feeding. Weaver *et al.* (1986) demonstrated that within *5 days of feeding* lactase activity reached 98 per cent efficiency, even in *preterm infants*. Peptidases are also at near adult levels of activity *at birth*. The capacity for glucose, water and salt absorption increases throughout *infancy and childhood*, with *older children and adults* absorbing twice the concentration of water at the same concentration of glucose as *younger infants* (Milla, 1983).

Dehydrated infants and young children are given commercially manufactured oral rehydration solutions containing carefully calculated concentrations of water, salt and glucose that optimize their capacity for absorption across the immature membrane. Home made solutions may be dangerous as overconcentration of glucose or salt may increase faecal fluid losses through the creation of an osmotic gradient pulling fluid into the gut lumen rather than facilitating absorption from the gut into the circulation.

Mechanical digestion in the small intestine

In the mature, small intestine there are well defined patterns of motility. *Preterm infants*, motor function is poorly coordinated. Infants of *26–29 weeks gestation* have disorganized patterns of motor activity. Immature fetal motor activity begins to develop between *weeks 30–33*, resembling the mature response from *week 34*. Motor activity in the fed state is less well researched, although from *35 weeks gestation* a relatively mature response is made (Bisset *et al.*, 1988, Milla, 1986). Maturation appears to depend on the integrated development of the smooth muscle, enteric nervous system and humoral environment (Bisset *et al.*, 1988).

The Large Intestine

Development of structure

The large intestine is approximately 40cm in length in the *term neonate*, in contrast to 150cm in adults (Weaver, 1991).

Chemical digestion in the large intestine

Until *28 weeks gestation* it is lined with villi and secretes brush border enzymes, though at a lower level than the small intestine. Colonic transport in *infants* has not been widely researched, but it appears that sodium absorption and anion exchange are poorly developed *at birth*, improving rapidly during the *first year of life* (Milla, 1983). Thus salt and water conservation is immature *at birth* giving rise to a relatively high stool output during *infancy*.

The gut is sterile in the fetus. Colonization with bacteria begins immediately after *birth* and proceeds rapidly throughout the *first few days*. Bacteria contribute to the hydrolysis and fermentation of undigested carbohydrates reaching the large intestine into short chain fatty acids, which can be used as an energy source. In *early infancy*, the most common colonic bacteria are Enterobacter, Bifidobacteria, Bacteriodes and Clostridium. The bacterial profile differs between infants fed on breast milk and those fed on formula feeds (see Chapter 10 for description of bacterial flora within the GI Tract). During weaning there is a gradual change to the adult pattern of gut flora with a wider range of microorganisms.

Mechanical digestion in the large intestine (see also 'defecation')

Up to *2 years of age*, incomplete neural maturation is demonstrated, with many immature ganglia. Maturation may not be complete until *5 years of age* (Israel, 1991).

Stool frequency is very variable throughout life, varying between individuals and according to diet. In the *first week of life* between one and nine stools are passed daily, reducing to one to seven stools from the *second to the twentieth week*. However, it is not unusual for healthy individuals to be outside this range. During the *first week of life*, there appears to be no difference in stool frequency between babies fed on breast milk or formula feeds. *After the first week*, breast fed babies tend to pass stools more frequently, which are larger and more fluid. After weaning, this difference disappears. High fibre and vegetarian diets produce bulkier stools in adults (Davies *et al.*, 1986; Kelsay *et al.*, 1978) and probably also in children. The early introduction of high fibre diets for children may result in under-nutrition due to the low energy density of such foods. Consequently fibre intake should be gradually increased during *pre-school years* with an accompanying increase in fluid intake (Wardley *et al.*, 1997).

Box 8.4   High Fibre Diets in Childhood

- Recommendations for high fibre diets for adults are not appropriate for infants and young children.
- The early introduction of high fibre diets for children may result in undernutrition due to the low energy density of such foods.

Consequently fibre intake should be gradually increased during pre-school years with an accompanying increase in fluid intake (Wardley et al., 1997).

Defecation

In *infancy and early childhood*, rectal distension promotes the relaxation of the external sphincter and defecation occurs as an involuntary act. However, as voluntary control of defecation is achieved, rectal distension promotes the contraction of the external sphincter, allowing defecation to be postponed until an appropriate time.

Achievement of voluntary control tends to be a gradual, learned process, during early childhood. Stools tend to become fewer and more solid during the *first year of life*. Around *15–18 Months of age*, the child begins to indicate that they have wet or soiled, and to recognize the urge to defecate. Many children develop bowel control around *18 months of age* and the upper age limit in western cultures is considered to be *2–3 years*, but other cultures vary. Sometimes control is apparently achieved much earlier, but this may be due to parents recognizing the child's defecation habits and putting the child on the pot at the appropriate moment, usually after a meal. Defecation is then due either to reflex conditioning or lucky timing, rather than true voluntary control (Murphy, 1991).

Immune Functions

The important immune functions of the gastrointestinal tract are discussed in Chapter 10.

Box 8.5   Breast Milk and Infant Formula

There is universal agreement that breast feeding provides the best source of nutrition for young babies. The composition of breast is designed for human infants in the following ways:

- The lowest protein concentration of any mammalian milk provides a low solute load for the infant's immature kidney.
- A high whey to casein ratio, which appears to be more easily digested than milk with a higher casein content (Inch, 1994), as a softer curd in formed in the stomach.
- A high proportion of fats provides a good energy source. The proportion of long-chain polyunsaturated fatty acids may be ideal for

promoting growth and development of the brain (Willatts *et al.*, 1998) (see Chapter 3).

- Carbohydrate is supplied mainly by lactose, which the infant is readily able to utilize. Minerals, such as iron, are present in relatively low concentrations in the easily absorbed form of lactoferrin (Inch, 1994).
- Fresh breast milk contains numerous non-nutritional factors, which make an important contribution to healthy development. Enzymes, such as breast milk lipase, aid digestion of specific nutrients. Important immunoglobulins, such as IgA, and other anti-bacterial molecules (detail of which can be found in chapter 10) offer significant protection against infection (Hamosh, 1996).
- Protection against gastrointestinal infection is also enhanced because milk fed from the breast is uncontaminated.
- Breast milk colonizes the intestine with bacteria, which compete favourably with pathogens such as e-coli (Newburg, 1999).
- Many growth factors, such as epidermal growth factor and hormones, such as pituitary, thyroid and adrenal hormones, are detectable in breast milk. These may promote maturation of the digestive, and other, systems (Aynsley-Green, 1991).

Although the relative contribution of each specific benefit is difficult to evaluate, overall, breast-fed infants are less likely to suffer from a wide range of disorders including wheezing and allergy (Burr *et al.*, 1993), respiratory tract illness (Wright *et al.*, 1989), otitis media (Duncan *et al.*, 1993), gastrointestinal infections in later childhood (Howie *et al.*, 1990) and sudden infant death syndrome (Ford *et al.*, 1993). There is a lower incidence of insulin dependent diabetes mellitus among children who were breast fed (Borch-Johnsen *et al.*, 1984; Virtanen *et al.*, 1993).

Infants who are not breast-fed require a modified formula milk. Formula milks have an overall nutritional composition similar to breast milk, although the precise amino acid, fatty acid, and micronutrient profiles may differ considerably from breast milk. The non-nutrient substances present in breast milk cannot currently be added to artificial formulas and it is of interest to note that in other species (calves and piglets) denial of colostrum leads to a high mortality rate (Weaver *et al.*, 1984).

Box 8.6   Weaning

Weaning may be defined as 'the process of expanding the diet to include foods and drinks other than breast milk or infant formula' (Department of Health, 1994). Weaning becomes necessary when the infant outgrows the nutritional provision of breast milk or infant formula. Current weaning recommendations in the UK (Department of Health, 1994) are that, for most infants, weaning should not be commenced before *4 months of age* and by *6 months of age* a mixed diet should be offered. Earlier weaning is generally discouraged for the following reasons:

- *Neuromuscular coordination* – Head control and development of feeding skills may not be adequate to cope with different textures.
- *Kidney function* may also be too immature to cope with the greater concentrations of solutes and reduced fluid volumes associated with weaning (see chapter 9).
- *Gastrointestinal function*- There is an increase in saliva, gastric and pancreatic enzymes and bile, between *4–6 months*.

Weaning should normally be underway by *6 months* as the energy and nutrient content of human or formula milks is unlikely to be adequate for the increasing needs of the infant (Lawson, 1994). In particular, the iron content of milk is unlikely to be adequate after the first *4–6 months*. Iron deficiency anaemia is the most common nutritional disorder of early childhood (Department of Health, 1994). The *4–6 month* period tends to be the time when infants become interested in putting things in their mouths and are likely to be tolerant to new textures. There are concerns that delaying weaning beyond this period may miss a 'critical period' of development and make introduction of solids later on more difficult (Stevenson and Allaire, 1991). However, the existence of a 'critical period' for weaning has not been proven (Milla, 1991). Although there is widespread professional agreement about the age of weaning, Foster *et al.* (1997) indicated that 91% of infants had received weaning foods before *4 months of age*.

Assessment of Gastrointestinal Function

Assessment of the gastrointestinal tract is outlined below in a top to toe structure with a primary focus on physiological aspects.

Mouth

Lips are examined for colour and skin integrity/turgor. Colour can provide indicators of anaemia if pale, or infection if reddened, while skin integrity/turgor can provide information about hydration, trauma to the mouth and, if dry, it may indicate persistent mouth breathing. In the *neonate* the lips are examined at birth for clefts.

Gums and oral mucosa are also inspected for colour, for the same reasons as the lips, and additionally moisture and general condition. Moisture again indicates hydration and inspection of the condition of the mucosa may reveal ulceration (which if persistent may indicate inflammatory bowel disease), Kopliks spots (small red spots with bluish-white centres in the mouth) in measles, oral vessicles in chickpox, or white plaques in the candida albicans infection commonly known as thrush. Inflammation of the gums may indicate gingivitis which is associated with poor dental hygiene.

Teeth are observed for the timing of eruption and shedding – delay occurs in some congenital disorders such as hypothyroidism. Once they erupt (see Figures 8.4 and 8.5), they are examined for condition, shape & colour. Some abnormal shapes are associated with specific diseases such as the notched incisors in congenital syphilis and peg shaped teeth in ectodermal dysplasias. Discoloration may occur with some drug therapy eg oral iron can stain teeth black.

Salivation is, as mentioned above, related to age with increased volumes after *3 months of age*, apparently decreasing once voluntary control of swallowing is achieved. Salivation may also increase in mumps and, in the *neonate*, bubbling saliva may indicate oesophageal atresia or tracheoesophageal fistula.

The palate is examined in the *newborn* for patency as cleft palate is a relatively common congenital anomaly, and in all ages for colour and shape. Petechiae – small round dark red spots caused by bleeding into the skin or mucous membranes) may be present in rubella.

Feeding

Assessment of gastrointestinal function in all children should start with a comprehensive assessment of daily nutritional intake, which should be analysed for the relative content of the major food groups and compared to the most recent guidelines available for the age group concerned. For example the Department of Health's (1994) guidelines on weaning and the weaning diet. Readers are refered to Wardley *et al.* (1997) and Thompson (1998) for more detail.

In *infancy* it is important to make an assessment of the type, frequency, volume and/or duration of milk feeds to ensure adequate intake of fluid and nutrients. With the first feeds, whether given by breast or bottle there is an opportunity to assess the infant's rooting, sucking and swallowing reflexes. There are numerous causes of swallowing difficulties, dysphagia, from the anatomical such as clefts, to neuromuscular eg, cerebral palsy and inflammatory or traumatic causes. See Bisset (1992, p. 492) for further detail.

In breast feeding the position of the infant feeding at the breast is important. Wardley et al. (1997) describe this as 'belly to belly' with the baby facing the breast, resulting in more effective 'latching on', although neonates do not form a tight seal with the breast until the necessary facial musculature has developed.

Vomiting reported during milk feeding needs to be assessed to establish the frequency, pattern and character of vomitus. Small quantities of feed are commonly passively regurgitated before the introduction of solid food and is termed 'possitting' or 'physiological' gastroesophageal reflux, attributed to the immaturity of the lower oesophageal sphincter (Thompson, 1998; Wardley *et al.*, 1997). Where larger volumes of milk are regurgitated the volume of feeds should be assessed, as the cause may be over feeding. Where active vomiting occurs this should be explored further.

Classically vomiting which is projectile and accompanied by visible peristal- sis and poor weight gain, is indicative of pyloric stenosis – congenital narrow- ing of the pylorus, the muscular outlet from the stomach. There are many more causes of vomiting in childhood, for more detail see Bisset (1992, p. 502).

The reaction and position of the baby after feeding should also be observed. Some *infants* with gastroesophageal reflux have been reported to twist the head to the side after feeds as a result of vagal stimulation (Sutcliffe, 1969 cited in Bisset, 1992).

Abdomen

Abdominal assessment is usually recorded using the nine sections described in surface anatomy. See any major anatomy and physiology textbook for a diagram. Assessment of the abdomen uses inspection, auscultation, palpation and percussion.

Inspection

Shape and contour may reveal distension or bulges – although it should be noted that children are naturally 'pot bellied' until around *5 years of age* as the pelvis is narrow and more abdominal contents and the bladder (when full) are therefore suprapubic. The abdomen should be seen to move with respiration. If absent, it may indicate abdominal distension, due to constipation, ascites (free fluid in the abdomen) or an inflammatory process such as peritonitis. Peristalsis is not usually visible, but as mentioned above may be seen in pyloric stenosis. The umbilicus should be examined as, in the *neonate*, there may be a discharge and inflammation indicating infection. In both the *neonate and the older child* a hernia may be visible. The position of the child should be observed as abdominal pain is often associated with the fetal position. Intermittent abdominal pain in *infants* is often attributed to infantile colic, which usually subsides after *3 months of age* (Bisset, 1992). Colic occurs in both breast- and bottle-fed babies, although in the breast-fed it has been attributed to inadequate intake of hindmilk, causing rapid gastric emptying and lactose overload (Woolridge and Fisher, 1988 cited in Thompson, 1998).

Exomphalos and gastroschisis will be immediately obvious as the bowel is visible outside the abdominal wall. Congenital anomalies require urgent medical and surgical investigation.

Auscultation

Bowel sounds, described as intermittent tinkling, crackling sounds, are normally heard over the whole abdomen (Forfar, 1992). These sounds increase with increased peristalsis, for example in obstruction such as pyloric stenosis or intussusception (the telescoping of one part of the bowel into another), and are absent with a paralytic ileus (absence of peristalsis) such as might occur in peritonitis (Forfar 1992) or when the baby fails to pass meconium (see under Anus below).

Palpation

Palpation of the abdomen can detect whether the abdomen is soft, hard or distended. It may identify hernias and masses such as the enlargement of the pylorus or a soft mass such as intussusception. Liver and spleen enlargement can be identified, although it should be noted that in *infants and children* the liver is normally 1cm below the costal margin (Forfar, 1992). Enlargement beyond this may indicate liver disease such as the bilary atresia mentioned earlier. Distension due to ascites may be detected by generating a 'fluid thrill' or through percussion (Forfar, 1992).

Anus

The anus can be assessed for the following:

- Presence – its absence indicates an imperforate anus;
- Position, in relation to normal – abnormal position may indicate other underlying structural abnormalities;
- Muscle tone – a reduction or absence of tone may be associated with spina bifida;
- Fissures (a cleft like defect) which may have resulted from passing a constipated stool or if accompanied by bruising or other signs of trauma, may indicate child abuse;
- Itching or scratching especially at night often caused by infection with threadworm;
- Inflammation or rashes – oral thrush is often accompanied by nappy rash – candida infection of the nappy area; and
- Patency, usually confirmed by the passage of meconium. Where this does not occur it is know as a meconium ileus and may be the result of a large segment Hirschprungs or cystic fibrosis (the result of thickened secretions in the gut).

Bowel Pattern

The frequency, consistency, colour and odour of stools should be assessed. The first stool – meconium, is dark green or tar coloured and is usually present in the *first three days after birth*, followed by transitional stools of increasing yellow colour over the remainder of the *first week of life* (Delahoussaye, 1994; Fuller and Schaller-Ayers, 2000). Breast-fed babies may then have frequent loose, yellow stools with a characteristic slightly sweet smell. Infants fed on formula have more solid, whiter stools with a more offensive smell indicative of the higher fat residue. Once mixed feeding is introduced the nature and consistency of all children's stools is related to dietary and fluid intake. The frequency of stools is discussed earlier and readers are reminded that there is considerable variation between individuals so the deviation from the individual's normal pattern should also be assessed. The presence of mucous or blood is abnormal and merits further examination. Diarrhoea is of particular note in the *infant and small child* as they have a reduced ability to retain fluids and are therefore more vulnerable to serious dehydration through such fluid losses. Although toddler diarrhoea occurring between *6 months and 5 years of age,* where the child passes increasingly fluid stools through the day often containing visible foods, is not usually associated with any failure to thrive. Its aetiology is unclear although there appear to be links with the later development of other gastrointestinal problems (Bisset, 1992).

Broad Areas of Asessment Related to Gastrointestinal Function

Some areas of assessment do not relate directly to one part of the gastrointestinal system but reflect the functioning of the system as a whole and can add significantly to information about the child's health status. Much of this information can be gathered from the history of the child and family. Asking about any family history of problems concerning the function of the gastrointestinal tract may reveal that other family members have had a disease that is known to have a familial pattern of inheritance, for example pyloric stenosis (Bisset, 1992) or late acquisition of continence. Concerning the individual child, their birth weight, length, head circumference and gestation are indicators of intrauterine growth and act as a baseline for later measurements. Assessment of growth is a useful measure of the efficacy of this body system – readers are referred to Hall and Elliman (2003) for recommendations on child health surveillance of which growth monitoring forms a part. Other areas for assessment include exposure to contaminated food or water as a result of recent travel or hygiene practices such as techniques for making up formula feeds and handwashing (Cusson, 1994).

Conclusion

Prenatal development of the digestive system is complex. *At birth*, healthy term infants are capable of feeding and of digesting and absorbing breast milk or a modified formula. However, many aspects of the system continue to mature during infancy. Progression to a mixed diet is not recommended before *4 months of age*. Maturation and feeding skills continue to develop throughout *early childhood* and this is reflected in the balance of food appropriate for each age group. Assessment of the gastrointestinal system can provide a wide range of information, which may elucidate either variations within normal parameters or more serious underlying disease. Generally the most commonly used assessment related to the digestive system during infancy and childhood is measurement of growth, the outcome of the functioning of the gastrointestinal system.

Review Questions

1. What structures of the gastrointestinal tract will already have started to develop by the time pregnancy can be confirmed?
2. During which stage of pregnancy does the majority of growth in the gastrointestinal system occur?
3. What features of the physiological development of the gastrointestinal tract underpin the recommendation not to commence weaning before 4 months of age?
4. When is it realistic to expect a child to be continent of faeces and why?
5. Outline the assessment of the gastrointestinal tract from top to toe.

Further Reading

Rutishauser, S (1994) *Physiology and Anatomy. A Basis for Nursing and Health Care.* Edinburgh: Churchill Livingstone. Chapter 6. Digestive System. This textbook takes an integrated functional approach to physiology and anatomy. It is well written and easy to read, supported by some excellent diagrams. This chapter is a good place to start if the reader is looking to develop an understanding of the basics of gastrointestinal functioning.

Larsen, W (1997) *Human embryology*, 2nd edn. New York: Churchill Livingstone.
Moore, K and Persaud, T (1998) *Before We Are Born*, 5th edn. Philadelphia: Saunders. Both of the above texts provide detailed explanations of the embryological development of the gastrointestinal tract.

Wardley, BL, Puntis, JWL and Taitz, LS (1997) *Handbook of Child Nutrition*, 2nd edn. Oxford. Oxford University Press. Provides further detail on a wide range of aspects of childhood nutrition. From recommended diets for children across the age range to feeding problems in infancy, diarrhoea, food allergy, obesity and dietary management of a range of metabolic and other chronic diseases.

Thompson, J M (ed.) (1998) *Nutritional Requirements of Infants and Young Children*. Oxford: Blackwell Science. This book takes a chronological approach to the topic for the first 5 years of life. Each age-related section addresses normal development of feeding, recommendations for that age group and common problems encountered.

Bisset, WM (1992) Chapter 11. Disorders of the alimentary tract and liver. In Campbell, AGM and McIntosh, N (eds), *Forfar and Arneil's Textbook of Paediatrics*, 4th edn. Edinburgh. Churchill Livingstone. This chapter provides further detail on abnormalities and diseases of the gastrointestinal tract. Specifically p. 492 provides further detail on causes of dysphagia whilst p502 provides detail on causes of vomiting in childhood.

References

Adamson, I, Esangbedo, A, Okolo, AA and Omene, JA (1988) Pepsin and its multiple forms in early life. *Biology of the Neonate*, 53(5), 267–73.

Alexander, R (1991) Prespeech and feeding. In JL Bigge (ed.), *Teaching Individuals with Physical and Multiple Disabilities*. New York: Macmillan.

Antonowicz, I and Lebenthal, E (1977) Developmental pattern of small intestinal enterokinase and disaccharidase activities in the human fetus. *Gastroenterology*, 72(6), 1299–1303.

Aynsley-Green, A (1991) Endocrine function of the gut in early life. In W Walker, P Durie, J Hamilton, J Walker-Smith and J Watkins, (eds), *Pediatric Gastrointestinal Disease*. Philadelphia: Decker.

Betz, CL, Hunsberger, M and Wright, S (1994) *Family-centered Nursing Care of Children*, 2nd edn. Philadephia. W.B. Saunders.

Bisset, WM (1992) Chapter 11. Disorders of the alimentary tract and liver. In AGM Campbell and N McIntosh (eds) *Forfar and Arneil's Textbook of Paediatrics*, 4th edn. Edinburgh: Churchill Livingstone.

Bissett, W, Watt, J, Rivers, R and Milla, P (1988) Ontogeny of fasting small intestinal motor activity in the human infant, *Gut*, 29, 483–8.

Borch-Johnsen, K, Joner, G, Mandrup-Poulsen, T, Christy, M, Zachau-Christiansen, B, Kastrup, K and Nerup, J (1984) Relation between breast-feeding and incidence rates of insulin-dependent diabetes mellitus. A hypothesis. *Lancet*, 2(8411), 1083–6.

Burr, ML, Limb, ES, Maguire, MJ, Amarah L, Eldridge, BA, Layzell, JC and Merrett, TG (1993) Infant feeding, wheezing and allergy: A prospective study. *Archives of Disease in Childhood*, 68(6), 724–8.

Cambell, AGM and McIntosh, N (eds) (1992) *Forfar and Arneil's Textbook of Paediatrics*, 4th edn. Edinburgh: Churchill Livingstone.

Cusson, RM (1994) Chapter 35. Altered digestive function. In CL Betz, M Hunsberger and S Wright *Family-centered Nursing Care of Children*, 2nd edn. Philadephia: W.B. Saunders.

Davies, GJ, Crowder, M, Reid, B and Dickerson, JW (1986) Bowel function measurements of individuals with different eating patterns, *Gut*, 27(2), 164–9.

Delahoussaye, CP (1994) Chapter 4 Families with neonates. In CL Betz, M Hunsberger and S Wright (1994) *Family-centered Nursing Care of Children*, 2nd edn. Philadephia: W.B. Saunders.

Department of Health (1994) *Weaning and the Weaning Diet. Report on Health and Social Subjects no.45*, London: HMSO.

Duncan, B, Ey, J, Holberg, CJ, Wright, AL, Martinez, FD and Taussig, LM (1993) Exclusive breast-feeding for at least 4 months protects against otits media, *Pediatrics*, 91(5), 867–72.

Ewer, AK, Durbin, GM, Morgan, MEI and Booth, IW (1994) Gastric emptying in preterm infants. *Archives of Disease in Childhood*, 71, F24–F27.

Fink, BR Martin, RW and Rohrmann, CA (1979) Biomechanics of the human epiglottis, *Acta Otolaryngology*, 87(5–6), 554–9.

Ford, RP, Taylor, BJ, Mitchell, EA, Enright, SA, Stewart, AW, Becroft, DM, Scragg, R, Hassall, IB, Barry, DM. and Allen, EM (1993) Breastfeeding and the risk of sudden infant death syndrome. *International Journal of Epidemiology*, 22(5), 885–90.

Forfar, JO (1992) Chapter 2. History taking, physical examination and screening. In AGM Cambell and N McIntosh (eds), *Forfar and Arneil's Textbook of Paediatrics*, 4th edn. Edinburgh: Churchill Livingstone.

Foster, K, Lader, D and Cheesborough, S (1997) *Infant Feeding 1995*. London: HSMO.

Fuller, J and Schaller-Ayers, J (2000) *Health Assessment. A Nursing Approach*, 3rd edn. Philadelphia: Lippincott.

Grand, RJ, Watkins, JB and Torti, FM (1976) Development of the human gastrointestinal tract. *Gastroenterology*, 70, 790–810.

Grybowski, JD (1965) The swallowing mechanism of the neonate. Esophageal and gastric motility. *Pediatrics*, 35, 445–2.

Hall, DMB and Elliman, D (eds) (2003) *Health for All Children*. 4th edn. Oxford. Oxford University Press.

Hall, JG, Froster-Iskenius, UG and Allanson, JE (1989) *Handbook of Normal Physical Measurements*. Oxford: Oxford University Press.

Hamosh, M (1996) Breastfeeding: Unravelling the mysteries of mother's milk. *Medscape Womens Health*, 1(9), 4.

Howie, PW, Forsyth, JS, Ogston, SA and Florey, CD (1990) Protective effect of breast feeding against infection. *BMJ*, 300(6716), 11–16.

Inch, S (1994) The importance of breastfeeding, In *The Growing Cycle: Child Mother Child*. London: National Dairy Council.

Israel, EJ (1991) The Intestines. In W Walker, P Durie, J Hamilton, J Walker-Smith and J Watkins (eds), *Pediatric Gastrointestinal Disease*. Philadelphia: Decker.

Iwayama, K and Eishima, M (1997) Neonatal sucking behaviour and its development until 14 months. *Early Human Development*, 47, 1–9.

Jaber, L, Cohen, IJ and Mor, A (1992) Fever associated with teething. *Archives of Disease in Childhood*, 67, 233–4.

Kelly, EJ, Lagopoulos, M and Primrose, JN (1993) Immunocytochemical localisation of parietal cells and G cells in the developing human stomach. *Gut*, 34(8),1057–59.

Kelly, E and Newell, S (1994) Gastric ontogeny: Clinical implications. *Archives of Disease in Childhood*, 71, F136–F141.

Kelsay, JL, Behall, KM and Prather, ES (1978) Effect of fibre from fruits and vegetables on metabolic responses of human subjects. *American Journal of Clinical Nutrition*, 31(7), 1149–53.

Lacroix, B, Kedinger, M, Simon-Assmann, P and Haffen, K (1984a) Early organogenesis of human small intestine: Scanning electron microscopy and brush-border enzymology. *Gut*, 25(9), 925–30.

Lacroix, B, Kedinger, M, Simon-Assmann, P, Rousset, M, Zweibaum, A and Haffen, K (1984b) Developmental pattern of brush border enzymes in the human fetal colon. Correlation with some morphogenetic events. *Early Human Development*, 9(2), 95–103.

Lang, S, Lawrence, C and Orme, R (1994) Cup feeding: an alternative method of infant feeding. *Archives of Disease in Childhood*, 71, 365–9.

Larsen, W (1997) *Human embryology*, 2nd edn. New York: Churchill Livingstone.

Lawson, M (1994) Feeding young children: Recommendations of the COMA Weaning Report. In National Dairy Council, *The Growing Cycle: Child Mother Child*. London: National Dairy Council.

Lebenthal, E and Lee, P (1980) Glucoamylase and disaccharidase activity in normal subjects and in patients with mucosal injury of the small intestine. *Journal of Pediatrics*, 97(3), 389–93.

Lebenthal, E, Lee, P and Heitlinger, LA (1983) Impact of development of the gastrointestinal tract on infant feeding. *Journal of Pediatrics*, 102(1), 1–9.

Macleod, A (1994) Parenteral nutrition. In V. Shaw. and M Lawson (eds), *Clinical Paediatric Dietetics*. Oxford: Blackwell.

Manson,W and Weaver, L (1997) Fat digestion in the neonate. *Archives of Disease in Childhood*, 76, F206–F211.

Marino, LR, Bacon, BR, Hines, JD and Halpin, TC (1984) Parietal cell function of full-term and premature infants: Unstimulated gastric acid and intrinsic factor secretion. *Journal of Pediatric Gastroenterology and Nutrition*, 3(1), 23–7.

McVerry, M and Collin, J (1998) Managing the child with gastrenteritis. *Paediatric Nursing* 10(8), 29–33.

Ménard, D (1994) Development of human intestinal and gastric enzymes. *Acta Paediatrica Scandanavia*, Suppl 405; 1–6.

Ménard, D, Monfils, S and Tremblay, E (1995) Ontogeny of gastric lipase and pepsin activities. *Gastroenterology*, 108, 1650–6.

Milla, PJ (1983) Aspects of fluid and electrolyte absorption in the newborn. *Journal of Pediatric Gastroenterology and Nutrition*, 2(Suppl.1), S272–S276.

Milla, P. (1986) The weanling's gut *Acta Paediatrica Scandanavia* Suppl 323; 5–13

Milla, P (1991) Feeding, tasting and sucking. In W Walker, P Durie, J Hamilton, J Walker-Smith and J Watkins, (eds), *Pediatric Gastrointestinal Disease*. Philadelphia: Decker.

Milla, P (1996) Intestinal motility during ontogeny and intestinal pseudo-obstruction in children. *Pediatric Clinics of North America*, 43(2), 511–32.

Moazam, F, Kirby, WJ, Rodgers, BM and McGuigan, JE (1984) Physiology of gastrin production in neonates and infants.*Annals of Surgery*, 199(4), 389–92.

Moore, K and Persaud, T (1998) *Before We Are Born*, 5th ed. Philadelphia: Saunders.

Moroz, SP, Espinoza, J, Cumming, WA and Diamant, NE. (1976) Lower esophageal function in children with and without gastroesophageal reflux *Gastroenterology*, 71(2), 236–41.

Murphy, M (1991) Constipation. In W Walker, P Durie, J Hamilton, J Walker-Smith, and J Watkins (eds), *Pediatric Gastrointestinal Disease*. Philadelphia: Decker.

Murray, RD, Kerznar, B, Sloan, HR, McClung, HJ, Gilbert, M and Ailabouni A (1986) The contribution of salivary amylase to glucose polymer hydrolysis in premature infants. *Pediatric Research*, 20(2), 186–91.

Newburg, DS (1999) Human milk glycoconjugates that inhibit pathogens. *Current Medical Chemistry*, 6(2),117–27.

Newell, SJ, Sarkar, PK, Durbin, GM, Booth, IW and McNeish, AS (1988) Maturation of the lower oesophageal sphincter in the preterm baby. *Gut*, 29(2), 167–72.

Nightingale, J (1994) Clinical problems of short bowel and their treatment. *Proceedings of the Nutrition Society*, 53, 373–91.

Nissen, E, Lilja, G, Matthieson, AS, Ransjo-Arvidsson, AB, Uvnas-Moberg, K and Widstrom, AM (1995) Effects of maternal pethidine on infants' developing breast feeding behaviour. *Acta Paediatrica*, 84(2), 140–5.

Nurko, S (1991) Esophageal motility. In W Walker, P Durie, J Hamilton, J Walker-Smith and J Watkin (eds), *Pediatric Gastrointestinal Disease*. Philadelphia: Decker.

Orlic, D and Lev, R (1977) An electron microscopic study of intrepithelial lymphocytes in human fetal small intestine. *Laboratory Investigation*, 37(6), 554–61.

Schmitz, J (1991) Digestive and absorptive function. In W Walker, P Durie, J Hamilton, J Walker-Smith, and J Watkins, (eds), *Pediatric Gastrointestinal Disease*. Philadelphia: Decker.

Schwartz, JL, Niman, CW and Gisel, EG (1984) Tongue movements in normal preschool children during eating. *American Journal of Occupational Therapy*, 38(2), 87–93.

Shaffer, E (1991) Hepatobiliary system: Structure and function. In W Walker, P Durie, J Hamilton, J Walker-Smith, and J Watkins (eds), *Pediatric Gastrointestinal Disease*. Philadelphia: Decker.

Siegal, M, Lebenthal, E and Krantz, B (1984) Effect of caloric density on gastric emptying in premature infants. *Journal of Pediatrics*, 104, 118–22.

Splinter, WM and Schreiner, MS (1999) Preoperative fasting in children. *Anesth. Analg.* 89(1), 80–9.

Stevenson, R and Allaire, J (1991) The development of normal feeding and swallowing. *Pediatric Clinics of North America*, 38(6), 1439–53.

Sutcliffe, J (1969) Torsion spasms and abnormal postures in children with hiatus hernia: Sandifer's Syndrome. *Progress in Pediatric Radiology*, 2, 190–7.

Thomas,B (1994) *Manual of Dietetic Practice*, 2nd edn. Oxford: Blackwell Scientific.

Thompson J M (Ed.) (1998) *Nutritional Requirements of Infants and Young Children*. Oxford. Blackwell Science.

Tomomasa, T, Hyman, PE, Itoh, K, *et al.* (1987) Gastroduodenal motility in neonates: Response to human milk compared with cow's milk formula. *Pediatrics*, 80, 434.

Touloukian, RJ and Smith, GJ (1983) Normal intestinal length in preterm infants. *Journal of Pediatric Surgery*, 18(6), 720–3.

Vanderhoof, J. (1995) Short bowel syndrome in children. *Current Opinion in Pediatrics* 7, 560–8.

Virtanen, SM, Rasanen, L, Ylonen, K, Aro, A, Clayton, D, Langholz, B, Pitkaniemi, J, Savilahti, E, Lounamaa, R and Tuomilehto, J (1993) Early introduction of dairy products associated with increased risk of IDDM in Finnish children. *Diabetes*, 42(2), 1786–90.

Wardley, BL, Puntis, JWL and Taitz, LS (1997) *Handbook of Child Nutrition*, 2nd edn. Oxford: Oxford University Press.

Warner, B and Ziegler, M (1993) Management of the short-bowel syndrome in the pediatric population. *Pediatric Clinics of North America*, 40(6), 1335–49.

Weaver, L (1991) Anatomy and embryology. In W Walker, P Durie, J Hamilton, J Walker-Smith, and J Watkins (eds), *Pediatric Gastrointestinal Disease*. Philadelphia: Decker.

Weaver, L, Laker, M and Nelson, R (1984) Intestinal permeability in the newborn. *Archives of Disease in Childhood*, 59, 236–41.

Weaver, L, Laker, M and Nelson, R (1986) Neonatal intestinal lactase activity. *Archives of Disease in Childhood*, 61, 896–9.

Wershil, B (1991) Gastric function. In W Walker, P Durie, J Hamilton, J Walker-Smith, and J Watkins (eds), *Pediatric Gastrointestinal Disease*. Philadelphia: Decker.

Widstrom, AM, Marchini, G, Matthiesen, AS, Werner, S, Winberg, J and Uvnas-Moberg, K (1988) Nonnutritive sucking in tube-fed preterm infants: Effects on gastric motility and gastric contents of somatostatin. *Journal of Pediatric Gastroenterology and Nutrition*, 7(4), 517–23.

Willatts, P, Forsyth, JS, DiModugno, MK, Varma, S and Colvin, M (1998) Effect of long-chain polyunsaturated fatty acids in infant formula on problem solving at 10 months of age. *Lancet*, 352(9129), 688–91.

Woolridge, M and Fisher, C (1988) Colic, 'overfeeding' and symptoms of lactose malabsorption in the breastfed baby: A possible artefact of feed management? *Lancet*, 2(8607), 382–4.

Wright, AL, Holberg, CJ, Martinez, FD, Morgan, WJ and Taussig, LM. (1989) Breast feeding and lower respiratory tract illness in the first year of life. *BMJ* 299(6705), 946–9.

CHAPTER 9

Control of Body Fluids in Childhood

Agnes Kanneh

Contents

- Overview of Renal Function
- Embryology and Maturation of the Urinary System
- Asessment of Renal Function
- Conclusion
- Review Questions
- Further Reading
- References

Learning Outcomes

At the end of this chapter you will be able to:

- Indicate the homeostatic roles of the kidneys.
- Provide an overview of the function of the kidneys.
- Describe the embryology and maturation of the urinary system.
- Explain why the kidneys are vulnerable to injury and disease.
- Integrate the above theory in the assessment of the child's urinary system.

Introduction

The kidneys, by the very nature of their architecture, are able to maintain the homeostasis of the blood chemistry and regulate fluid volume in health. These processes are dependent on accurate formation of the urinary system in prenatal life, and ongoing maturational processes from birth to adulthood. In order to explore the influence of the developing urinary system on the health of the child, this chapter begins by briefly reviewing the whole of the urinary system. This is followed by an overview of the embryology of the urinary system and the maturational processes occurring during childhood. From this basis the assessment of effective function is presented.

Overview of Renal Function

Homeostasis of body fluids and blood chemistry is the key biological role of the kidneys in the maintenance of health and cellular integrity in the child. This is achieved through three major roles: regulation of blood pressure, volume and pH; excretion of metabolic wastes, toxic and inert agents or chemicals; and synthesis of erythopoetin, renin, prostaglandin and the active form of vitamin D. These roles are accomplished through the formation of urine, which is achieved through three renal processes namely:

1 Filtration of blood;
2 Tubular reabsorption of essential components of the glomerular filtrate; and
3 Secretion of unwanted, toxic or metabolic waste products in urine.

The following are essential for these functions:

- an intact and functional neuro-endocrine pathway;
- an effective systemic blood pressure and renal autoregulation of blood flow;
- an effective circulating blood volume to maintain an adequate renal perfusion;
- a net filtration pressure created by the pressure gradient between transcapillary hydrostatic and oncotic pressures;
- a healthy and adequate renal surface area to facilitate ultrafiltration of blood;
- a selectively permeable glomerular basement membrane; and
- free flow of the formed urine into the bladder with an effective micturition process.

For a fuller explanation of renal function please refer to any good anatomy and physiology textbook, eg, Martini (2001) (see 'Further Reading' section at the end of this chapter).

Embryology and Maturation of the Urinary System

A pre-requisite for renal function is the correct and timely formation of the renal structures in the embryo.

Genetic Basis of Renal Development

The Hox and Pax genes, located on the short arm of chromosome 11 are involved in the initiation of renal development. They encode the information necessary for the induction and survival of renal mesenchymal cells (embryonic connective tissue derived from the mesoderm), and the proliferation of nephron precursor cells. Wilm's Tumour suppressor gene (WT1) is indicated to be necessary for the induction and survival of renal connective tissue cells.

Mutation of the Hox-2 and Pax-2 genes are implicated in renal abnormalities eg, Potter's sequence in which the kidneys fail to develop. The WT1 gene mutation is linked to the loss of tumour-suppression function and subsequent formation of Wilm's tumour (Levy and Kramer, 1999).

Embryology of the Renal System

Cells of the intermediate mesoderm undergo a series of inductive signaling that serves to organize the renal architecture accomplishment in a carefully controlled, regulated, sequential and progressive manner, which for descriptive purposes produces three renal structures:

1 Pronephros (Fore kidney);
2 Mesonephros (Middle kidney); and
3 Metanephros (Permanent kidney).

In mammals, the first two structures are transient with little excretory capacity but are, nonetheless, critical to the formation of the metanephros, the permanent kidney (Gomez and Norwood, 1999).

The pronephros – week 4

The pleural term pronephroi is used here as the two kidneys grow simultaneously. They are derived from cells of the intermediate mesoderm, which at first represent several pairs of solid segmentally arranged cell clusters in the cervical region on the embryo. Their formation subsequently induces growth of tortuous tubular ducts called pronephric ducts. These ducts possess buds at their terminals, are initially attached to the pronephric cell clusters, but eventually form complete fusion with the ducts. Thereafter, the ducts elongate, extending from the cervical region of the embryo to its tail end by the process of cell migration. The epithelium of the pronephric duct and its derivatives act as an inducer to determine the differentiation, shape and form of the proceeding kidneys. The pronephroi, in essence, can be viewed as the rough draft copy of the kidneys and in humans degenerates by the end of the *fourth week* without fulfilling their excretory roles (Polin and Fox, 1998) (see Figure 9.1).

The mesonephros – middle of week 4

As the pronephric tubules degenerate, their midportion induces a new set of kidney tubules in the adjacent tissue. This inductive process leads to the formation of approximately 30 mesonephroi, described as large, elongated excretory organs which extend from the upper thoracic to the upper lumbar region of the embryo. The elongated cell clusters become hollowed out into vesicles. The vesicles in turn flatten, stretch and twist to form the mesonephric tubules (see Figure 9.1). Further transformation causes them to grow out towards the mesonephric duct and open into it as they approach it. The tubules rapidly grow in length, form S-shaped loops and acquire a tuft of capillaries that emerge as the glomeruli. An intriguing process ensues whereby

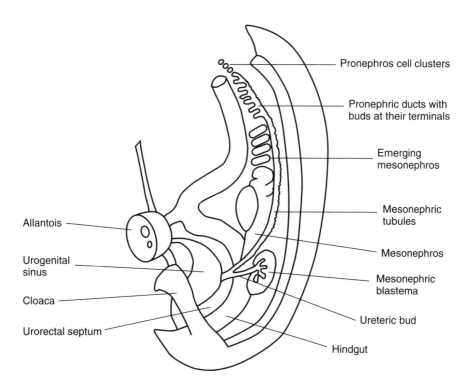

Figure 9.1 The Pronephros, which Originates from the Intermediate Mesoderm

the branches grow towards each other until their ends meet, creating the tangled ball of capillaries called glomeruli. When each glomeruli reaches the medial end of a mesonephric tubule, it makes an indentation, analogous to a closed fist making a punch into an oblong-shaped dough. This is the genesis of the glomerulus and Bowman's capsule which transforms into a cup-like structure, hogs the glomerulus and creates the renal corpuscle. The mesonephroi possess excretory capacity and function briefly in the human embryo. They are the second draft copy of the kidneys in humans but remain the definitive kidneys in fish and amphibians. Regression of the mesonephric tubules is complete in females and any existing remnant to date has no known function. In the male, the mesonephric tubules become the ductus deferens and efferent ducts of the testes (Sadler, 2000).

The metanephros – week 5

The metanephroi are the mammalian permanent or 'true' kidney. The metanephric mesenchyme is the connective tissue that is genetically programmed to form nephrons but, it requires additional inductive signals from the ureteric bud to permit it to differentiate. The tips of the ureteric buds express the RET genes, experimentally shown to be critical to the development of kidneys and ureters. In *week 5* of embryonic life, the ureteric bud grows outward from the mesonephric duct, elongates and penetrates the metanephric mesoderm (see Figures 9.2 and 9.3). Making this contact induces the mesenchyme to become epithelial cells, adhere together and thicken. The ureteric bud and its branches form epithelia of the collecting ducts, renal pelvis, ureter and bladder trigone. The metanephric mesenchyme on the other hand differentiates into the glomerulus, proximal tubule, loop of Henle and interstitial cells (Gilbert 1997). About 20 per cent of the nephrons are formed by *12 weeks* of gestation, 30 per cent by *20 weeks* and human nephrogenesis is complete by *36 weeks* of gestation when the nephrons reach their upper limit of 1 million. Nephrogenesis continues to be part of human development only in preterm babies. Postbirth renal growth is now believed to involve only the elongation of the proximal tubules and loops of Henle (Colón and Ziai, 1985; Ichikawa, 1990).

Box 9.1 Prenatal Development of the 'True' Kidney

- The metanephroi or mammalian permanent or 'true' kidneys begin to develop in the *fifth week* of gestation.
- Metanephric mesenchyme forms the nephrons when inductive signals are received from the ureteric bud.
- The ureteric bud and its branches form the epithelia of the collecting ducts, renal pelvis, ureter and bladder trigone.

- About 20 per cent of the nephrons are formed by *12 weeks* gestation, 30 per cent by *20 weeks* and human nephrogenesis is complete by *36 weeks* gestation when the nephrons reach their upper limit of 1 million.
- Postnatal renal growth is now believed to involve only the elongation of the proximal tubules and loops of Henle.
- Urine production starts soon after glomerular capillary differentiation, at about *12 weeks* gestation.

Significant development is therefore taking place within the first trimester of pregnancy.

The renal pelvis and calyces

On contact with one another, the metanephric mesenchyme induces the ureteric bud to elongate and branch dichotomously (into two branches). The initial single ureteric bud remains the ureter. Its first bifurcation (division into two branches) forms the renal pelvis, and collapse of the next four generations form the minor calyces of the collecting system (Barratt *et al.*, 1999; Moore and Persaud, 2000) (see Figure 9.4).

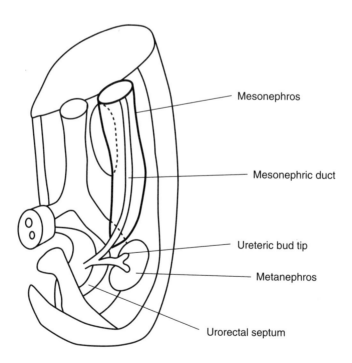

Figure 9.2 The Mesonephros at 6 Weeks

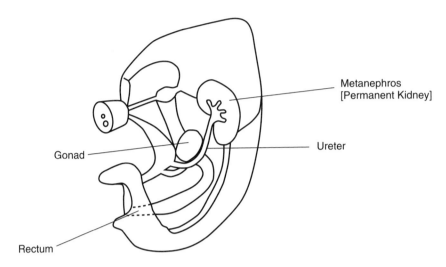

Figure 9.3 The Metanephros at 12 Weeks

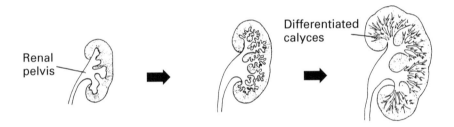

Figure 9.4 Progressive Differentiation of the Metanephros to Produce the Renal Pelvis and Calyces

The glomerulus and Bowman's capsule

Here, the tips of the collecting tubules induce clusters of mesenchymal cells in the metanephric mesoderm to form aggregates and condense into metanephric tissue caps (see Figure 9.5). These aggregates epithelialize and become renal vesicles. They then proceed from this vesicular stage to become comma-shaped, then s-shaped tubules by a process called cleft involution at both curving ends of the comma. The most proximal end of the tubules undergo angiogenesis (the formation of blood vessels). At the most distal end of the S-shape, an open connection is made with the collecting tubules, establishing passage from the Bowman's capsule to the collecting duct.

Continuous lengthening and coiling of the tubules result in the formation of the proximal convoluted tubules, loop of Henle, distal convoluted tubules and the macula densa. Capillaries grow into the proximal ends of the S-shaped

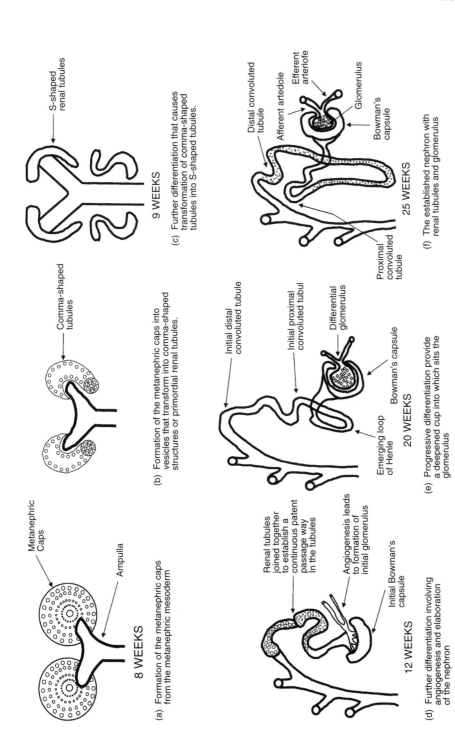

Figure 9.5 Differentiation of the Nephrons to Produce the Glomerulus and Renal Tubules

tubules and differentiate into glomeruli. Urine production starts soon after glomerular capillary differentiation, about *12 weeks* in embryonic life.

Fetal kidneys are subdivided into lobes that are externally visible. The lobulation disappears as the nephrons increase and grow until *36 weeks* in utero. At first, the kidneys are in the pelvic region and lie close to each other. As the fetal abdomen and pelvis grow, the kidneys ascend and become abdominal organs, moving further apart, and attaining their adult position. Ascent of the kidneys stops when they reach and touch the inferior aspect of the adrenal glands, around the *12th week* of embryonic life. They eventually become retroperitoneal on the posterior abdominal wall (Sadler, 2000).

The urinary bladder – by week 12

The bladder originates mostly from the vesicular part of the urogenital sinus, the cranial part of which expands to become the urinary bladder. The transitional epithelium of the inner bladder is derived from embryonic endoderm. At first, the bladder is continuous with the allantois. This vestigial structure soon constricts and transforms into a thick fibrous cord called the urachus, extending from the bladder apex to the umbilicus, represented in the adult by the medium umbilical ligament (see Figure 9.6).

The distal portion of the mesonephric duct is incorporated into the bladder as it enlarges to form the trigone of the bladder. The base of the bladder undergoes traction due to the pull exerted by the ascending kidneys. This causes the ureteric openings to move superolaterally so that the ureters enter obliquely through the base of the bladder. As time progresses, the lining of the trigone is replaced by endodermal epithelium which finally lines the whole of the urinary bladder to become the resilient, distensible transitional epithelium.

The bladder in infants and young children is an abdominal organ. It begins to enter into the pelvis major at approximately *6 years* of age and enters the pelvis minor at *puberty*.

Failure of the lower abdominal wall to grow contributes to the pathology of bladder extrophy (Modi, 1999).

Box 9.2   Bladder Position in Infants and Young Children

- The bladder in infants and young children is an abdominal organ and when full it can be palpated above the symphysis pubis.
- It begins to enter into the pelvis major at approximately *6 years* of age.
- The bladder enters the pelvis minor at *puberty*.

Suprapubic aspiration of urine can be carried out while the bladder remains abdominal to obtain an uncontaminated sample of urine in the critically ill child where urinary tract infection is suspected or needs to be eliminated. As it is an unpleasant procedure, it would not normally be carried out on any child when a sample can be obtained by other means or at a later time.

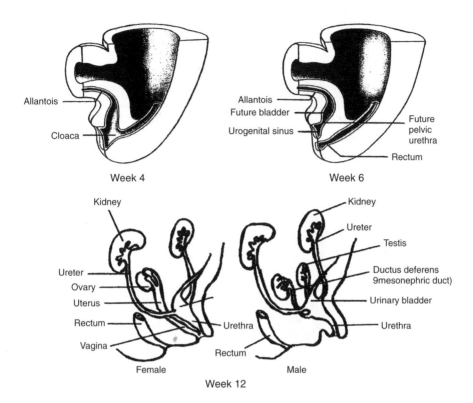

Figure 9.6   Development of the Bladder and Urethra between
Weeks 4 and 12

Source: Reprinted from *Human Embryology*, Larsen, copyright 1993, with permission
from Elsevier.

The urethra – by week 12

The epithelium of most of the male urethra and that of the whole female
urethra originates from the endoderm of the urogenital sinus, the surrounding connective tissue and smooth muscle tissue derived from the mesoderm.
In the male, the phallus elongates to become the penis. As this process occurs,
a groove appears in the middle of the phallus called the urethral groove, lined
with endodermal cells this develops into the urethral plate. Along the side
walls of the urethral groove, folds of tissue develop termed urogenital folds
which move towards one another and fuse to become the penile urethra. See
Figure 9.7 for cross sectional representation of this development.

Incomplete fusion of the penile urethral can result in hypospadias, when
the opening of the urethra is on the underside of the penis.

Ectodermal cells of the glands penis penetrate inwardly in the midline to
form a short cord which hollows out into the external urethral meatus.

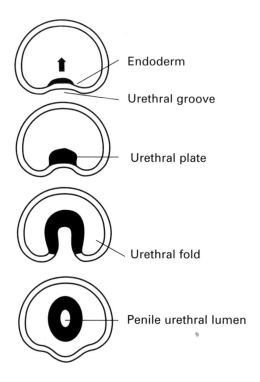

Figure 9.7   Development of the Male Urethra

Source: Reprinted from *Human Embryology*, Larsen, copyright 1993, with permission
from Elsevier.

Multiple buddings occur, invade the surrounding mesenchyme and become
the prostate gland. The pelvic part of the urogenital sinus gives rise to the
prostatic and membraneous urethra (Moore and Persaud, 2000).

The Kidneys in Postnatal Life

Nature has it in such a way that the structural and functional maturation of
the kidneys parallels the metabolic demands of the growing child. In utero
renal function relates not so much to homeostatic activities in the fetus but to
the maintenance of amniotic fluid volume. From birth onwards, the child's
biological functions set in motion adaptive mechanisms for survival in
extrauterine life. Here, the structural, neuro-endocrine, renal tubular function
and micturition are reviewed (Gomez *et al.*, 1999; Ichikawa, 1999; Jones and
Chesney, 1999). See Figures 9.8 to 9.10 for the normal anatomy of the renal
system.

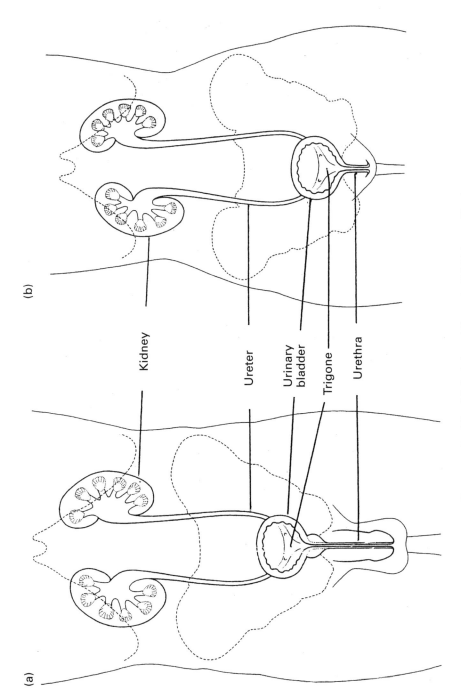

Kidney

Ureter

Urinary
bladder

Trigone

Urethra

(a)

(b)

Figure 9.8   The Male (a) and Female (b) Urinary Systems

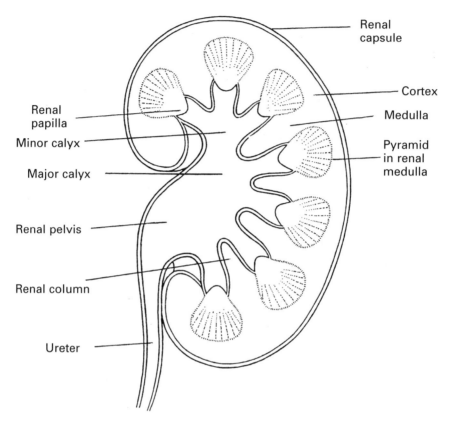

Figure 9.9   The Structure of the Kidney

Structural features

The anatomical dimensions and characteristics of the neonatal kidney are very different from that in the adult. Renal growth in *infancy* and *childhood* occurs as a result of hyperplasia of connective tissue until *6 months* and an increase in vascularization and hypertrophy of the existing renal tissues. The mean glomerular diameter in the neonate is approximately 100 µm *at birth* and progressively increases through *childhood* to reach *adult* size of approximately 300 µm in diameter. A striking finding in the *neonatal* kidney is the physical underdevelopment of the proximal tubules in relation to the corresponding glomeruli. Its mean length is about 2 mm, a tenth of the adult length of 20 mm. The glomeruli in the deeper cortex are larger in size than those in the more superficial regions. The layers of the glomerular capillary walls differentiate synchronously to form the mature filtration barrier (see Figure 9.11). Immature glomerular basement membranes *(GBM)* are less selective in their permeability than mature ones. The glomeruli have less fenestrae (window like openings), a lower hydrostatic pressure and reduced renal plasma flow. The

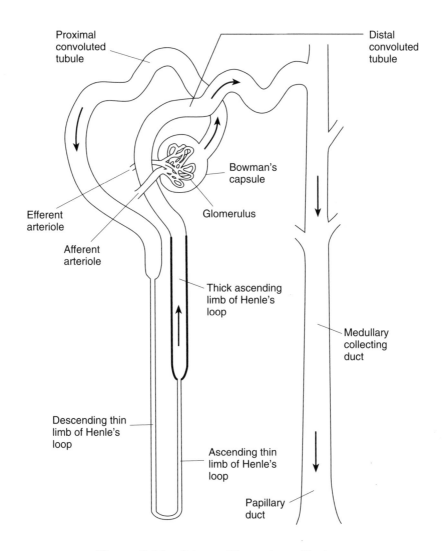

Figure 9.10   Schema Illustrating a Nephron

smallest and least mature glomeruli are found in the outer cortex and have the shortest and least coiled proximal tubules.

Renal blood flow and the glomerular filtration rate (GRF)

Blood supply to the kidneys develops between *weeks 6 to 8*. The initial renal arteries are branches of the common iliac arteries and receive the blood supply when they reach their higher level from the aorta. The permanent renal arteries originate from the aorta between T_{12} and L_2. The *fetal* kidneys receive

256

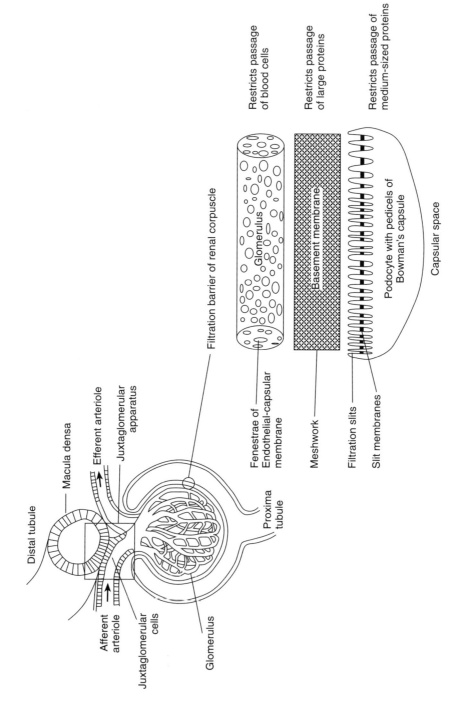

Distal tubule

Macula densa

Efferent arteriole

Juxtaglomerular apparatus

Afferent arteriole

Juxtaglomerular cells

Glomerulus

Proxima tubule

Filtration barrier of renal corpuscle

Glomerulus

Basement membrane

Podocyte with pedicels of Bowman's capsule

Capsular space

Fenestrae of Endothelial-capsular membrane

Meshwork

Filtration slits

Slit membranes

Restricts passage of blood cells

Restricts passage of large proteins

Restricts passage of medium-sized proteins

Figure 9.11   Schema Illustrating the Ultrastructure of the Filtration Barrier of the Glomerulus

3 per cent of the cardiac output, rising to 20 to 30 per cent *after birth*, facilitated by the fall in the renal vascular resistance (Modi, 1999).

Birth signals a dramatic increase in renal blood flow (RBF) and the GFR because peripheral vascular resistance (PVR) decreases by about 25 per cent but, in comparison with adults, RBF is still low and PVR is still high. During the *first 24 hours after birth*, GFR measurement reflects the status of renal function in prenatal life as neonates need at least 24 hours to adapt their GFR to extrauterine life. Factors which limit the GFR in the *neonate* are as follows (Avner *et al.*, 1990):

1 low renal blood flow, secondary to high renal vascular resistance;
2 low arterial perfusion, hence low intraglomerular capillary hydrostatic pressure;
3 small glomerular capillary surface area;
4 low water permeability of glomerular capillaries; and
5 high red blood cell volume.

GFR doubles during the *first two weeks of life*. This is brought about both by haemodynamic and structural reasons. It continues to rise, reaching adult values by *1 year*. GFR *postbirth* is mainly due to lengthening of the superficial cortical nephrons (Gomez *et al.*, 1999).

Box 9.3   Glomerular Filtration Rate

- Glomerular filtration rate (GFR) doubles during the *first two weeks of life*, in part because blood flow to the kidneys increases.
- GFR continues to rise, reaching adult values by *1 year*.
- Increases in GFR after *birth* is mainly due to lengthening of the superficial cortical nephrons (Gomez *et al.*, 1999).

The limited GFR makes the neonate vulnerable to fluid overload. When feeding orally the baby will be able to limit its own fluid intake to some extent. Consequently this risk is greatest for those neonates receiving fluids through other routes.

Sodium potassium ATPase activity

Sodium-potassium ATPase ($Na^+ K^+$ ATPase) pump activity is observed to be lower in the *neonatal period*, with a parallel increase in sodium (Na^+) absorption as age progresses, especially at the *weaning period*. The fractional Na^+ excretion is relatively high in *neonates* in relation to the increase in GFR, gradually decreasing over the first *6 to 12 months* of postnatal life. The *full term infant* is able to maintain the positive sodium balance necessary for growth in health, on a relatively low Na+ intake such as that in breast milk for instance. The ability of the distal tubule to handle a sodium load is at first imperfect, having only 70 per cent of the full capacity of load delivered in early neonatal life in health, gradually increasing to 85 per cent by the end of the *second week*.

The reasons for this inability are:

- the low GFR;
- the greater proportion of renal blood flow to juxtamedullary nephrons (those near the medulla) having longer and efficient loops of Henle;
- the active renin angiotensin aldosterone system (a cascade of hormones, which results in peripheral vasoconstriction, Na+ and therefore water reabsorption); and
- elevated plasma aldosterone level, independent of renin or angiotensin II levels (Jones and Chesney, 1999).

The renal response to sodium load increases progressively during *infancy* and reaches that of *older children* by the *end of the first year*. An increased activity of the Na+ K+ ATPase pump causes an over secretion and accumulation of fluid in the tubular cells.

When the pump is positioned on the apical rather than basolateral surface of the renal tubular cells, a sodium and thus a fluid drive towards the apical surface results, producing polycystic kidneys (MacDonald *et al.*, 1999).

Box 9.4 Renal Response to Sodium

- At birth the ability to handle a sodium load is imperfect, at only 70 per cent of the full capacity in *early neonatal life* in health, gradually increasing to 85 per cent by the end of the second week.
- The *full term infant* can maintain the positive sodium balance necessary for growth in health, on the relatively low Na+ intake in breast milk.
- The initially high sodium excretion in the *neonate* gradually decreases over the the first *6 to 12 months* of postnatal life.
- The renal response to sodium load increases progressively during *infancy* and reaches that of *older children* by the *end of the first year*.

Infants are vulnerable to sodium overload if fed overconcentrated formula or other high solute feeds. They should therefore be weaned onto solids at the recommended time (DoH, 1994), using the recommended weaning diet, to prevent inadvertent complications which can lead to fatalities, which are sometimes reported in the media.

Other transport mechanisms

Glucose: *Neonates* have a reduced reabsorption and an increase excretion of glucose thus, glycosuria is more common among neonates. The membranes become less 'leaky' as the child grows older because there are: an increase in the number of apical carrier proteins; a more favourable electrochemical gradient; reduced turnover of transporter proteins; and reduced fluidity in tubular membranes. The cumulative effect is an increased capacity for renal tubular glucose reabsorption (Avner *et al.*, 1990).

Amino Acids: The *neonatal* kidneys show a reduced reabsorption and an increased excretion of amino acids. Generally, urinary amino acids are higher in *neonates* than in adults. The reasons proposed are:

- the differences in the renal tubular structures;
- decreased rate of efflux of amino acids in the existing transporter systems from the cell into the circulation; and
- nonspecific maturational differences in the cell membrane or cell metabolism.

Thus, *young infants* are less able to reabsorb amino acids, making them very vulnerable and less able to adapt to the adverse effects of malnutrition (Avner *et al*., 1990).

Organic acids: The capacity to excrete hydrogen ions is mature in healthy *full term neonates* after *age one month* but, tubular excretion of organic acids is limited in *young infants* for the following reasons:

- the low GFR;
- anatomical immaturity leading to low tubular secretory surface area, offering a limited surface area for transport of various substances;
- poor access of organic acids to tubular transporting membranes;
- low number of transporting sites per unit tubular surface area;
- incomplete development of metabolic processes that provide energy for acid transport; and
- preponderance of blood flow to deep cortical nephrons during early infancy.

The tubular excretion of weak acids increases progressively with age, and reaches adult levels between *1 and 3 years of age*.

Incomplete renal proximal tubular reabsorption of bicarbonate increases the risk of metabolic acidosis (Jones and Chesney, 1999).

Urine concentration in childhood

In the *neonate*, there is a progressive increase in the tubular reabsorption of sodium. This is partly due to the increased tubular response to aldosterone.

Neonatal urine is diluted *at birth* but the ability to concentrate urine develops in the *first month* of life as the loop of the Henle lengthens, the medulla increases its urea concentration capacity and an increased tubular response to antidiuretic hormone (AHD) occurs. The capacity for *neonates* to concentrate urine is limited *at birth*, gradually increasing as age progresses. This is attributed to several factors:

- low GFR;
- short collecting ducts and loops of Henle, diminishing effectiveness of counter current multiplier mechanism;
- incomplete reabsorption of solute in the water impermeable ascending loop of Henle;
- low levels of ADH, and low urinary cylic AMP levels causing medullary hyporesponsiveness to ADH;
- elevated intra renal prostaglandin E_2; and
- increased total sodium and expanded extra-cellular volume *at birth*.

Water deprivation tests show a maximal urine osmolality to 680 mOsm/Kg only, as opposed to 1200 mOsm/Kg in the adult. ADH levels gradually rise over the *first three months* in postnatal life. The renal medullary architecture is still incompletely formed and animal studies have shown that urine concentration ability of the kidney during maturation correlates with structural changes. As indicated previously, the distal tubules in *young infants* are relatively insensitive to ADH. This mandates a greater intake of fluid thus, a larger production of urine is required to excrete any given solute load. Renal concentration mechanism reaches adult levels by *1 to 2 years of age* (Yared and Ichikawa, 1998). See Table 9.1 for the changes in urine osmolality from *birth to adulthood*.

Table 9.1   Age-related Urine Osmolality

Age	Urine osmolality mOsm/ Kg H_2O
3 days	515
6 days	663
10 days–1 month	896
1–2 months	1054
2–12 months	1118
14–18 years	1200

Box 9.5   Urine Concentration in Childhood

- Neonatal urine is diluted *at birth* but the ability to concentrate urine develops in the *first month* of life as the loop of the Henle lengthens, the medulla increases its urea concentration capacity and an increased tubular response to antidiuretic hormone (ADH) occurs.
- ADH levels gradually rise and the tubular response to ADH increases over the *first 3 months* of postnatal life, further increasing concentration ability.
- *Young infants* therefore produce more urine to excrete a given solute load and a need a greater intake of fluid to maintain fluid balance.
- The renal concentration mechanism reaches adult levels by *1 to 2 years of age.*

Young infants and *children under 2 years of age* are vulnerable to dehydration and solute overload with decreased fluid intake.

The Process of Micturition

Micturition is the act of urination, the voiding or passing of urine (McPherson 1999). It is a simple spinal reflex under both conscious and unconscious control from the brain and is characterized by the following phases:

1 The filling of the bladder – under sympathetic nervous system control.
2 The desire to pass urine – under parasympathetic nervous system control.
3 Awaiting a socially acceptable location and or preparation for the act e.g. adjusting clothing – involving the higher centres, cerebral cortex, hypothalamus and brainstem, plus movement capacity.
4 The initiation of sphincter relaxations and bladder contraction.
5 Complete emptying of the bladder.

Figure 9.12 provides a view of the basic anatomy of the urinary bladder and Figure 9.13 provides an overview of the pathways involved in the micturition reflex.

Patterns of childhood micturition:

- Full term, breastfed infant passes 20 ml/24 hours in *Days 1–2.*
- This increases to 200 ml/24 hours by *day 10* of post natal life.
- 30 per cent of newborns pass urine *during or soon after birth.*
- 92 per cent in the *first 24 hours* of birth.
- 98 per cent of neonates pass urine in the *first 48 hours* after birth.

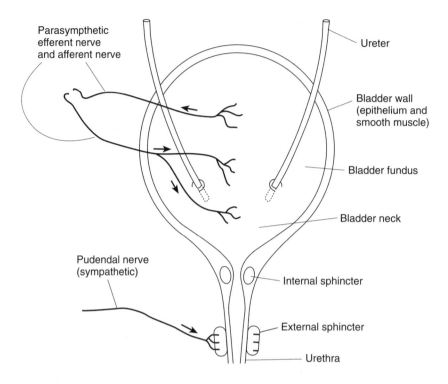

Figure 9.12   Basic Anatomy of the Urinary Bladder Including Parasympathetic and Sympathetic Innervation

Note: The area of the fundus at which the ureters enter the bladder is referred to as the trigone.

- Children of both sexes between *5 and 14 years* pass urine about 4 to 8 times per day.

Healthy *neonates* excrete between 15–30 ml/Kg of urine every 24 hours or pass 1 to 3 ml/Kg/hour. Within *1 month of birth*, urine output increases to approximately 5 ml/Kg/hour, depending on the solute load delivered to the kidneys, or plasma osmolality.

   Oliguria (abnormal low volume of urine as expected by age) is said to exist when urine output is *less than 1ml/Kg/hour*. Uronephrological investigations are indicated when the *neonate* fails to pass urine within *72 hours of birth*. Usually severe dehydration is the likely cause of oliguria in *infants* but, in the normovolaemic infant, intrinsic renal failure or obstruction to urinary flow has to be considered. A weak or intermittent urine stream in boys is suggestive of bladder outflow obstruction (Guignard and Drukker, 1999).

In sleep, the normal sphincter control mechanism is inhibited until the

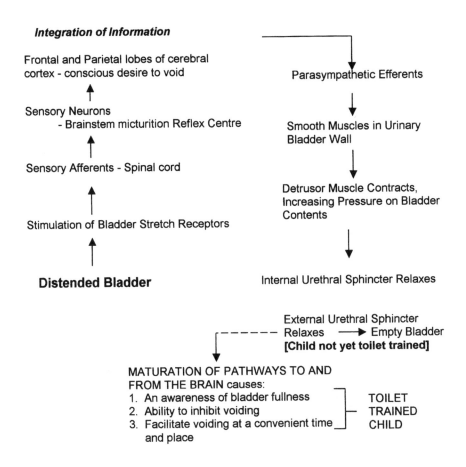

Figure 9.13   Schema Illustrating the Operational Pathway in the
Micturition Reflex

Source: Silverthorn (2001).

cerebral neurones have been activated through the afferent neurones from the detrusor muscle, indicating that the bladder is full. Once the cortical centres have been activated, the child usually awakens to empty their bladder. Maturation of bladder voiding occurs *between 1½ and 4½ years of age*. In *infancy*, the bladder wall responds to a small amount of urine and contracts to expel the urine it contains thus, urine expulsion is automatic. From *1½ to 2½ years of age*, the child develops an awareness of wanting to void but can retain urine for short periods only before voiding. The volume of urine passed at a time increases with age as the child gains control of the diaphragm, abdominal and perineal muscles in the initiation of voiding. Bladder control continues to improve from there onwards, leading to dryness in the day, followed by dryness at night (Abrams,1997).

Detrusor Stability in UK Children

- 77 per cent gain cortical awareness during sleep by *3 years;*
- 90 per cent by *5 years;* and
- 98 per cent by *15 years.*

Girls seem to attain detrusor stability earlier than boys (Payne, 1991). Day time bladder control starts at approximately *18 months.* The child is usually out of nappies during the day at *2½ years* of age and at night between *3–5 years.* Bowel control is achieved during the day and night by *3 years of age.*

These processes occur spontaneously in most children but for some, micturition on a voluntary basis is not achieved readily hence, the phenomenon of enuresis (Attard-Montalto and Saha, 1999; Rudolph and Levene, 1999).

Urinary bladder capacity is estimated at 30 mls for each age in years plus 30 mls. Thus *a 5-year-old* bladder can hold 180 ml of urine $(30 \times 5) + 30 = 180$ ml. The primary functions of the urinary bladder are to allow for adequate (age-related) storage capacity at low pressure and efficient emptying capacity. The physiological process that allows this involves the brain, brainstem, spinal cord, bladder detrusor muscle and external urethral sphincter. These structures work together in a well coordinated manner to establish and maintain urinary continence (Abrams, 1997).

Box 9.6 Calculating Bladder Capacity

Urinary bladder capacity is estimated at 30 mls for each year of age plus 30 mls.

Example:
a 5-year-old's bladder can hold: $(30 \times 5) + 30 = 180$ ml of urine.

Urinary continence

Urinary continence denotes the ability of the individual to retain the contents of the bladder until conditions are appropriate for voiding (Dorlands, 2000). Acquiring urinary continence is a very important milestone for the child and a fulfilling achievement for the family. For the child however, continence is acquired with the following prerequisites:

1 maturation of the nervous system;
2 an intact and healthy neuromuscular pathway of related organ systems;
3 effective filling, storage and emptying of bladder;
4 acquisition of cognitive, psychomotor and motivational skills by the child; and

5 application and integration of the affective elements of child rearing into the toilet-training process by family or carers (Abrams, 1997).

Assessment of Renal Function

Assessment of renal function is important as the renal system is particularly vulnerable to disease during childhood. There are several reasons for this vulnerability. The intricate and delicate structure and architecture of the nephrons, their blood supply and ureters make them vulnerable to physical as well as chemical trauma. The kidneys have an increased metabolic demand, with the potential to become overwhelmed if faced with extreme physiological or pathological challenge. The excretory role of the kidneys ensures that most toxic agents in the blood are delivered to the kidneys to be eliminated.

Drug therapy in the child should be implemented with extreme care in terms of types, dosages and intervals of administration to protect the immature kidneys from potential toxic effects.

In addition, the kidneys are considered as vital organs so they thus bear the effects of other systemic organ malfunction. Functionally, capacity in terms of GFR is not reached until towards the *end of infancy*, and the structural components at *preschool age*. As a result the kidneys of children, in particular the very young are vulnerable to disease and damage in extreme demands.

As renal tissue structural growth takes place in the early years, any disease processes, in particular reflux uropathies suppress renal growth (Barratt *et al.*, 1999).

For all these reasons, the child's diet, especially in *infancy* should be managed carefully so that the immature kidneys are not over-burdened with solutes. Any disease processes eg, urinary tract infection should be managed effectively to minimize or prevent long-term impairment.

Assessment of renal function should therefore be comprehensive, including history taking from the child, where old enough to contribute, and his/her parents/carers, the assessment of the physical appearance of the child, recording of vital signs, patterns of voiding and bowel action, and the examination of the constituents of urine. Each of these areas of assessment are discussed below. This is followed by tables summarizing the laboratory and clinical tests available to augment assessment of the child's renal function.

History taking

The child's life history begins with conception, therefore events related to the *prenatal, perinatal* (within 7 days of birth) as well as *neonatal* (first 28 days/first month of life) should be included in the history taking. Such information is usually recorded in the medical/nursing notes of the child. Analysis of this history enables the children's nurse to distinguish the normal from the abnormal. The concern of parents should be noted and considered carefully. This may include areas related to poor weight gain, poor feeding or excessive weight gain in particular around the waist band, bed wetting, undue restlessness in *an infant/neonate*, abnormal urine colour or smell. The family history and a detailed history of voiding should be obtained from the older child or from the parent.

Physical appearance

Malaise, lethargy, pallor and irritability are indicative of early infection and cardiovascular collapse in sepsis. Lassitude, anorexia and vomiting are associated with ureamia (accumulation of urea in the blood). Physical examination may reveal an abdominal mass. It can also exclude other anomalies and systemic infection.

Appearance of skin and mucous membranes.   A dry inelastic skin with decreased turgor (elasticity) can be indicative of moderate to severe dehydration. A pale skin, mucous membranes, conjunctiva and nail beds can be related to the anaemia of chronic renal disease. So is a skin that has lost its lustre, or one that is itchy. In health, red blood cell turnover is maintained by the growth factor erythropoetin (EPO) produced by the renal peritubular cells in response to hypoxia or reduced erythrocyte mass. On production, EPO stimulates the bone marrow erythroid stem cells to divide and mature, thus raising the erythrocyte level and correcting any anaemia. Anaemia or renal failure occurs because of failed or impaired action of the peritubular cells in maintaining erythrocyte homeostatis (Pugh *et al.*, 1993).

Oedema: Generalized, periorbital or ankle oedema in a toddler can be indicative of renal disease, in particular nephrotic syndrome (a disease characterized by damage to glomerular basement membranes resulting in increased losses of protein in the urine). This can also be exhibited as unexpected rapid weight gain especially in *infants*. In health, the oncotic pressure produced by plasma proteins, in particular albumin, helps to keep plasma water in the capillaries. Heavy proteinuria in nephrotic syndrome causes hypoproteinaemia. The fall in plasma protein reduces the oncotic pressure, causing fluid to enter in excess and remain in the interstitial space, producing the oedema (Cotran *et al.*, 1999).

Vital Signs

Pyrexia in which the core temperature is above 37.5°C or hyperpyrexia, in which the core temperature is above 38.5°C suggests the presence of pyrogens in the child's body which has reset the hypothalamic thermostat at a higher level. These include inflammatory mediators such as interleukins and prostaglandins produced in acute cystitis or pyelonephritis.

Tachycardia, an abnormally raised heart rate relative to age observed at recording the apex beat or pulse rate, accompanies inflammation or infections eg, urinary tract infection (UTI). It raises the child's metabolic rate reflected in the increased workload on the heart in an effort to meet the extra energy demand of the tissue cells.

Tachypnoea, an abnormally raised respiratory rate, usually accompanies tachycardia as the heart and the lungs work in harmony in meeting the extra energy demand on the tissue cells in the case of infection or inflammation within the body. The only exception here are *neonates*, whose compensatory mechanisms may be blunted because of organ system immaturity and thus exhibit bradycardia and hypothermia in infection.

Blood pressure

Renal scarring, whether congenital or acquired as a result of UTI with vesi-coureteric reflux (VUR), back flow of urine from the bladder into the ureters, confers significant risk of hypertension and it can take years or even decades to manifest (Hellerstein, 2000). Unlike adults, blood pressure (BP) levels considered as hypertensive have not yet been correlated to cardiovascular morbidity or mortality for children. Thus, definitions are based on epidemiological data rather than illness outcome studies. Nonetheless, 60–80 per cent of children with secondary hypertension have renal parenchymal damage, polycystic kidneys and posterior urethral valves causing reflux of urine into the young kidneys. Also, 10 per cent of children with renal scarring have been estimated to become hypertensive by the age of *adolescence* or *young adulthood*. The pathological basis of this hypertension is due to increased production of renin which activates the renin–angiotensin–aldosterone system, ultimately causing increased peripheral vascular resistance and the subsequent hypertension (Bullock, 1998).

Prevention of UTIs which result in renal scarring is the most likely way to prevent hypertension due to reflux nephropathy and children with renal scarring should receive ongoing blood pressure monitoring. Fundal examination by an ophthalmoscope may show papiloedema, swelling of the optic disc, as a complication of the hypertension (Hellerstein, 2000).

Convenient estimates for systolic and diastolic BP for the 95th centile as offered by Trompeter and Barratt (1999, p. 323) are as follows:

$$\text{Age 1–5 years} \quad = \quad \frac{115}{75} \ \text{mm Hg}$$

$$\text{Age 5–10 years} \quad = \quad \frac{125}{80} \ \text{mm Hg}$$

$$\text{Age 10–15 years} \quad = \quad \frac{135}{85} \ \text{mm Hg}$$

Here the experience of the practitioner or the clinician in both communication skills, as well as the technical skills in recording the BP are of extreme importance in order to facilitate accurate recording.

Patterns of voiding and bowel action

Patterns of voiding and bowel action should be observed and a thorough history taken to assess:

- frequency;
- urgency;
- day or night wetting, enuresis after 5 *years* of age;
- quality and volume of stream;
- any straining on voiding;
- volume of voided urine; and
- any soiling or constipation.

These might suggest poor bladder function due to UTI or congenital anomalies. Enlargement of the bladder can be visible or ascertained on skilful abdominal examination.

Examination of the characteristics of urine

Physical and chemical examination of freshly passed or collected urine can reveal disorders of the urinary system. Table 9.2 shows the physical characteristics of urine in health, abnormal findings on urinalysis, and clinical significance of the abnormal findings.

Tables 9.3 and 9.4 present a summary of microscopy and biochemical assessments of childhood renal function (Avner *et al.*, 1990; Barratt *et al.*, 1999; Linne and Ringsrud, 1999). These are the most common methods of assessment beyond urinalysis. However, if indicated by the findings from such tests, children's renal structure and/or function may also be assessed using an expanding variety of technological tools:

- Renal ultrasonography to assess renal anatomy;
- Micturating cystourethorgram to evaluate the bladder structure and function;
- Diethylenetriamine pentaacetic acid (DTPA) scans, which provide radionuclide imaging of the kidneys to assess renal blood flow and function;
- Dimercaptosuccinic acid (DMSA) scans, which visualize the functioning renal parenchyma;
- Magnetic recording imaging (MRI) providing detailed anatomical information; and
- CT scans, which also provide anatomical information of the kidney and surrounding abdominal tissues.

Table 9.2 Childhood Urinalysis

Characteristics	Normal Findings	Abnormal Findings and their possible Implications
Colour	Pale yellow to amber due to presence of urochrome, a yellowish pigment containing urobilin Pale = Dilute urine eg, neonates Amber = Concentrated urine eg, early morning or urine of older children	Very pale = Dilute urine: • Increased volume due to increased or excessive fluid intake or fluid over-load • Damaged/shortened LOH in pyelonephritis, hydronephrosis or reflux • Renal impairment due to inability to concentrate urine eg, renal disease in sickle cell disease Dark yellow or orange-red = Concentrated urine: • Fluid deficit where the kidneys conserve body water to maintain home-ostasis eg, poor intake or dehydration
Transparency	Clear when fresh. Cloudy when allowed to stand and means no visible particulate is present due to normal urate crystals	Turbid or very cloudy • White blood cell casts in urinary tract infection • Presence of pus cells • The presence of mucus as in some chronic inflammatory disease • Renal transitional or squamous epithelial cells, bacteria, semen • Contamination with faecal matter or powders and antiseptics
Specific Gravity Neonate Older Child Adult	1.002–1.008 1.002–1.030 1.003–1.035	Fixed specific gravity • Loss of the ability by the kidneys to concentrate urine eg, end-stage renal failure Low specific gravity in older children • Passage of large volumes of dilute urine eg, diabetes insipidus or exces-sive fluid intake High specific gravity • Reduced fluid intake with renal compensation • Dehydration eg, gastroenteritis • In diabetes mellitus where glycosuria causes increased urine specific gravity

Table 9.2 (Cont.)

Characteristics	Normal Findings	Abnormal Findings and their possible Implications
pH Neonate Thereafter	5–7 4.5–8 (Average ~ 6)	Decreasing pH is seen in conditions resulting in metabolic acidosis as hydrogen ions are lost in the urine.
Smell/Odour	Ammoniacal or faintly aromatic due to the presence of volatile acids. Bacterial action breaks down urea to produce ammonia when urine is allowed to stand	Putrid or foul smell • Heavily infected urine by bacteria gives this unpleasant smell but only indicative if the urine is fresh. Bacteria causes the decomposition of proteins [putrefaction] which causes the foul, unpleasant smell. • Contamination by infected vaginal discharge can similarly cause this odour
Protein	Less than 150 mg/Day loss in urine considered normal Mainly albumin, usually due to immature renal structures	Proteinuria over 1000 mg [1g]/Day • Considered pathological especially if accompanied by oedema eg, nephrotic syndrome • Persistent proteinuria in the presence of sterile urine is indicative of renal function impairment. • Healthy, intact glomerular filtration barrier should not leak protein in urine due to molecular size of proteins and diameter of apertures in filtration barrier. • Suggestive of glomerular or tubular damage or infection. • Transient or mild proteinuria occurs in children with febrile illness, and following extreme exercise • Consistent microalbuminuria is an early sign of renal complication of diabetes mellitus • Adolescents may show orthostatic proteinuria, in which proteinuria is evident in long time vertical position but disappears in the horizontal position. It is proposed to be caused by pressure on the renal veins on standing.

Table 9.2 *(Cont.)*

Characteristics	Normal Findings	Abnormal Findings and their possible Implications
Glucose Glucose is the preferred substrate for cerebral neurons and does not need insulin to enter into their cells	Plasma glucose 8–11 mmol/l = renal threshold Transport proteins in renal tubular membranes become exhausted, causing glucose to spill over in urine.	Glycosuria = Presence of glucose in urine Renal threshold [plasma glucose >11 mmol/l] exceeded eg, diabetes mellitus • Test assesses metabolic rather than renal disease • Diabetes mellitus is the most common cause of glycosuria, in which the accompanying hyperglycaemia exceeds the renal threshold and causes glycosuria • Gluconeogenesis from systemic corticosteroid therapy or extreme metabolic stress eg, sepsis
Ketones 1 Acetone 2 Acetoacetate acid 3 Beta hydroxy-butyrate 'Cerebral neurons can use ketones as an energy source in starvation or diabetes mellitus'	Products of fat metabolism	Ketonaemia or Ketonuria If more fat than normal is metabolized, the body is unable to utilize all the ketone bodies which are then excreted in the urine. Ketosis = combination of increased ketones in both blood and urine • In Diabetes mellitus the body is unable to use carbohydrate as a primary energy source and compensates by turning to fat catabolism • In starvation the body is depleted of glycogen stores and must resort to using fat as an energy source • Ketosis is also seen in severe dehydration, fever, vomiting and diarrhoea

Table 9.2 (Cont.)

Characteristics	Normal Findings	Abnormal Findings and their possible Implications
Blood	0–2 red blood cells per high-power field in the concentrated sediment (0.2/hpf) Contamination by menstrual flow or discolouration by strong dyes such as rhubarb must be excluded in older females or children respectively. Ingestion of beetroot and certain food colouring can cause red discolouration.	Red = Blood or haem derived pigments; urates or uric acid; drugs or food stuffs Haematuria = presence of red blood cells in urine confirmed by dipstick or laboratory test • Caused by bleeding or disease from any part of the urinary system • Necessary to determine the site of bleeding eg. glomerular bleeding accompanied by red cell casts • There may be little correlation between the extent of renal disease and degree of haematuria • Can be indicative of polycystic kidneys • Trauma or inflammation of the urinary tract can also cause haematuria
Bilirubin Should be tested on fresh urine.	Bilirubin breaks down rapidly on exposure to light, or oxidation to biliverdin on exposure to room air, turning it to green colour.	Yellow-brown or green-brown = bilirubin, a highly coloured bile pigment related to jaundice if present. Urine foams when shaken and the foam has a vivid yellow colour. • Characteristic and alarming to the experienced assessor • Indicative of liver disease as in biliary cannaliculi obstruction, hepatitis or common bile duct obstruction • Presence in urine requires further investigation as may appear in the urine before evidence of clinical jaundice

Table 9.3 Urine Microbiology

Test	Normal Findings	Abnormal Findings and their Implications
Microbiological studies Urine is a good medium for bacterial growth. Confirms presence or absence of bacteria in the urine. • (Hansson and Jodal, 1999; Turner and Haycock, 2002)	• In health, the periurethral area is normally colonized by endogenous microflora • Disturbance of these can occur eg, antibiotic therapy • Enterobacteria forms part of the microbial flora in the nappy age or encopretic child • Thus children 0–5 years of age, especially females are susceptible to UTI • Examined macroscopically and microscopically • Culture to detect and identify any bacteria present • Tested for antibiotic sensitivity or resistance	Sterile urine = 2,894 micro organisms Bacteriuria ≥ 50,000 CFU/ml (colony-forming units = CFU) Bacteria count of 100,000 CFU per millimeter of urine is a significant bacteriuria. Urinary Tract Infection: ⊆ More than 10 WBCs/ml ⊆ Or pure growth of more than 100 000 CFU/ml of midstream or clean catch specimen ⊆ Or Catheter Urine of more than 10 000 CFU/ml • Bacteria present at time of collection will continue to multiply • Specimen must therefore be sent to the laboratory or kept under the appropriate conditions • Urine should be sterile within 24 hours of antibiotic therapy in UTI • Mass screening for bacteriuria in infancy has been debated. It seems to mainly detect innocent bacteriuria episodes and is not recommended. Symptomatic children should be investigated • Pyuria, presence of pus in the urine, with absent bacterial growth on urine culture should raise suspicion of renal or urinary tract tuberculosis

Table 9.4 Biochemical Assessment of Renal Function

Test	Normal Findings	Abnormal Findings and their possible Implications
Plasma Creatinine Derived from the turnover of phosphocreatinine in muscle and excreted in urine At a steady state it is a direct reflection of lean skeletal muscle mass	Plasma creatinine Infant: 18–35 umol/l Child: 27–62 umol/l Adolescent 44–88 umol/l • The normal plasma concentration increases with age as muscle mass increases with growth • It is high at birth due to diffusion across the placenta from the mother and the low GFR, but decreases fairly rapidly and plateaus at 7–14 days • Small muscle mass leads to low levels eg, in some women and in children	Low Plasma Creatinine • Abnormally low in wasting and starvation and corticosteroid therapy because of protein degradation High Plasma Creatinine • Increase in muscle metabolism sees a small increase following vigorous exercise • Increased muscle bulk elevates plasma creatinine • Increased in reduced renal perfusion, glomerular nephritis, and obstructive uropathy (See Brocklebank in Addy, 1994 for Glomerular Filtration Rate GFR)
Plasma Urea It is a major metabolite of protein metabolism	Plasma urea Neonate: 1.0–5.0 mmol/l Infant: 2.0–7.0 mmol/l Child: 2.5–6.5 mmol/l • Reflects protein intake and renal excretory capacity	High Plasma Urea • Pre-renal causes – Impaired renal perfusion producing reduced urine flow • Dietary causes – High Protein diet because excess amount is not stored in the body • Increased catabolism – High stress states, extreme starvation in which protein is broken down and also increased gluconeogenesis by the stress hormones

Table 9.4 (*Cont.*)

Test	Normal Findings	Abnormal Findings and their possible Implications
	• It involves the release of ammonia, a very toxic agent which is detoxified by the liver to produce urea on the deamination of amino acids • Kidney excretes 90 per cent of the urea produced and rest is lost through the skin or gastrointestinal tract • Inferior to creatinine, as 50 per cent filtered at the glomeruli is passively reabsorbed via the renal tubules	• Renal uraemia – Can be caused by an outflow obstruction, pressure on the renal tubules which enhances back-diffusion of urea, causing plasma urea to rise Low Plasma Urea • In malabsorption syndrome or starvation as there is less protein/amino acids for the liver to deaminate
Plasma Sodium Predominantly an extracellular cation	Plasma sodium 130 – 150 mmol/l	Hypernatraemia – Plasma sodium >150 mmol/l • Sodium excess with weight loss suggestive of dehydration in which there is a deficit in total body water e.g. diarrhoea and vomiting • Sodium excess with weight gain suggestive of sodium and water overload • Child abuse with salt poisoning in very rare cases

Table 9.4 *(Cont.)*

Test	Normal Findings	Abnormal Findings and their possible Implications
		Hyponatraemia – Plasma sodium <130 mmol/l
		• Overhydration with hypotonic fluid as in iatrogenesis in intravenous fluid therapy involving the administration of hypotonic solutions
		• Sodium depletion as a complication of loop diuretic therapy
		• Sodium depletion with weight loss or static weight suggests low sodium intake
		• Salt losing disease eg, congenital adrenal hyperplasia
Potassium Predominantly an intracellular cation	Plasma potassium 3.5 – 5.6 mmol/l Plasma levels influenced by exchanges within the fluid compartments	Hyperkalaemia – Plasma potassium > 5.6 mmol/l
		• Difficult cannulation, venepuncture or delay in processing blood specimens may produce elevated measurements
		• Excessive tissue damage, bruising
		• Tissue breakdown resulting in redistribution of potassium within compartments e.g. from intravenous administration of old red blood cells or from excess release in the extracellular fluid space as in tissue injury caused by trauma or tumour lysis in cancer chemotherapy
		• Dehydration
		• Renal failure
		• Metabolic acidosis
		• Excess intake, as in iatrogenesis for example
		Hypokalaemia – Plasma potassium < 3.4 mmol/l
		• Diarrhoea: Potassium depletion through stool and urine
		• Diuretics eg, frusemide
		• Metabolic alkalosis

Conclusion

The kidneys of the urinary system fulfil their homeostatic role by regulating the blood chemistry, body fluids and electrolytes. To do this, they need to be healthy in structure as only then can they carry out their regulatory, excretory and synthetic roles in the quest for homeostasis. Functional genes are essential in directing the activities that occur in embryonic formation of the kidneys and the rest of the structures that constitute the urinary system. They are prone to embryological errors as their formation is intricate and complex. After birth, growth and maturational processes ensue to enable the structures to acquire adult functional competence and capacity to sustain life. The very nature of their structure makes the kidneys prone to disease and damage and as vital organs they are affected by pathology involving other organ systems such as the heart. This vulnerability to damage means that any threat of disease should be investigated so that prompt, appropriate and effective treatment can be started and follow-up care ensured.

Review Questions

1 Which genes are involved in renal development and for what do they encode?
2 Outline the intrauterine development of the true kidneys.
3 What are the key steps in the development of the bladder in both sexes?
4 Outline the three key roles of the kidneys in the process of maintaining homeostasis of the blood chemistry and body fluids.
5 Describe the physical characteristics of urine in a healthy child.
6 Explain the clinical significance of abnormal findings in urinalysis.
7 Explain why the kidneys of children are prone to disease and damage.

Further Reading

Barratt, TM, Avner, ED, Harmon, WE (1999) *Pediatric Nephrology*, 4th edn. Baltimore: Lippincott, Williams and Willkins. An evidence-based, comprehensive and international reference text edited by experts, of extreme value to the practitioner in paediatric nephrology.

Martini, FH (2001) *Anatomy and Physiology*. Upper Saddler River: Prentice Hall. The latest publication by a credible author. The content is coherent, comprehensive and addresses current theory on renal physiology and some key areas of pathophysiology, very readable and review questions student friendly.

Moore, KL and Persaud, TVN (2000) *The Developing Human. Clinically Oriented Embryology*, 7th edn. Philadelphia: WB Saunders. A reliable embryology text by outstanding authors, well versed and established in the area, very readable and the clinical focus of chapters extremely useful to practitioners.

References

Abrams, P (1997) *Urodynamics*, 2nd edn. London: Springer.

Addy, DP (1994) *Investigations in Paediatrics*. London: Harcourt Brace Publishing.

Atala, A and Bauer, SB (1999) Chapter 57. Bladder dysfunction. In TM Barratt, ED Avner and WE Harman (eds), *Pediatric Nephrology*. Baltimore: Lippincott Williams and Wilkins.

Attard-Montalto, S and Saha, V (1999) *Paediatrics*. Edinburgh: Churchill Livingstone.

Avner, ED, Ellis, D, Ichikawa, I *et al.*, (1990) Chapter 5. Normal neonates and the maturational development of homeostatic mechanisms. In I Ichikawa I (ed.), *Pediatric Textbook of Fluids and Electrolytes*. Baltimore: Williams and Wilkins

Barratt, TM, Avner, ED and Harman, WE (1999) *Pediatric Nephrology*. Baltimore: Lippincott Williams and Wilkins.

Bullock, BL (1998) *Pathophysiology Adaptation and Alterations in Function 4th Edition*. Philadelphia: Lippincott.

Colón, AR and Ziai, M (1985) *Pediatric Pathophysiology*. Boston: Little, Brown and Company.

Cotran, RS, Kumar, V and Collins, T (1999) *Robbins Pathologic Basis of Disease*, 6th edn. Philadelphia: WB Saunders.

Department of Health (1994) *Report on Health and Social Subjects 45. Weaning and the Weaning Diet. Report of the Working Group on the Weaning Diet of the Committee on Medical Aspects of Food Policy*. London. HMSO.

Dorlands, NW (2000) *Dorlands Illustrated Medical Dictionary*. 29th edn. Philadelphia: WB Saunders.

Dyball, REJ, Navaratnam, V and Tate, PA (1999) Chapter 9. Basic embryology and embryological basis of malformation syndrome. In JM Rennie and NRC Roberton *Textbook of Neonatology*, 3rd edn. Edinburgh: Churchill Livingstone.

Gilbert, SF (1997) *Developmental Biology*, 5th edn. Sunderland: Sinauer Associates Inc.

Gomez, RA and Norwood, VF (1999) Recent Advances in Renal Development. *Current Opinion in Pediatrics*, April, 11(2), 135–40.

Gomez, RA, El-Dahr, S and Chevalier, RL (1999) Chapter 5. Vasoactive Hormones. In TM Barratt, ED Avner and WE Harman (eds), *Pediatric Nephrology*, 4th edn. Baltimore: Lippincott Williams and Wilkins.

Goodenough, U (1984) *Genetics*. 3rd edn. Philadelphia: Saunders College Publishing.

Guignard, JP and Drukker, A (1999) Second International Symposium on Perinatal Nephrology. *Pediatric Nephrology*, April, 13(3), 265–6.

Hansson S and Jodal ULF (1999) Chapter 52 Urinary Tract Infection. In TM Barratt et al. (eds) *Pediatric Nephrology 4th Edition*. Baltimore: Lippincott Williams and Wilkins.

Hellerstein, S (2000) Long-term Consequences of Urinary Tract Infections. *Current Opinion in Pediatrics*, April, 12(2), 125–8.

Ichikawa, I (ed.) (1990) *Pediatric Textbook of Fluids and Electrolytes*. Baltimore: Williams and Wilkins.

Jones, DP and Chesney, RW (1999) Chapter 4. Tubular function. In TM Barratt, ED Avner and WE Harman (eds), *Pediatric Nephrology*, 4th edn. Baltimore: Lippincott Williams and Wilkins.

Levy, JB and Kramer, SA (1999) Chapter 59. Renal tumours. In TM Barratt, ED Avner and WE Harman (eds), *Pediatric Nephrology*, 4th edn. Baltimore: Lippincott Williams and Wilkins.

Limwongse, C, Clarren, SK and Cassidy, SB (1999) Chapter 25. Syndromes and malformations in the urinary tract. In TM Barratt, ED Avner and WF Harman (eds), *Pediatric Nephrology*, 4th edn. Baltimore: Lippincott Williams and Wilkins.

Linne, JJ and Ringsrud, KM (1999) *Clinical Laboratory Science: The Routine Techniques*. 4th edn. St Louis: Mosby.

MacDonald, RA, Watkins, SL, Avner, ED (1999) Chapter 27 Polycystic Kidney Disease. In TM Barratt *et al.* (eds), *Pediatric Nephrology 4th Edition*. Baltimore: Lippincott Williams and Wilkins.

Martini, FH (2001) *Anatomy and Physiology*. Upper Saddler River: Prentice Hall.

McPherson, G (1999) *Black's Medical Dictionary 39th Edition*. London: A & C Books.

Modi, N (1999) Chapter 39. Renal function, fluid and electrolyte balance and neonatal renal disease. In JM Rennie and NRC Roberton (eds), *Textbook of Neonatology*, 3rd edn. Edinburgh: Churchill Livingstone.

Moore, KL and Persaud, TVN (2000) *The Developing Human: A Clinically Oriented Approach*, 7th edn. Philadelphia: WB Saunders.

Payne, S (1991) Childhood Enuresis. *Postgraduate Update*, December, 855–63.

Polin, RA and Fox, WW (1998) *Fetal and Neonatal Physiology*. Philadelphia: WB Saunders.

Pugh, CW; Maxwell, PH; Nicholls, LG *et al.* (1993) Inducible operation of the erythropoietin 3 enchances in different cells lines. In C Bauer *et al.* (eds), *Erythropoietin Molecular Physiology and Clinical Applications*. New York: Marcel Dekker Inc.

Rudolph, M and Levene, M (1999) *Paediatrics and Child Health*. Oxford: Blackwell Science.

Sadler, TW (2000) *Langman's Medical Embryology*, 8th edn. Philadelphia: Lippincott Williams and Wilkins.

Silverthorn, DU (2001) *Human Physiology: An Integrated Approach*, 2nd edn. Upper Saddle River: Prentice Hall.

Trompeter, RS and Barratt, MT (1999) Chapter 18. Clinical evaluation. In MT Barratt, ED Avner and WE Harman (eds), *Pediatric Nephrology*, 4th edn. Baltimore: Lippincott Williams and Wilkins.

Turner, A and Haycock, G (2002) Renal disease. In: J Strodsant and D Field (eds), *Handbook of Paediatric Investigations*. London: Churchill Livingstone.

Vander, AJ (1995) *Renal Physiology*, 5th edn. New York: McGraw Hill.

Watkins, SL and McDonald, RA (1999) Chapter 24. Renal dysplasia, hypoplasia and miscellaneous cystic disease. In TM Barratt, ED Avner and WE Harman (eds), *Pediatric Nephrology*, 4th edn. Baltimore: Lippincott Williams and Wilkins.

Woolf, AS (1995) Clinical impact of the biological basis of renal malformations. *Seminars In Nephrology*, 15(4), July, 361–72.

Yared, A and Ichikawa, I (1998) Chapter 146. Postnatal development of glomerular filtration. In RA Polin and WW Fox (eds), *Fetal and Neonatal Physiology*, 2nd edn. Philadelphia: WB Saunders.

CHAPTER 10

Protecting the Body from Infection During Childhood

Edward Purssell

Contents

- Infectious Diseases
- The Human Immune System
- Non-specific/Innate System
- Specific Immunity
- The Immune Response to Infection – Key Features of Assessment

- Conclusion
- Review Questions
- Further Reading
- References

Learning Outcomes

At the end of this chapter you will be able to:

- Explain the importance of infectious disease as a cause of morbidity and mortality around the world, including some of the new and emerging diseases.
- Describe the development and function of key components of the immune system.
- Consider the importance of maintaining the child's own bacterial flora, the protection of the integrity of the skin and mucous membranes.
- Explain passive and active immunization.
- Describe some of the common effects of infection on the child and relate to the assessment of the child.

Introduction

This chapter examines the mechanisms involved in protecting the child from infection. Although two systems are considered, the innate/non-specific immune system and the specific/adaptive immune system, in reality they interact to form a highly integrated protective mechanism. The non-specific immune system comprises the most basic host defence systems and allows for a rapid response to micro-organisms and other antigens. In addition to physical protective mechanisms, it also includes chemicals that degrade bacteria, and a number of phagocytic cells that ingest and destroy micro-organisms and antigens.

The specific immune system is based around a number of specialized cells that are able to identify individual micro-organisms and antigens and launch a tailored response against the specific organism. Moreover specific immunity has a memory that allows a more vigorous response to subsequent exposures to the same micro-organism or antigen.

Most of the focus of this chapter is on the differences in the immune system between adults and children. Much of what we know about the immune system is based on animal studies and although knowledge is expanding, there is also a lot that we do not know about the human immune system, especially the immune system in children.

Infectious Diseases

Infectious diseases are a major source of morbidity and mortality around the world, particularly so in the developing world. Deaths occur despite there being cost-effective treatments available, such as oral rehydration fluid for diarrhoeal diseases and vaccinations for a number of common infectious diseases. In the developed world, infectious disease is more commonly a cause of morbidity than mortality. However worldwide, new and re-emergent diseases continue to appear – HIV, new variant CJD, and antibiotic-resistant bacteria have all become problems that need to be tackled.

Growth in travel and tourism increases spread of disease, while changes in lifestyle, climate and industry may also predispose to new infectious disease (Epstein, 2000). Our ability to treat viral illnesses remains poor, with seasonal epidemics of influenza and other respiratory viruses, HIV, and a number of other viruses all contributing to significant morbidity in children.

Advances in medical treatments mean that very low birth weight children are now surviving, as are children with primary immune deficiencies and those who have treatments for conditions such as cancer and autoimmune diseases that suppress the immune system. Such children may be particularly vulnerable to infectious diseases. It is, therefore, important that health care professionals understand the importance of infection as a cause of morbidity and mortality and the natural defences that the body has to prevent infection.

The Human Immune System

The immune system is a highly complex and integrated system of defensive cells and substances. For clarity, the immune system is broken down into component systems, the non-specific/innate and specific/adaptive immune systems. However in practice the different parts of the immune system are inseparable. The two systems work synergistically to enhance effectiveness of the immune response – the innate mechanisms stimulate the specific immune system to respond and, in turn, the specific system utilizes the mechanisms of the innate system to eliminate pathogens from the body. The key features of the immune system are outlined in Table 10.1.

Table 10.1 Key Features of the Immune System

	Non-specific/innate	*Specific/adaptive*
Components	Skin	Antibodies in blood, on skin
	Mucosa	and mucosal surfaces
	Anti-microbial chemicals	
	Cytokines	Cytokines
	Complement	
	Phagocytes (macrophages	
	and neutrophils)	Lymphocytes
	Natural killer cells	
Memory	No memory for repeated exposure to antigens.	Memory for repeated exposure permits increase in speed and intensity of response.
Features	Provides immediate defence to infection. Prevents attachment and growth of pathogens and provides mechanisms for removal of pathogens.	Develops later in the time course of infection. Two types of response are involved: • the production of antibodies, (the humoral responses). This is effective against extracellular micro-organisms and toxins. • the cell-mediated responses involving T lymphocytes and providing defence against intracellular micro-organisms

Non-specific/Innate System

These mechanisms are present from birth. They are the most basic immune responses and include:

- physical and chemical barriers at epithelial surfaces;
- phagocytic and natural killer (NK) cells;
- inflammation; and
- cytokine activity.

Some of these mechanisms are a constant presence in the body eg the physical and chemical barriers, but other mechanisms are initiated by the presence of microbes or microbial structures, such as membranes and bacterial cell wall components.

Physical and Chemical Barriers

The first defensive mechanism that potential pathogens must overcome is the intact surfaces of the skin and mucous membranes, including the normal micro-organisms that live in these areas. Epithelial surfaces produce substances that maintain the pH and an environment conducive to the growth of the normal flora. They also produce peptides (defensins) in response to cytokines that are able to act as anti-microbial agents.

The skin

Intact skin provides an effective barrier by virtue of its impermeability and the constant removal and renewal of the outermost layer of dead cells. Pathogens are therefore normally unable to infect this layer. *At birth* the infant's skin is sterile, but it is quickly colonized by bacteria and fungi, gained initially from the mother's vagina and anal area. *After birth*, the external environment and other people become important sources of colonization. The initial colonization does not necessarily reflect the stable colonization pattern that emerges later to constitute the normal flora for that individual.

The normal flora have a role in preventing the growth of pathogens by competing for substrate on which the micro-organisms live as well as in some cases producing antimicrobial substances to fend off the competition. Some of the micro-organisms that make up the normal flora metabolise fatty acids and sebum to produce an acid pH of around 5.5 (Mims *et al.*, 1995) which can further inhibit growth of potential pathogens.

There are a number of differences in the skin of *infants* that reduce the protection provided by the skin. These include the lack of a stable skin flora, the lower free fatty acid content of the immature skin, the higher pH (around 6.6), and sebaceous glands that do not function until *puberty*. The smaller body surface area of *babies*, and less developed ecological niches might increase the ability of bacteria to be spread from one area to another through handling (Carr and Kloos, 1977).

The skin flora develop rapidly over the first few months, with increasing numbers and varieties of *Staphylococcus* and *Micrococcus* species. In the early teenage years there is a marked increase in *Propinonibacterium acnes*. This species of bacteria acts on sebum, causing the inflammation that leads to acne (Mims *et al.*, 1995).

Normally the skin flora are commensal, meaning that they are neither harmful nor beneficial to the host organism. They can however be pathogenic in certain circumstances where the immune system is not functioning well or where there is a route of entry through the skin such as in those with prosthetic implants, intravascular catheters, and wounds. For example, *Staphylococcus epidermis* is commonly found as a constituent of skin flora, but is becoming an increasing problem as a cause of intravascular catheter infection.

The gastrointestinal tract

Throughout its length, the gastrointestinal tract offers different environments and mechanisms of protection against infection.

The mouth provides a moist, warm environment that has plenty of nutrients and a neutral pH. Teeth and mucous membranes provide surfaces for the adhesion of micro-organisms. Aggregations of bacteria on the surface of the teeth form a thin film of dental plaque containing bacteria. These bacteria ferment sugar in the diet causing the local pH to fall and subsequent loss of minerals from the teeth, dental caries and tooth decay (Marcott and Lavoie, 1998; Theilade, 1990). The mucous membranes of the mouth are subject to rapid and constant loss of cells due to desquamation, caused by movement of the mouth, the action of eating and by saliva washing over the mucous membranes. There are also significant numbers of defensive neutrophils present in the normal mouth environment. Glycoproteins – known as mucins are contained within mucus and are able to trap micro-organisms. As cells are lost, so are the bacteria that are attached to them.

Saliva contains a number of protective factors including lysozyme, an enzyme that hydrolyses bacterial cell walls, and lactoferrin, a glycoprotein that binds iron and so deprives bacteria of the iron that they need to grow and multiply. Many body secretions, including saliva, mucous and tears also contain immunoglobulin A (IgA), which is the major immunoglobulin (or antibody) in secretions from mucosal surfaces (Male *et al.*, 1996). The role of immunoglobulins will be discussed later. The mucous membranes are easily damaged, and this may result in inflammation and ulceration.

In *adults* and *older children*, the stomach contains few micro-organisms due to the very low pH and rapid flow of food through it (Mackic *et al.*, 1999). Although there is an initial burst of acid production *after birth*, thereafter *newborn infants* initially produce only small amounts of gastric acid, with full amounts not being produced until *2–3 weeks after birth* (Hill, 1990). This makes them vulnerable to colonization with pathogenic organisms, particularly in the first few days when their normal gastrointestinal flora is not fully established. This is exacerbated by the relaxed nature of the pylorus in *infants*, which allows bacteria from food direct access into the upper ileum (Hill,

1990). This risk is reduced in breast fed babies by the anti-infective components of breast milk or by the use of sterile artificial feed.

As the gastrointestinal tract continues, the numbers of micro-organism increase, with the largest number being found in the colon. Here numbers are typically 10^{10} to 10^{11} per gram of bowel contents (Mackie *et al.*, 1999). This flora, which remains relatively stable, is inhibitory towards other micro-organisms through physically blocking new species and possibly through the production of inhibitory substances (eg, some strains of *E. coli* produce a substance called colicin). The mucosal layer is constantly replenished. Physical removal is caused by peristaltic contractions, the action of food and faecal matter.

At birth the gastrointestinal tract is sterile and, although colonization begins immediately, the development of stable flora takes time. The flora of the gastrointestinal system depends subsequently on the diet. The high lactose content of breast milk favours colonization with *Bifidobacterium* spp., and the low buffering capacity of breast milk leads to a lower pH, reducing colonization with some of the pathogens that may cause diarrhoea. Breast-feeding exposes the infant to a large number of micro-organisms, both from those in the milk and from the skin flora of the breast and nipple (Mackie *et al.*, 1999).

A large number of micro-organisms will enter the gastrointestinal tract with food. As solids are introduced the flora of the gastrointestinal tract changes. The change is more pronounced in breast-fed babies, as the flora becomes more like those of artificial formula fed infants (Orrhage and Nord, 1999).

In addition to these mechanisms described within the gastrointestinal and respiratory tracts, a number of defences and substances are also found. These include phagocytic cells, complement and other chemicals, immunoglobulins and lymphocytes. These mechanisms are more fully described in the next section.

Box 10.1   Breast Feeding and the Immune System

Breast-fed babies appear to get fewer gastrointestinal and respiratory infections than formula-fed babies (Howie *et al.*, 1990).There are several contributing reasons for this:

1. Breast-milk contains a number of immunologically helpful substances such as IgA, maternal lymphocytes, lactoferrin, fibronectin and lysozyme. IgA has a role in lining the infant gastrointestinal tract providing protection until the infant produces its own.
2. Growth factors in breast milk may have a role in maintaining the protective role of the intact gastrointestinal mucosa.
3. Breast milk promotes the growth of a normal gut flora (Emmett and Rogers 1997; Mackie *et al.*, 1999).
4. Unhygienic preparation and storage of artificial formula may lead to infections.

Respiratory tract

The respiratory tract consists of a number of different environments, ranging from the heavily colonized upper respiratory tract, to the lungs which are normally sterile. The hairs in the nose provide a filtering action, but this is insufficient to filter many pathogenic organisms. Mucus secreted from goblet and sub-epithelial cells trap micro-organisms and this is then transported away from the lower respiratory tract by the action of the ciliated cells. In *infants* the length of the respiratory tract is shortened, increasing the risk that micro-organisms will enter the lungs. The alveoli of the lungs contain macrophages that are able to phagocytose particles or organisms that obtain access to the lungs.

In the upper respiratory tract *staphylococcal* spp. are the most common bacteria in the first few months, but by the age of *6 months* a diverse flora has developed (Harrison *et al.*, 1999). Viral infections of the upper respiratory tract may predispose to bacterial infection because they damage epithelial cells, impair the immune system, cough reflex and ciliary structure, and cause secretions to accumulate (Korppi, 1999). Tobacco smoke damages mucociliary function at a time of growth and immune immaturity and passive exposure may predispose *young children* to lower respiratory tract infections.

The respiratory tract is also protected by immunoglobulins, primarily IgA and IgG, although in the respiratory tract levels of IgA are low in the *infant*. IgG is transferred from the mother in utero, but declines after *3 to 6 months* (Burrows *et al.*, 1995). Airway secretions also contain a variety of chemicals – anti-microbial substances such as:

- defensins (Wilmott *et al.*, 2000), which are active against bacteria and fungi;
- lactoferrin, which reduces the bio-availability of iron essential for bacterial growth;
- collectins, which are able to bind allergens and antigens; and
- complement components, which stimulate inflammation such as the increased production of mucous and attraction of phagocytic cells to the site of inflammation.

The urinary tract

Sterility in the bladder is maintained by the regular passing of urine which helps to prevent micro-organisms ascending the urethra and so any interference with micturition may predispose to urinary tract infections (Mims *et al.*, 1995).

Most bacteria causing such infections originate from the bowel and the risk of infection is higher in *infants* because of their inability to maintain their own hygiene, and the relatively short urethra. The latter is particularly problematic in girls.

Box 10.2   Factors Influencing Vulnerability to Infection

Whether an individual succumbs to an infection depends on a number of complex interrelated factors. These include the nature of the infecting organism, the size of the dose, what methods it employs to circumvent the defence mechanisms of the body, the ability of the intended target to prevent attachment and growth of the invading organism and effectiveness and efficiency of the target at eliminating the organism.

The physical and chemical factors described have a key role to play in preventing the attachment and growth of potentially damaging micro-organisms to the surfaces of the body.

Cells of the Innate/Non-specifc Immune System

Phagocytic cells

Phagocytosis is the method by which a number of cells of the immune system are able to ingest and destroy micro-organisms. A number of cell types have phagocytic potential, including neutrophils, monocytes, macrophages, eosinophils and basophils. The sequence of events involved in the phagocytic killing of bacteria is outlined below.

1 Receptors on the membranes of phagocytes recognize microbial products. (Figure 10.1 a) This triggers biochemical processes that increase cell motility and induce the cells to migrate from the blood through the endothelium (diapedesis) (Rosales and Brown, 1993). The phagocytic cell moves towards the antigen, from an area of low concentration of chemokines (a type of cytokines) to an area of higher concentration. This is known as chemotaxis. Chemokines are produced by a wide range of cells.

2 The phagocytic cell can bind to the microbe directly, (Figure 10.1b) This binding process is enhanced if the microbe is coated with 'opsonins'. Antibodies, complement molecules and some of the proteins found in plasma can act as effective 'opsonins'. Phagocytes produce protrusions known as pseudopodia (Figure 10.1c,d) which gradually engulf the antigen and encloses it in a membrane bound vesicle known as a phagosome. (Figure 10.1e)

3 The phagosome fuses with the cellular granules known as lysosomes. (Figure 10.1e) These contain enzymes such as elastase, which breaks down microbial proteins, together with enzymes that lead to the production of reactive oxygen intermediates (Male *et al.*, 1996) and nitric oxide – these substances being chemicals that are able to destroy the microbe. One of the enzymes involved in this process, myeloperoxidase, is responsible for

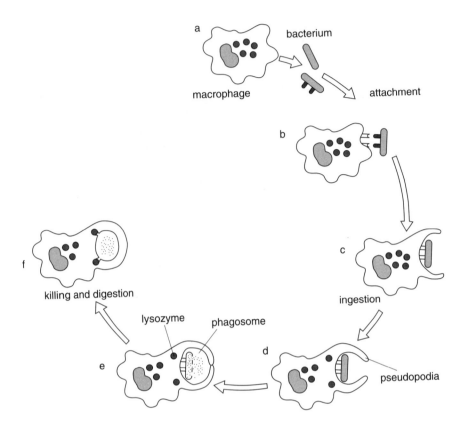

Figure 10.1   The Process of Phagocytosis

Source: Reprinted from *Introducing Immunology*, 2nd ed, Staines N, *et al.*, copyright 1999, with permission from Elsevier.

the characteristic green colour of pus. It produces hypochlorite (the active compound of household bleach) for hydrogen peroxide and chloride ions. These substances lead to the killing of the microbe (Figure 10.1f).

4 The toxic compounds involved in phagocytosis can also be secreted, killing microbes outside of the cell. These products are capable of causing tissue damage. Abscesses containing pus – a mixture of destroyed tissue, and neutrophils – is an example.

Neutrophils, the most numerous phagocytic cells, are produced in large numbers in the bone marrow. Neutrophil function in *young infants* is often less efficient than that in adults and older children. The absolute number of neutrophils may be lower. Those that are present are less effective at egress from the circulation and the subsequent phagocytosis and killing of pathogens (Kanwar and Cairo, 1993). *Pre-term infants* are at a particularly high risk, as the circulating neutrophil count at *22 weeks gestation* is only around $0.1–0.2 \times 10^9$ per litre, compared to $5–8 \times 10^9$ per litre at term (Christensen, 1989). *At birth* there is a temporary rise in the neutrophil count, before it settles at a lower level.

A reduction in the number of neutrophils is known as neutropenia. Neonates are particularly susceptible to neutropenia following infection as the result of the increased consumption of neutrophils that occurs when fighting an infection, alongside a decrease in the production of neutrophils (Kanwar and Cairo, 1993). In this age group neutropenia may indicate sepsis, even without other signs of infection. The definition of neutropenia varies, some defining it as a neutrophil count of less than 1×10^9 per litre and some less than 0.5×10^9 per litre. Whatever level is used, a neutrophil count of less than 1×10^9 per litre will predispose to infection.

Mononuclear cells and macrophages are named according to their characteristics and location in the body. In the blood they are known as monocytes, while those found in the tissues are known as macrophages. Mononuclear cells in some areas of the body undergo specific differentiation to fulfil a particular role (Winkelstein *et al.*, 1998). Dendritic cells have the ability to present antigens to T lymphocytes which in turn are able to direct a specific immune response. This process will be discussed in the next section.

Macrophages are highly phagocytic, more so than blood monocytes, as they have a larger number of receptors on their cell surface, are more metabolically active and possess a greater number of degradative enzymes (Male *et al.*, 1996). They are also able to present antigens to other parts of the immune system (in much the same way that dendritic cells can) and secrete a large number of cytokines, (chemical messengers between parts of the immune system). Some of these are described later. Although situated in the tissues, macrophages travel to the site of infection at a slower rate than neutrophils, but are more phagocytic than neutrophils. They are, therefore, less important in the immediate response to infection (Winkelstein *et al.*, 1998).

Basophils, along with the related cells in the tissues, known as mast cells, are important as mediators of the inflammatory response. Eosinophils are normally found in the blood but like neutrophils can migrate into inflamed or infected tissues. Their main purpose is the secretion of toxic substances which equip them to kill extracellular and large organisms such as helminths and other multicellular parasites (Male *et al.*, 1996).

Natural Killer cells are large lymphocytes that kill virus-infected or malignant cells. They do not respond to specific antigens but respond to cells lacking normal cell markers. MHC (Major Histocompatibility Complex) class I molecules are normally present on the outside surface of all nucleated cells. Many viruses and some malignancies cause a loss of these molecules and Natural Killer cells are able to detect this. By releasing the toxic contents of intracellular granules, they can lyse the infected or malignant cell. NK cells also secrete an interferon, IFN-γ, an important cytokine that stimulates macrophages to kill phagocytosed microbes.

Chemical Components

Complement

The complement system is important in both innate/non-specific immunity and in specific immunity. Complement consists of a number of proteins that form a cascade, commencing with activation and ending in products that act as:

- opsonins (substances that increase phagocytosis);
- chemoattractants (chemicals that attract cells of the immune system to the site of infection); and
- a membrane attack complex, which leads to cell lysis.

This cascade of reactions can be initiated by two major routes, one the 'classical pathway' is activated by complexes of antibody with their target protein (antigen) and is, therefore, a mechanism of humoral immunity. The 'alternative pathway' is activated by microbial cell components and is, therefore, an innate, non-specific mechanism.

Cytokines

Cytokines are proteins secreted by the cells of both the innate and adaptive immune system that carry messages between the cells of the immune system thereby helping to control the immune responses (Male *et al.*, 1996). The nomenclature of cytokines is complex due to their large number and the fact that although their names have been based on the cellular sources, some of them can be synthesized by a number of different cells. Cytokines can have different functions depending on which cell they bind to and can interact with other cytokines to modify (enhancing or antagonising) their effect. They are produced in response to microbes and antigens and can bind to membranes of target cells initiating new functions in that cell. Cytokines can act on a wide range of different cell types and can cause systemic effects if produced in large enough quantities. For example in septic shock, TNFα and IL-1, produced in response to widespread infection, are believed to be important mediators of the symptoms of shock. Table 10.2 shows some important cytokines involved in host defence.

The levels of some cytokines in *children* are different from those of adults. Some, such as IL-4 and IL-6 increase with physical growth, other cytokines including TNFα are found in higher levels in children than in adults. Others such as IFN-γ exist at similar levels in children and adults (Lilic *et al.* 1997; Sack *et al.*, 1998). The result of this is not only a different level of response, but a qualitatively different response (Pollard *et al.* 1999). Cytokine production develops with age. However, there is significant variation between individuals (Lilic *et al.*, 1997) and although cytokines can be found in the *fetus* further research is needed to understand their role during these early stages of development.

Table 10.2 Some Important Cytokines

Cytokine	Class	Major cell source	Main functions
Interleukin-1 (IL-1)	Monokine	Monocytes	Wide range of effects stimulating cells to fight infections. In low concentrations it stimulates local inflammation and in high concentrations leads to fever, synthesis of acute phase proteins (serum proteins produced by the liver and involved in the innate immune resonse) and muscle wasting. It does not by itself cause septic shock.
IL-2	Lymphokine	Lymphocytes	IL-2 acts as a growth factor to promote the growth of the same cells that produce it. In high concentrations it can enhance apoptosis (cell suicide) in T cells affected by antigen. IL-2 increases the growth of NK cells and they become more cytotoxic. IL-2 also enhances B-lymphocytes to produce antibodies.
IL-4	Lymphokine	Lymphocytes	IL-4 encourages B-lymphocytes to produces IgE and the growth of mast cells. It is also important in the growth of T helper (T_H2) lymphocytes that specialize in responding to allergens and helminths.
IL-6		Many cell types including activated mononuclear, phagocytes, endothelial cells and fibroblasts.	IL-6 helps to stimulate the production of acute phase proteins and the antibody producing cells.
IL-8	Chemokine	Leukocytes and tissue cells such as endothelial cells, and fibroblasts.	Neutrophil chemotaxis to site of infection

Table 10.2 (*Cont.*):

Cytokine	Class	Major cell source	Main functions
Tumour necrosis factor α (TNFα)	Monokine/ lymphokine	Activated mononuclear phagocytes.	TNFα recruits neutrophils and monocytes to the infection site and activates these cells to eliminate microbes. In moderate quantities it causes fever through acting on the hypothalamus to increase synthesis of prostaglandins. It also causes production of acute phase proteins such as C reative protein (which activates complement/acts as an opsonin), fibrogen and serum amyloid protein (which activates leukocyte chemotaxis, phagocytosis and adhesion to endothelial cells) Prolonged production of TNFα suppresses appetite leading to muscle and fat wasting and inhibits release of fatty acids from lipoproteins. In high concentrations TNFα inhibits vascular contractility and smooth muscle tone leading to hypotension and shock. It also causes intravascular thrombosis and very low glucose levels.
IFNα	Interferon	Macrophages	Promotes antiviral mechanisms in a wide range of cells by helping to prevent viral replication in uninfected cells and in the identification and lysis of virus infected cells.
IFN-γ	Interferon	Lymphocytes	Has a number of effects including increasing the ability of antigen presenting cells to be recognized by T lymphocytes and promoting the growth of T helper lymphocytes (T_H1) that kill cells infected with virus and intracellular infections. Causes fever.

Cytokines are secreted into the local area but can result in systemic effects through general inflammation and over activation of the immune system, as well as acting upon their specific cellular target. They are responsible for many of the clinical signs of infection. Fever may be seen as a negative side effect but some constituents of the immune system may be enhanced by the presence of fever (Blatteis, 1986), for example interferon production and activity (Kluger, 1991). Innate responses such as polymorphonuclear migration to the site of infection and function upon arrival may also be enhanced in the presence of high temperature (Kluger, 1991). The theory of overall immunological enhancement by fever is not universally accepted and contrary evidence exists in some cases (Blatteis, 1986).

Box 10.3   Inflammation

Inflammation is a normal response to tissue damage or infection. The outward signs of inflammation – rubor, calor, tumor and dolor– are signs of the following underlying processes:

- The inflamed area is red (rubor) and warm (calor) due to vasodilation and consequent increased local blood supply.
- Swelling (tumor) also results from vasodilation, but also because of the presence of exudate that collects due to increases in capillary permeability, which also allows cells of the immune system to leave the circulation and gain access to the injured or infected area. This relates to the process of diapedesis.
- Pain (dolor) occurs due to tissue distension caused by the build-up of exudate and the presence of pain-mediating substances (Mims *et al.*, 1995).

The inflammatory response is the result of a highly complex network of chemicals and physiological changes that may be initiated by one of a number of different pathways.

Either direct tissue damage, the action of antigen binding with IgE on mast cells or the activation of the complement cascade can all cause the release of histamine and other inflammatory substances from mast cells. In addition to this, platelets and a number of white blood cells release prostaglandins, which along with kinins from the plasma cause vasodilation, increases in the permeability of local blood vessels, and pain.

The inflammatory response might, at first appear to be deleterious but does serve a number of useful purposes. Pain is an indicator of injury and this together with swelling, can lead to immobilization which in some circumstances may enhance healing. The inflammatory exudate

---

attracts white blood cells to the site of the inflammation, dilutes bacterial toxins, obstructs the spread of bacteria and encourages the carriage of antigen, via drainage through the lymphatic system, to the lymph nodes where a specific immune response can be initiated (Weir and Stewart, 1997).

Specific Immunity

Specific immunity has defining features that differentiate it from the non-specific immunity discussed previously. These are:

1 Antigens elicit a response that is specific for that particular antigen. The immune system is incredibly diverse so that it is capable of responding to a huge variety of different antigens, and most microorganisms consist of a number of different antigens. Because the response is specific for each antigen it develops over time as the body is exposed to new antigens. The specific immune response is coordinated by T helper lymphocytes.
2 It has memory which allows an improved response, both in terms of speed and intensity, when an antigen is met for a second or subsequent time.

There are two types of specific immunity:

- Humoral immunity is effective against extra-cellular micro-organisms and involves antibodies produced by plasma cells derived from B lymphocytes.
- Cell-mediated immunity involves cytotoxic T lymphocytes and is effective against intracellular micro-organisms.

The components of the specific immune system are described briefly followed by key elements of the immune response. The features that are most relevant to children are discussed but a full description of the complex mechanisms involved are beyond the scope of this book. Suggestions for further reading are given at the end of this chapter.

Lymphocytes

Lymphocytes arise from stem cells in the bone marrow in *children and adults*, and in the liver of the *fetus*. After production, B-lymphocytes mature in the bone marrow and T-lymphocytes mature in the thymus. The mature lymphocytes then circulate in the bloodstream or congregate in the secondary lymphoid system. During maturation and development, lymphocytes acquire the following properties:

- able to respond to a specific antigen;
- non-responsive to self;
- a functional role; and
- are found in sufficient numbers.

During the maturation process they acquire specificity for a particular antigen. The process by which this is reached is still not fully understood, but it appears that a limited number of genes can be recombined to produce a wide range of antigen receptors.

These antigen receptors are expressed on the surface of the lymphocyte. Where antigen receptors are not expressed on the lymphocyte, or where these antigen receptors show high affinity for self-molecules, the cell concerned is destroyed through a process known as apoptosis, or programmed cell death. This ensures that the lymphocytes that are produced do not react highly against self-molecules which could lead to autoimmunity, where the immune system attacks the body. A number of diseases in children are thought to be the result of autoimmunity, including some types of diabetes, aplastic anaemia and systemic lupus erythematosus. About 10^9 different lymphocytes are produced each capable of identifying a unique antigen. The potential to meet the full range of antigens develops at around *24 weeks of gestation*, but they continue to develop over the remaining 15 weeks (Schelonka *et al.*, 1998).

Two important subsets of T lymphocytes develop within the thymus:

1 T-helper lymphocytes regulate the immune response by stimulating other cells of the immune system, such as cytotoxic T lymphocytes and B lymphocytes. They are sometimes referred to as CD4 cells because they carry CD4 surface molecules.
2 Cytotoxic T lymphocytes kill cells that are infected with intracellular micro-organisms, particularly viruses. These cells carry *CD8* surface markers.

An expansion of lymphocyte numbers occurs at *1 week after birth* for T lymphocytes, and about *6 weeks* for B cells. Prior to this the main type of lymphocyte is the NK cell, which then declines in relative importance (de Vries *et al.*, 2000). So although the *premature and newborn infant* is capable of mounting a specific immune response, the effector cells are not fully mature, leaving the neonate at risk of infection. This means that the passive transfer of specific immunity through the transfer of immunoglobulins via the placenta and breast milk have an important role in protecting the *fetus and the new born infant*.

Lymphoid Tissue

Lymphoid tissue includes the sites for production and maturation of the lymphocytes (the bone marrow and thymus), the lymphatic vessels that drain lymph from the tissues and the secondary lymphoid tissues (see Figure 10.2).

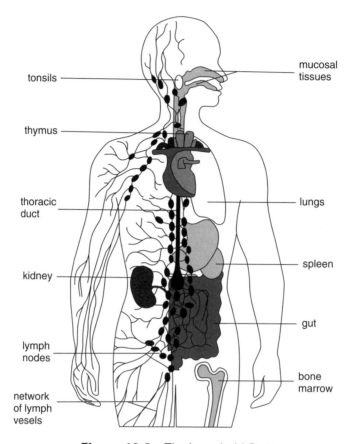

Figure 10.2   The Lymphoid System

Reprinted from *Introducing Immunology*, 2nd ed, Staines N, *et al.*, copyright 1999, with permission from Elsevier.

Secondary lymphoid tissue is found widely in the body including:

1 Lymph nodes;
2 Spleen; and
3 Mucosal, gut and skin associated lymphoid tissue (sometimes referred to as MALT, GALT, and SALT respectively).

These tissues contain a large number of lymphocytes, and so increase contact between antigens and the specific lymphocyte that can recognize them.

The lymphoid tissues form a relatively large proportion of the body of an *infant* and young child peaking at *puberty*, following which it declines to adult levels (Tanner, 1989). The thymus atrophies following puberty. By this age the maturation of the T lymphocyte population is almost complete, and activity in the thymus declines.

Peyers patches (organized lymphoid tissue in the mucosal of the gastrointestinal tract) develop from about *11 weeks* and their number increases from about 45 at *24 weeks gestation* to 80–120 at *birth* (Cornes, 1965). The number continues to double until it reaches a peak at during *adolescence* after which there is a decline during adult life.

The Immune Response

Babies and young children have a high rate of infection but their response to infection and to immunization is usually appropriate and adequate. Therefore, it is perhaps more useful to think of the immune system as naïve rather than immature (Cummins and Thompson, 1997). The immune response can be thought of in terms of:

• the recognition of antigen by the cells of the specific immune system;
• activation of these and other immune system cells;
• elimination of the micro-organisms by the host; and
• memory of the infection.

Recognition of antigen

Every cell in the body carries molecules that identify the cells as belonging to the body. The cells of the immune system are capable of distinguishing the cells of the body – 'self' from foreign or 'non-self' cells (see Figure 10.3). This

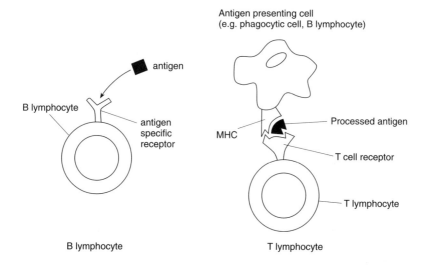

Figure 10.3 Antigen Recognition by Lymphocytes

Note: The receptors are not drawn to scale with the cells. They are shown larger than scale for clarity.

ensures that in normal circumstances the immune cells do not destroy the cells of the body. The recognition of 'self' from 'non-self' relies on the presence of Major Histocompatability Complex (or MHC) molecules, proteins found on the cell surfaces of all of the body cells. MHC class l molecules are found in all nucleated cells. MHC class II molecules are produced by a smaller range of cells, known as antigen presenting cells. These include macrophages, Langerhans cells, dendritic cells, and B lymphocytes.

The other important element in the recognition of cells as non-self is the maturation process of the immune cells as detailed above in the description of lymphocytes. This ensures that each lymphocyte is capable of responding through an antigen specific receptor molecule on the surface of the cell.

In Figure 10.3 both the B and the T lymphocyte have antigen specific receptors but the T lymphocyte is only capable of binding to the antigen when it is presented in conjunction with the MHC class 2 molecule. So T lymphocytes respond only to antigens on cell surfaces and not soluble antigens as B lymphocytes are capable of doing.

Activation

In order to become effective, lymphocytes need to not only be able to recognize the antigen as above but also to be stimulated by either microbial products directly or a product of the innate immune system such as cytokines or complement. Thus the importance of both the innate/non-specific and specific systems working together to produce an effective immune response.

Once activated by both these signals, the lymphocytes respond in a number of ways:

- By producing a variety of new proteins. These include cytokines which stimulate growth and differentiation of lymphocytes and other immune cells.
- By proliferation – clonal expansion- of the cells specific to that antigen that initiated the response. Thus more lymphocytes are produced that are capable of identifying and responding to the micro-organism that poses a potential threat to the body.
- By differentiation of a portion of the antigen-specific lymphocytes so that they become effective at eliminating the antigen either through the production of antibodies or the secretion of cytokines that activate other cells to eliminate the micro-organism.

Box 10.4   The Link Between Exposure to Infections and Later Allergy

It has been proposed that there is a link between the increased incidence of asthma and the reduction in childhood infections (Illi et al., 2001;

Strachan, 1989). The mechanism for this is that the T helper (T_H) lymphocytes can differentiate into two subsets, which produce different cytokines and lead to a different type of response. The T_H1 response is effective against intracellular pathogens such as bacteria and viruses. The T_H2 response involves the activation of mast cells and eosinophils which are effective against helminths and extracellular parasites. These T_H2 responses are also known to be implicated in allergy and atopy. At birth the T_H2 responses predominate with the T_H1 responses maturing later together with the T_H2 responses being suppressed under the influence of exposure to common infections. Thus the reduced number of childhood infection under modern, hygienic conditions may lead to a maintained T_H2 predominance into later life, resulting in increased allergic responses and asthma.

Elimination of the micro-organism

Cell mediated immunity: acts against intracellular microbes (see Figure 10.4). The cells that are responsible for this form of action are the cytotoxic T lymphocytes. This occurs because MHC class I molecules are produced within cells, they pick up and display fragments of the protein being produced in that cell (these fragments are known as peptides). These are then displayed on the outside of the cell. If host proteins are being produced, the MHC class I molecules will therefore be presenting host peptides, however if the cell is producing viral proteins because of infection, some will present viral peptides. This can be recognized by cytotoxic T lymphocytes which will kill the virally infected cell, preventing the production of more viruses.

The action against an intracellular organism within other cells is through the release of cytotoxic substances by the cytotoxic T lymphocyte, resulting in lysis and death of the target cell. This process relies on the close physical presence of the infected cell to the attacking lymphocytes. It is thought that significant amounts of the damage done in some viral infections is due to the immune system destroying infected cells, and the release of cytokines leading to the activation of the macrophages and stimulation of inflammation which attracts further immune resources into the area and causes inflammation.

Humoural immunity: Immunoglobulins (antibodies) are produced by plasma cells derived from B lymphocytes, which like T lymphocytes, are specific for an individual antigen, and the antibodies that they produce are similarly specific for that antigen (see Figure 10.5). These are produced as a result of the presentation of foreign peptides in association with MHC class II molecules that are found on antigen-presenting cells. These molecules, unlike MHC class I, present proteins taken up by phagocytic cells. These are degraded within the cell, and again displayed on the outside of the cell. T-helper lymphocytes are

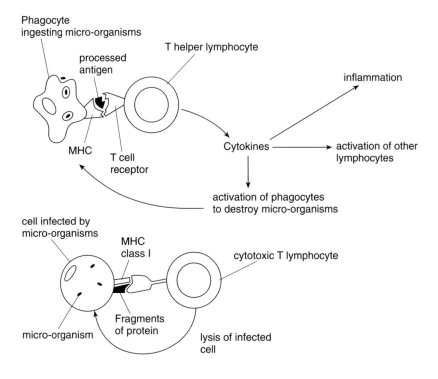

Figure 10.4   Cell-mediated Immunity

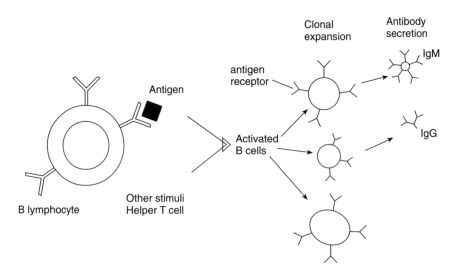

Figure 10.5   Humoral Immunity

able to recognize this, and can activate an immune response, including the production of antibody. Once activated the B lymphocyte is capable of producing antibodies which act by binding to the antigen, thus reducing any damage that it can cause. This is possible because they can:

- clump or agglutinate antigens, thus preventing or minimizing damage and making pathogens which express them easier for phagocytes to destroy;
- make the pathogen more attractive to phagocytes (called opsonization); and
- reduce damage by binding to the active part of the antigen, and in so doing neutralizing it.

Some of the important classes of immunoglobulin are shown in Table 10.3. In the *fetus*, IgG crosses the placenta by active transport from *14 weeks*

Table 10.3   Classes of Immunoglobulin and their Immunological Role

Immunoglobulin class	Role of immunoglobulin
IgA	Secretory, found on mucosal surfaces
IgD	Bound to B cells, very little circulating
IgE	Bound to mast cells and basophils, important in inflammatory response and allergic asthma.
IgG	Major circulating immunoglobulin. Important in secondary (memory) response
IgM	First antibody produced in response to an antigen

gestation onwards, although this increases markedly in the *third trimester*. At birth the baby has adult levels of IgG, but these then decline. Although IgG production starts in the newborn baby long before maternal IgG is lost completely, there is a period at about three months of age when IgG levels are particularly low. IgG, IgA and IgM secreting cells can be identified in the *25 week fetus* in response to uterine acquired infections (Stoll *et al.*, 1993) but adult levels of these main immunoglobulins are reached at around *a year* for IgM, *2 years* for IgG, and even longer for IgA (Weir and Stewart, 1997). However breastmilk contains IgA, so that levels may be boosted by breast-feeding.

There are different classes of IgG produced, which reach mature levels at different times. Those subclasses that respond to protein antigens attain adult levels by the age of *3 to 4-years* whereas those that respond to polysaccharide antigens do not mature fully until *8 to 10 years* of age. These latter antigens are known as T-independent antigens, and the response to these is particularly poor in children *under the age of 2 years*. This is a major reason why organisms that have important polysaccharide antigens cause significant childhood disease. These include Haemophilus influenza type B, Streptococcus pneumoniae and Neisseria meningitidis which cause meningitis, pneumonias and septicaemia (Goldblatt, 1998).

Secondary response: The secondary response will be illustrated with reference to antibody production, but the same principle applies throughout the adaptive immune system. When the immune system first meets an antigen, there is a lag phase of varying length in immunoglobulin production while the appropriate B lymphocytes for that antigen multiply (this is known as clonal expansion) and differentiate into plasma cells that begin to secrete antibodies (see Figure 10.6). Subsequent challenges by the same antigen are met with a much quicker response, and a much higher level of antibodies.

This more rapid secondary response happens because some of the B cells that were activated the first time the antigen was encountered have remained as memory cells, and can proliferate and start secreting antibodies much more quickly than they were able to on first exposure. The type of antibody secreted also varies, in initial infections the response is primarily IgM, a large molecule, the smaller IgG being produced later. In secondary responses, IgG is produced straight away and because it is smaller it can be produced in much greater amounts. Because of this, the presence of significant amounts of IgM is sometimes used as a marker of a recent infection.

It is this feature that is utilized in the process of artificial immunization where the first antigen challenge is provided in the form of antigen whose virulence or toxicity is eliminated or controlled. This stimulates the

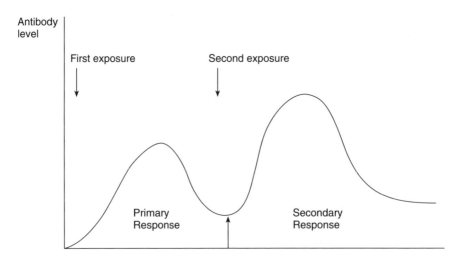

Figure 10.6 Primary and Secondary Immune Response

production of memory cells and hence permits a rapid elimination of the antigen on subsequent exposure. Some examples are given in Table 10.4.

Table 10.4 Examples of Different Types of Vaccine

Type of vaccination	Examples	Clinical notes
Toxoids, are bacterial toxins which have been inactivated	Tetanus, diphtheria	Uses modified toxin to stimulate antibody production.
Killed vaccines, use micro-organism that have been killed	Pertussis, injected polio	May need a number of doses to achieve full effect.
Subunit vaccines, use specific antigen fragments from bacteria	Pneumococcus, Haemophilus influenzae b	Use individual or multiple antigens rather than complete organisms.
Live vaccines, use micro-organisms that are attenuated, ie, had their pathogenicity removed	Oral polio vaccine (OPV), BCG, MMR	May be inappropriate for immunosuppressed children.

Most vaccinations are given to all children, according to a set schedule. Others, such as hepatitis B, are only given to certain high-risk groups (in this case babies of mothers who have tested positive for the virus). In some cases multiple doses may be needed to achieve a sufficient and long-lasting response. The first immunisations are given at around *2 months*. However some immunizations may be delayed because the antibody levels may already be high in the infant due to the acquisition of immunoglobulins from the mother. This is because this may reduce the effectiveness of the vaccine.

These vaccinations stimulate antibody production by the body and are known as active immunizations. Passive immunization involves the acquisition of formed antibodies either naturally through placental transmission, breast milk or artificially through injection. Because the recipient does not actively produce antibodies themselves and hence no memory lymphocytes are produced, passive immunity gives only short-term protection.

Vaccinations and the developing immune system

When designing a vaccination programme, a balance must be struck between giving the vaccine as soon as possible to protect *infants*, and allowing the immune system sufficient time to mature and so providing the best possible protection. The vaccine also has to stimulate the immune system in the optimal way, for example, if the vaccine is to protect against a virus, it would have to stimulate the cell-mediated immune system, while retaining some antibody response. If the pathogen is a bacteria, then an antibody response is more important. Finally a method of administration has to be found that is practical and acceptable to parents and children. Not all vaccines can be mixed in the same syringe, or given at the same time, and experience suggests that giving lots of single vaccines is not practical. Most of the vaccines that have used have been live attenuated vaccines, this means that they look and behave like the pathogen they are designed to protect against, while not being pathogenic. The advantage of these vaccines is that to the immune system, they look and behave like the real pathogen. The oral polio vaccine is a very good example of a live vaccine, because it is ingested orally (like the wild-type virus) and so it stimulates the immune system in the gastrointestinal tract, which is the right part of the immune system for protection against polio. Killed vaccines, which are used when a safe and effective live vaccine cannot be produced, do not usually produce such a good immune response.

There are a number of vaccines that remain problematic. Some bacteria are covered in a polysaccharide coat, which gives them some protection from the immune system. Although vaccines can be made from polysaccharides, these molecules are poorly immunogenic in young children *under the age of 2 years*. The solution to this is to conjugate (or bind) the polysaccharide to a protein carrier. This technique was used with the Haemophilus influenzae type b and meningococcus C vaccines. Organisms that mutate rapidly, such as HIV and influenza, are also difficult to vaccinate against because their antigens change, while vaccines against RSV and rotavirus were withdrawn due to side effects.

The Immune Response to Infection – Key Features of Assessment

Most infections in children are minor and self-limiting, requiring no active treatment. However, a few will be more serious, and it is, therefore, important to differentiate those that require treatment from those who do not.

The immune system interacts with all the systems of the body. This purpose of this section is to help readers identify the ways that the presence of infection may be revealed within these systems. The mechanisms that lead these symptoms are discussed.

In general the symptoms of infection are those involved in the process of inflammation. Signs of inflammation are as follows:

- redness;
- pain;
- swelling;
- heat; and
- loss of function

These symptoms can be seen within the various body systems as detailed in Table 10.5.

Table 10.5 Effects of Inflammation on the Body Systems

System and symptom	Observation	Underlying mechanisms
Gastrointestinal System (see also Chapter 8) Diarrhoea and vomiting	Changes in the frequency, volume and consistency of stools. Stool colour and smell may also change. Presence or absence of mucuous or blood may be significant. Blood may indicate invasive infection.	The mechanisms for the production of diarrhoea vary with the infecting agent They include: • Alteration in the balance between absorption and secretion in the gastro-intestinal tact leading to an increase in fluid in the intestinal lumen (eg cholera). Mucosal damage leading to an inflammatory process. This leads to increased permeability and leakage of tissue fluids. • Virus multiplication may occur particularly in the tips of the villi, reducing the capacity to absorb fluid.
Skin	Presence of rashes – colour. Distribution over the skin and mucuous membranes, profile of the rash (eg, raised, flat), size of the individual marking. Skin colour – pallor and flushing Integrity of skin surface – presence of wounds, scars and lesions. Location, colour, type of wound, stage of healing.	Rashes may be caused by micro-organisms, toxins or antigens localized in skin blood vessels. Petechial rashes typical of meningococcal disease are the result of small bleeds from capillaries caused by the bacteria, while those found in allergic responses are localised inflammatory responses Macules and papules involve inflammation in the dermis. Vesicles and pustules form when the inflammatory fluids accumulate in the superficial layers of the skin. In the mucuous membranes vesicles break down to form ulcers. It is not always clear why certain diseases have such a characteristic distribution of rashes across the body. Flushing of the skin can be caused by cytokines and prostaglandins produced by the body in response to infection. Breaks in the skin surface provide opportunities for the adhesion and growth of pathogenic bacteria, which can provoke an inflammatory response involving redness, swelling and pain
Cardiovascular	Heart rate Perfusion of body extremities.	Increased rate due to raised metabolism. Poor perfusion – Vasodilation results in a larger intravascular space, and blood volume may be decreased by loss of fluid through the capillary epithelium. This mismatch between blood and intravascular volume decreases peripheral perfusion as blood is redirected towards vital organs.
Respiratory	Rate of respiration. Presence of sputum. Secretions from mucosa. Red and swollen fauces.	Mucosa become inflamed and swollen with increased secretions. These may become yellow or green coloured indicating the process of phagocytosis and cell destruction. In the smaller airways of young children inflammation can impede breathing, and cause hyperinflation or collapse of the lungs.

Table 10.5 (Cont.):

System and symptom	Observation	Underlying mechanisms
Systematic effects	Fever. Lethargy/consciousness level. Loss of appetite Pain.	Fever and lethargy caused by the production of inflammatory cytokines and prostaglandins produced as part of the immune responses (especially IL-1, IFNγ, TNF). The significance of temperature as an indicator of serious bacterial infection diminishes with age. (Baker, et al., 1987). In infants aged 8–12 weeks, the degree of fever is positively related to the incidence of such infections (Bonadio et al., 1994). Lethargy and dysphoria are mostly caused by cytokines produced in response to the infections, especially TNFα, IL-1 and IFNγ. Infants with serious bacterial infections often do not present in this way, possibly due to their immature neurological system (Bonadio et al., 1994). In older children there is a stronger relationship between symptoms such as impaired quality of cry, reaction to parents, colour, hydration and responsiveness, and septicaemia, but this is not significant enough to be of clinical use (Teach and Fleisher, 1995). Cytokine production and pressure caused by local oedema causes stimulation of pain pathways.
Special senses	Appearance function	Infection and inflammation of the eye and ear can cause pain and infiltration and accumulation of debris of infection (pus). This accumulation in the middle ear reduces movement of the bones and transmission of impulses. Frequent and chronic inflammation can lead to loss of elasticity and impairment of function.
Genitourinary system	Frequency of micturition Volume Odour and colour of urine	Cytokine production and inflammation leads to stimulation of the nerve pathways of the bladder causing frequency and pain. Infection of the urine causes egress of phagocytes into the urine and the turbidity associated with urine infections.
Lymphoid tissue	Swelling of lymph glands	Increased activity of the glands as the rate of lymph flow increases. The concentration of white blood cells increases because of recruitment into the lymph nodes from the blood and division of the cells.

Laboratory Tests

A wide variety of laboratory tests are available to support the clinical examination. They seek to identify two main aspects – first the causative agent and second the way in which the body is responding to the infection. The following list represents only a small sample of wide range of laboratory tests.

- *Full blood count* the white cell count will generally be raised during infection, with an increase in immature cells seen under the microscope. A differential count shows the numbers and proportions of each white cell type. Neutropenia might indicate an immune deficiency, although neutropenia and thrombocytopenia can also occur following infection, and a particular increase in lymphocytes may indicate viral infection.
- *ESR* – the erythrocyte sedimentation rate is reduced in infection as the result of increased viscosity due to the production and release of anti-infective products into the blood.
- *Cerebrospinal fluid* – can be tested biochemically to identify glucose level (low in bacterial meningitis and normal in viral meningitis), and protein which is raised in all forms of meningitis. Micro-organisms can be identified as can the presence of white blood cells.
- *Blood cultures*. Blood is normally sterile, so the presence of any micro-organism is abnormal, although contaminant organisms may enter the blood sample from the skin
- *Acute phase proteins* – these are produced in response to inflammation, the most commonly tested being c-reactive protein (CRP), which is raised in bacterial infection.
- *Urine* – microscopy and culture can identify both micro-organsims as a causative agent and also the presence of white blood cells indicative of the body's response to infection.
- *Stool* – can be investigated for bacteria, viruses, and ova and parasites. Stool samples always contain large numbers of faecal flora.

Box 10.5 Assessment

The assessment process involves collating a number of sources of information that include:

- history of growth and development, likely exposure to pathogens and the nature and time course of the symptoms;
- physical examination to identify the presence and impact of the inflammatory process on the body; and
- laboratory findings that give information related to the presence of pathogens and the body's response to infection.

Conclusion

The immune system is a complex and highly integrated system that allows the body to respond to the threat of infection from pathogenic micro-organisms ever present within our normal environment. Some of these pathogens may be initially repelled through innate/non-specific systems that prevent their attachment and growth. Chemicals and phagocytic cells play an important part in this process as does the presence of the normal flora.

The adaptive/specific immune system is involved slightly later in response to infection and involves lymphocytes and the their products. The infant is born with the capacity to respond to the vast majority of these antigens. The lymphocytes develop this capacity in the maturation process that occurs in utero. Importantly too this process of maturation also programmes the lymphocytes to be relatively non-responsive to the self antigens – the molecules that make up the infant's own body. Without this process the immune system would identify the body's own cells as a threat, leading to damage.

At birth, while the infant has a competent immune system, they lack the experience of infection and it is this experience which helps develop the immune response further by the production of memory cells. These memory cells allow for a rapid response to any subsequent exposure to the same pathogen and effective elimination of the threat before the individual becomes aware of it. Artificial immunization is effective in preventing infection as it promotes the production of memory cells.

Elimination of the pathogen is achieved through the cell-mediated or humoral systems and the involvement of mechanisms of the innate immune system. This complex array of different parts of the immune system are orchestrated primarily by the cytokines.

The inflammatory signs of increased redness, warmth, swelling and pain can be identified in the body's response to infection and this provides the basis for observational assessment. Additional information can be provided through the use of laboratory tests.

Review Questions

1 Describe how the normal flora develops in the gastrointestinal tract.
2 Identify two important cytokines and describe their role.
3 Explain the process of maturation of the lymphocytes and why it is important.
4 How does immunization work to prevent serious illness in the individual child?
5 What are the signs of inflammation and how might they be identified in a particular body system?

Further Reading

Davies, EG, Elliman, DAC, Hart, CA, Nicoll, A and Rudd, PT (2001) *Manual of Childhood Infections*, 2nd edn. London: WB Saunders. This is the standard UK text on paediatric infectious diseases. It is very accessible for clinicians and has general background reading as well as an infection by infection guide to the treatment and public health implications of each.

Roitt, I, Brostoff, J and Male, D (2001) *Immunology*, 6th edn. London: Mosby. This is only one of many good immunology books. This is an accessible and well-known text now in its sixth edition.

Gould, D and Brooker, C (2000) *Applied Microbiology for Nurses.* Basingstoke: Palgrave-Macmillan. Microbiology books aimed at nurses have traditionally over simplified things, this book strikes a balance between accessibility and depth of coverage. More advanced readers may like to look at a more specialist microbiology book however.

Tortora, GJ, Funke, BR and Case, CL (2001) *Microbiology: An Introduction*, 7th edn. San Francisco, CA: Benjamin Cummings. A general microbiology text that gives a good introduction to the principles of the subject. Includes a CD ROM.

Department of Health (1996) *Immunization Against Infectious Disease.* London: HMSO. Sometimes known as 'the green book' this is the standard UK text on immunisation, although it is very dated now and is due for an update soon. Some chapters have been updated and are available on the Department of Health website.

Kassianos, GC (2001) *Immunization, Childhood and Travel Health.* Oxford: Blackwell. Comprehensive manual on the use and administration of vaccines. In the absence of an update to the 'green book' would serve as the main reference manual for nurses giving vaccines.

Websites

Public Health Laboratory Service (PHLS): http://www.phls.co.uk Collects and publishes data on infectious diseases in the UK. In particular look for the Communicable Disease Report link.

Centers for Disease Control and Prevention (CDC): http://www.cdc.gov

The American version of the PHLS. Website contains a huge amount of information and links to other sites.

World Health Organisation and UNAIDS For an international view on healthcare and *HIV/AIDS*: http://www.who.int and http://www.unaids.org

References

Baker, DM, Fosarelli, PD. and Carpenter, RO (1987) Childhood fever: Correlation of diagnosis with temperature response to acetminophen. *Pediatrics*, 80(3), 315–18.

Blatteis, CM (1986) Fever: Is it beneficial? *The Yale Journal of Biology and Medicine*, 59, 107–16.

Bonadio, WA, Smith, DS and Sabnis, S (1994) The clinical characteristics and infectious outcomes of febrile infants aged 8 to 12 weeks. *Clinical Pediatrics*, 33(2), 959.

Burrows, PD, Schroeder, HW and Cooper, MD (1995) B-cell differentiation in humans. In T Honjo and FW Alt (eds), *Immunoglobulin Genes*. London: Academic Press, 3–31.

Carr, DL and Kloos, WE (1977) Temporal study of the Staphylococci and Micrococci of normal infant skin. *Applied and Environmental Microbiology*,34, 673–80.

Christensen, RD (1989) Hematopoiesis in the fetus and neonate. *Pediatric Research*, 16(6), 531–5.

Cornes, JS (1965) Number, size and distribution of Peyer's patches in the human small intestine.*Gut* , 6, 225–9.

Cummins, AG and Thompson FM (1997) Postnatal changes in mucosal immune response: A physiological perspective of breast feeding and weaning. *Immunology and Cell Biology*, 75, 419–29.

Curfs, JHAJ, Meis, JFGM and Hoogkamp-Korstanje, JAA (1997) A primer on cytokines: Sources, receptors, effects, and inducers. *Clinical Microbiology Reviews*, 10(4), 742–80.

De Vries, E, De Bruin-Versteeg, S, Comans-Bitter, M, De Groot, R, Hop, WCJ, Boerma, JM, Lotgering, FK and Van Dongen, JJM (2000) Longitudinal survey of lymphocyte subpopulations in the first year of life. *Pediatric Research*, 47(4), 528–37.

Emmett, PM and Rogers, IS (1997) Properties of human milk and their relationship with material nutrition. *Early Human Development*, 49 (suppl), S7–S28.

Epstein, PR (2000) Is global warming harmful to health? *Scientific American*, 283(2), 36–43.

Goldblatt, D (1998) Immunisation and maturation of the immune responses. In S Plotkin, F Brown and F Horaud (eds), *Preclinical and Clinical Development of New Vaccines. Dev Biol Stand.*, Basel: Karger, vol 95, 125–32.

Harrison, LM, Morri, JA, Telford, DR, Brown, SM and Jones, M (1999) The nasopharyngeal bacterial flora in infancy: Effects of age, gender, season, viral upper respiratory tract infection and sleeping position. *FEMS Immunology and Medical Microbiology*, 25, 19–28.

Hill, MJ (1990) Factors controlling the microflora of the healthy upper gastrointestinal tract. In MJ Hill and PD Marsh (eds), *Human Microbial Ecology*. Boca Raton, FL: CRC Press, 57–85.

Howie, PW, Forsyth, JS, Ogston, SA, Clark, A and du Florey VC (1990) Protective effects of breast feeding against infection. *British Medical Journal*, 300;11–16.

Illi, S, von Mutius, E, Laus, Bergmann, R, Niggemann, B, Sommerfeld, C, Wahn, U and the MAS group (2001) Early childhood infectious diseases and the development of asthma up to school age: a birth cohort study. *BMJ*, 322, 390–5.

Kanwar, VS and Cairo, MS (1993) Neonatal neutrophil maturation, kinetics, and function. In JS Abrahamson and JG Wheeler (eds), *The Neutrophil*. Oxford: IRL Press, 1–21.

Kluger, MJ (1991) Fever: role of pyrogens and cryogens. *Physiological Reviews*. 71(1), 93–127.

Korppi, M (1999) Mixed viral-bacterial pulmonary infections in children. *Pediatric Pulmonary*, 19 (suppl),110–12.

Lilic, D, Cant, AJ, Abinun, M, Calvert, JE and Spickett, GP (1997) Cytokine production differs in children and adults. *Pediatric Research* 42(2), 237–40.

Mackie, RI, Sghir, A and Gaskins, HR (1999) Developmental microbial ecology of the neonatal gastrointestinal tract. *American Journal of Clinical Nutrition*, 69 (suppl), 1035S–1045S.

Male, D, Cooke, A, Owen, M, Trowsdale, J and Champion, B (1996) *Advanced Immunology*, 3rd edn. London: Mosby.

Marcott, H and Lavoie, MC (1998) Oral microbial ecology and the role of salivary immunoglobulin A. *Microbiology and Molecular Biology Reviews*, 62, 71–109.

Mims, C, Dimmock, N, Nash, A and Stephen, J (1995) *Mims' Pathogenesis of Infectious Disease*, 4th edn. London: Academic Press.

Orrhage K, and Nord, CE (1999) Factors controlling the bacterial colonization of the intestine in breastfed infants. *Acta Paediatr Suppl*, 430, 47–57.

Pollard, AJ, Galassini, R, van de Voort, EMR, Hibberd, M, Booy, R, Langford, P, Nadel, S, Ison, C, Kroll, JS, Poolman, J and Levin, M (1999) Cellular immune responses to Neisseria meningitidis in children. *Infection and Immunity*, 67(5), 2452–63.

Rosales, C and Brown, J (1993) Neutrophil receptors and modulaiton of the immune response. In JS Abrahamson and JG Wheler (eds) *The Neutrophil*. Oxford: IRL Press, 23–62.

Sack,U, Burkhardt, U, Borte, M, Schadlich, H, Berg, K and Emmrich, F (1998) Age-dependent levels of select immunological mediators in sera of healthy children. *Clinical and Diagnostic Laboratory Immunology*, 5(1), 28–32.

Schelonka, RL, Raaphorst, FM, Infante, D, King, E, Teale, JM and Infante, AJ (1998) T cell receptor repertoire diversity and clonal expansion in human neonates. *Pediatric Research*, 43(3), 396–402.

Strachan, DP (1989) Hay fever, hygiene and household size. *BMJ*, 299, 1259–60.

Stoll, BJ, Lee, FK, Hale, E, Schwartz, D, Holmes, R, Ashby, R, Czerkins, C, Nahmas, AJ (1993) Immunoglobulin secretion by the normal and the infected newborn infant. *J Pediatrics*, May, 122(5 Pt 1), 780–6.

Tanner, JM (1989) *Foetus into Man*, 2nd edn.Ware: Castlemead.

Teach, SJ and Fleisher, GR (1995) Efficacy of an observation scale in detecting bacteremia in febrile children three to thirtysix months of age, treated as outpatients. *Journal of Pediatrics*, 126, 877–81.

Theilade, E (1990) Factors controlling the microflora of the healthy mouth. In MJ Hill and PD Marsh (eds), *Human Microbial Ecology*, Boca Raton, FL: CRC Press, 1–56.

Weir, DM and Stewart, J (1997) *Immunology*, 8th edn. New York: Churchill Livingstone.

WHO (1999) *Reducing Obstacles to Health Development*. Geneva: WHO.

Winkelstein, A, Sacher, RA, Kaplan, SS and Roberts, T (1998) *The White Cell Manual*, 5th edn. Philadelphia: FA Davis.

Wilmott, RW, Khurana-Hershey, G, Stark, JM (2000) Current concepts on pulmonary host defense mechanisms in children. *Current opinion in pediatrics 2000*, 12, 187–93.

Index